Clinically Oriented

Anatomy

Clinically Oriented
Anatomy

Clinically Oriented

Anatomy

Jnanesh S Rayapati MBBS MD DFM

Associate Professor of Anatomy
MSU-GEF International Medical School
MS Ramaiah, Bangalore campus
Bangalore, Karnataka, India

Formerly
Assistant Professor of Anatomy and Histology
St Matthews University School of Medicine
Grand Cayman, Cayman Islands
British West Indies

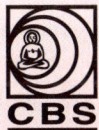

CBS

CBS Publishers and Distributors Pvt Ltd

New Delhi • Bengaluru • Pune • Kochi • Chennai
Mumbai • Kolkata • Hyderabad • Patna • Manipal

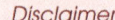

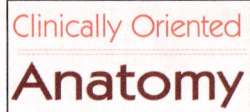

Clinically Oriented
Anatomy

ISBN: 978-81-239-1875-4

Copyright © Author and Publishers

First Edition: 2010
Reprint: 2013

Published by Satish Kumar Jain for

CBS Publishers & Distributors Pvt Ltd
4819/XI Prahlad Street, 24 Ansari Road, Daryaganj, New Delhi 110 002, India.
Ph: 23289259, 23266861, 23266867   Fax: 011-23243014   Website: www.cbspd.com
e-mail: delhi@cbspd.com; cbspubs@airtelmail.in

Corporate Office: 204 FIE, Industrial Area, Patparganj, Delhi 110 092
Ph: 4934 4934   Fax: 4934 4935   e-mail: publishing@cbspd.com; publicity@cbspd.com

Branches

• **Bengaluru:** Seema House 2975, 17th Cross, K.R. Road,
  Banasankari 2nd Stage, Bengaluru 560 070, Karnataka
  Ph: +91-80-26771678/79   Fax: +91-80-26771680   e-mail: bangalore@cbspd.com
• **Pune:** Bhuruk Prestige, Sr. No. 52/12/2+1+3/2 Narhe, Haveli
  (Near Katraj-Dehu Road Bypass), Pune 411 041, Maharashtra
  Ph: +91-20-64704058, 64704059, 32342277   Fax: +91-20-24300160   e-mail: pune@cbspd.com
• **Kochi:** 36/14 Kalluvilakam, Lissie Hospital Road, Kochi 682 018, Kerala
  Ph: +91-484-4059061-65   Fax: +91-484-4059065   e-mail: cochin@cbspd.com
• **Chennai:** 20, West Park Road, Shenoy Nagar, Chennai 600 030, Tamil Nadu
  Ph: +91-44-26260666, 26208620   Fax: +91-44-42032115   e-mail: chennai@cbspd.com

Representatives

• **Mumbai** 0-9833017933   • **Kolkata** 0-9831437309   • **Hyderabad** 0-9885175004
• **Patna** 0-9334159340   • **Manipal** 0-9742022075

Printed at Magic International Private Limited, Greater Noida, UP

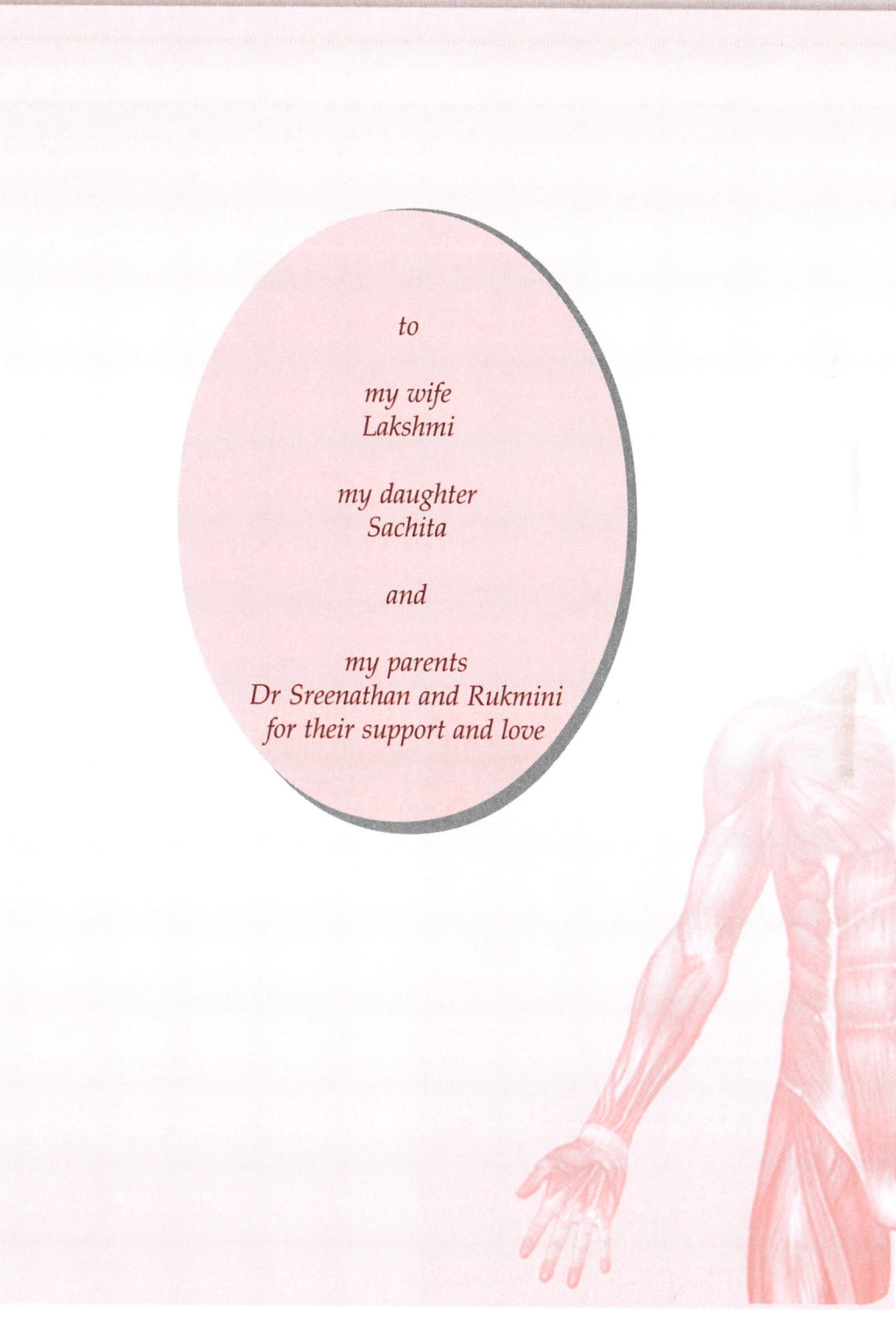

to

my wife
Lakshmi

my daughter
Sachita

and

my parents
Dr Sreenathan and Rukmini
for their support and love

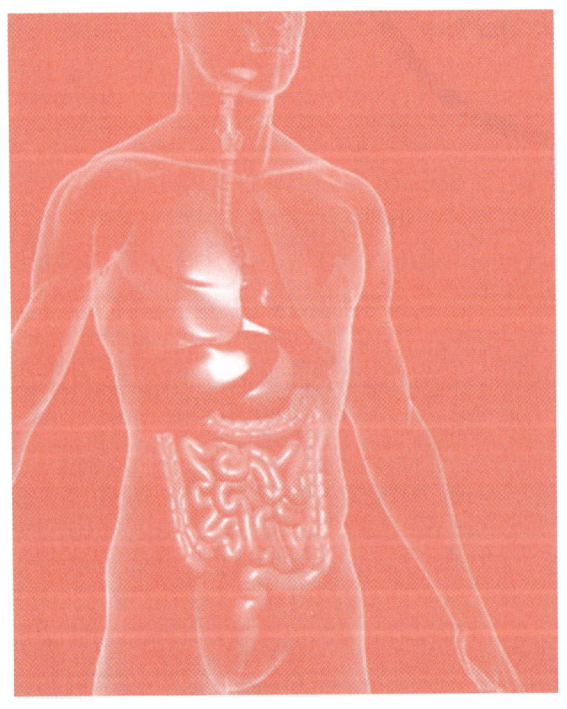

Preface

The main aim of this book is to provide a concise yet sufficient material on clinical anatomy. It is written in simple language in a point format. Unnecessary details have been omitted. Facts of clinical importance have been highlighted in distinctive colour.

I hope that this book will be of benefit to undergraduate, postgraduate (graduate) students preparing for examinations as a rapid review. It will be helpful as a review book for students preparing for exams like USMLE, PLAB and All India PG Entrance Examinations. The book focuses on material that is most likely to be tested in these examinations.

The book provides enough information for those wishing to refresh their knowledge of anatomy. I shall be grateful to the readers for their suggestions to improve the book.

Jnanesh S Rayapati

Acknowledgements

I am grateful to my father Dr RN Sreenathan, formerly Dean of Students Affairs, Chairman, Department of Anatomy, St Matthews University School of Medicine, Grand Cayman, for his help in the production of this book. I wish to acknowledge Dr Sandhya Belwadi, Professor, Department of Microbiology and Dr YJ Visweswara Reddy, Head, Department of Medicine, PES Medical College, Kuppam, for their encouragement. I am indebted to Mr SK Jain, Managing Director, Mr YN Arjuna, Publishing Director, and Mr Deepak Rao of CBS Publishers & Distributors, for their cooperation. I am grateful to Mr RK Majumdar for his wonderful illustrations.

Jnanesh S Rayapati

Contents

1 General Anatomy

- *Human anatomy* deals with the structure of the body.
- *Anatomy* = cutting up (Greek word). It is a wide field of study.
- *Dissection* = cut into two (Latin word). It is a technique.
- Anatomy is the basic foundation for the field of medicine.
- It introduces most of the medical terminologies.

SUBDIVISIONS OF ANATOMY

1. *Cadaveric anatomy* is studied on dead bodies usually with naked eye (gross anatomy).
   a. *Regional anatomy:* Body is studied in parts such as upper limb, lower limb, etc.
   b. *Systemic anatomy:* Body is studied system-wise such as:
      - Skeletal system (osteology).
      - Muscular system (myology).
      - Articular system (arthrology).
      - Vascular system (angiology).
      - Nervous system (neurology).
      - Respiratory, digestive, urogenital and endocrine system (splanchnology).
      - Locomotor system includes osteology, arthrology and myology.

2. *Living anatomy* is studied on living humans:
   - Inspection.
   - Palpation.
   - Percussion.
   - Auscultation.
   - Endoscopy (bronchoscopy, gastroscopy, etc.).
   - Radiography.
   - Electromyography.

3. *Embryology (developmental anatomy):* Prenatal (before birth) and postnatal (after birth) developmental changes in an individual.

4. *Histology (microscopic anatomy):* Study of the structure with the aid of microscope.

5. *Surface anatomy (topographic anatomy):* Study of deeper structures in relation to the skin surface projection. Important in clinical and surgical fields.

6. *Radiographic anatomy:* Study of deeper organs by plain and contrast X-rays.

7. *Comparative anatomy:* Human anatomy compared to that of other animals.

8. *Applied anatomy (clinical anatomy):* Application of the anatomical knowledge to the medical and surgical field.

ANATOMICAL TERMINOLOGY

Terms of Position

Anatomical Position

"Anatomical position" represents the basis from which all directions and directional concepts will be developed.

Please note that the subject is standing erect with his eyes looking forward, arms at his side, the palms of the hands facing forward and feet beside each other (Fig. 1.1).

Throughout the course of study, all structures or organs in the body are described in relation to the anatomical position. It is generally assumed that a student of anatomy remembers this basic concept each time a structure is encountered in the course of study.

In the dissection hall, the cadaver is kept on the table in supine or prone position. However, when description of a structure and its relation is to be given, it should be explained in terms of its location in the body in anatomical position. If we do not realize and practise this basic, the subject of anatomy becomes a big puzzle.

- *Erect* is standing up.
- *Recumbent* is lying down.
- *Prone* is lying face down.

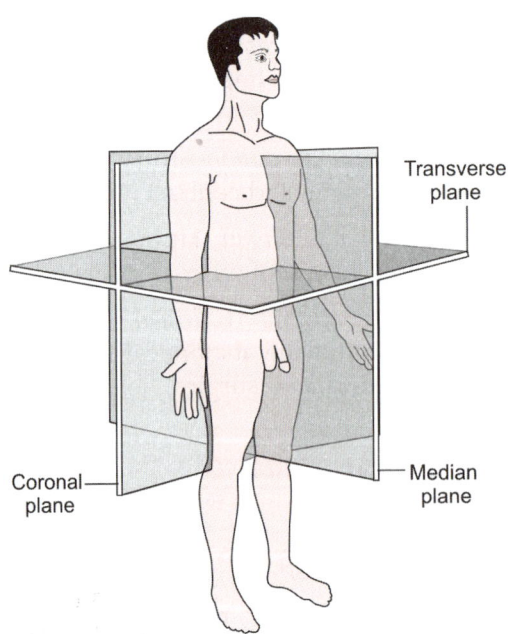

Fig. 1.1: Use of some anatomical terms and body planes

- *Supine* is lying down, face upwards.
- *Lateral recumbent* is lying on the side. A patient found "left lateral recumbent" is lying down on the left side.
- *Lithotomy position* is lying supine with the hips and knees fully flexed and thighs apart.

Anatomical Planes

1. *Median (midsagittal plane) vertical plane:* Divides the body or an organ into left and right halves (Fig. 1.1).
2. *Sagittal plane:* Plane parallel to the median plane.
3. *Coronal plane*: Vertical plane that divides the body or organ into anterior and posterior parts. It is at right angles to the median plane (Fig. 1.1).
4. *Transverse (horizontal) plane*: Divides the body or organ into superior (upper) and inferior (lower) portions (Fig. 1.1).
5. *Oblique plane*: Any other plane.

Sagittal plane	Divides body into left and right parts.
Median plane	Divides body into equal left and right halves.
Coronal plane	Divides body into anterior/posterior.
Transverse plane	Divides body into superior/inferior.

Other Terms Commonly Used

- Anterior—towards front.
- Posterior—towards back.
- Superior—towards head.
- Inferior—towards feet.
- Medial—towards the median plane.
- Lateral—away from the median plane.
- Anterosuperior, anteroinferior, postero-superior, posteroinferior, anterolateral, anteromedial, etc. are terms used in combination (Fig. 1.2).

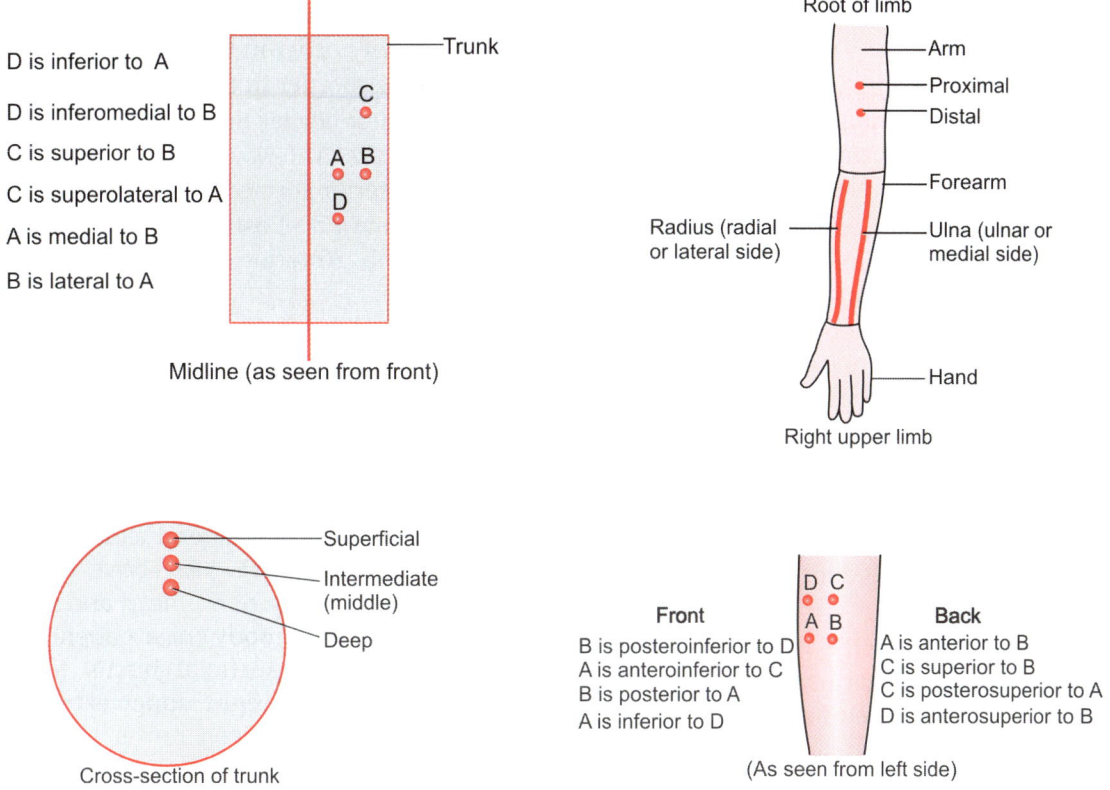

Fig. 1.2: Use of various anatomical terms

The anterior surface is the front, and the posterior surface is the back.

- Interior or inner.
- Exterior or outer.
- Invagination or inward protrusion.
- Evagination or outward protrusion.
- Superficial or towards the surface.
- Deep or away from the surface and inwards (Fig. 1.2).

Superior	Inferior
Cranial/Rostral	Caudal
Anterior	Posterior
Ventral	Dorsal

Proximal	Distal
Medial	Lateral
Superficial	Deep
External	Internal

- There are eight pairs of directional concepts to define. *Left* and *right*, always refers to the patient's left or right. To the left or right of the midline, moving away from it or back toward it, is a concept that defines lateral or medial.

- *Lateral* being farther from the midline, medial being closer to the midline (Fig. 1.2).

- *Superior* is closer to the head than inferior which is closer to the feet (simply stated higher or lower) (Fig. 1.2).
- *Superficial* and *deep* are "measurements" of depth from the surface of the skin, and do not need much explanation (Fig. 1.2).
- *Bilateral* and *unilateral* are used to describe structures or occurrences in the body. Eyes, for example are bilateral (one on either side of the midline) whereas some organs are unilateral (only on one side, e.g. the spleen). A patient might be a bilateral amputee (having lost both legs) or might be experiencing unilateral paralysis secondary to a stroke.
- *Ipsilateral* of the same side.
- *Contralateral* of the opposite side.
- *Ipsilateral* and *contralateral* refer to the same side or different sides.

The following terms are commonly used in embryology, but sometimes in gross anatomy:

- *Ventral* and *dorsal* refer to the anterior and posterior aspects of the torso. These two terms are also useful to describe aspects of the feet and hands, but more specifically the ventral (inferior) aspect of the foot is referred to as plantar and the ventral (anterior) aspect of the hand as palmar.
- *Cranial* or *rostral* towards the head.
- *Caudal* towards the tail.

Terms used for Limbs

- *Proximal* and *distal* refer to directions or relationships between different structures or aspects of the extremities (upper and lower limbs) (Fig. 1.2).
- *Proximal* nearer the trunk.
- *Distal* away from the trunk.
- For example, the elbow is proximal to the wrist, and the elbow is distal to the shoulder.

- *Radial* outer border in the upper limb.
- *Ulnar* inner border in the upper limb.
- *Tibial* inner border in the lower limb.
- *Fibular* outer border in the lower limb.
- *Flexor surface*: Anterior surface in the upper limb. Posterior surface in the lower limb.
- *Extensor surface*: Posterior surface in the upper limb. Anterior surface in the lower limb.
- *Palmar* (volar) referring to the palm of the hand.
- *Plantar* towards the sole of the foot.

A patient might have pain that originates in an area just superior to the left ear, travels over the superior aspect of the skull and travels down the contralateral aspect of the upper torso (pain starts just above the left ear, goes over the top of the head and down the right side of the body) or a patient may have sustained superficial burns to the medial aspect of the right upper extremity, with superficial and deep burns to lateral aspect of the ipsilateral lower extremity (superficial burns to the inside of the right upper limb and superficial and full thickness burns to the outside of the right lower limb).

That is medical terminology, cool, ok?

Terms used for describing Movements

- *Flexion* reduces joint angle. Approximation of flexor surfaces.
- *Extension* increases joint angle. Approximation of extensor surfaces.
- *Abduction* moves away from body midline.
- *Adduction* moves closer to body midline.
- *Medial rotation* inward rotation toward midline on the body.
- *Lateral rotation* outward rotation away from midline on the body.
- *Circumduction* combination of the above movements.
- *Pronation* forearm rotation so that the palm faces down.

- *Supination* palm faces anterior or up.
- *Protraction* segment glides anteriorly (forward protrusion).
- *Retraction* segment glides posteriorly.
- *Inversion* inward (medially) rotation of the sole of the foot.
- *Eversion* outward (laterally) rotation of the sole of the foot.
- *Dorsiflexion* bringing toes toward tibia (on heel).
- *Plantar flexion* point/plant toes so that toes are at a lower level and heel is at a higher level.

Movements across Joints

Flexion/Extension	Toward anterior/posterior or decrease/increase angle respectively.
Abduction/ Adduction	Away from/toward midline respectively.
Medial rotation/ Lateral rotation	Movement along longitudinal axis turning anterior side toward/ away from midline respectively.
Circumduction	Windmill action that combines all the above.

SKIN

- The term integument refers to skin (epidermis and dermis) and associated appendages (sweat glands, sebaceous glands, hair and nails) (Fig. 1.3).
- It is considered to be the largest organ in the body.

Functions

1. To protect the body from injury, water loss and infection.
2. It plays a role in sensory reception (has sensory receptors).
3. Excretion.
4. Thermoregulation (temperature).
5. Maintenance of water balance. Epidermis is devoid of blood vessels and receives its nourishment from blood vessels in dermis by diffusion.

CLINICAL ASPECTS

- *Psoriasis* results from an increase in the number of proliferating cells in epidermis. This results in greater epidermal thickness and continuous turnover of the epidermis.
- *Albinism/vitiligo* occurs due to absence of melanin characterized by white patches.
- *Skin cancers*—Exposure to the sun's ultraviolet (UV) rays appears to be the most important factor.
- *Burns*—Patient suffers from evaporative water loss.
- *Infections*—Due to loss of respective skin functions.
- *Boil* is infection involving the hair follicle and sebaceous gland.
- *Sebaceous cysts* result from blockade of sebaceous duct.
- *Skin grafting* is done to replace lost skin. It may be split thickness skin grafting or full thickness skin grafting.

Fascia

- Fascia is connective tissue.
- It is of 2 types: Superficial and deep.
- Superficial fascia is between deep fascia and skin. It is loose, fatty connective tissue. It is also called hypodermis or subcutaneous tissue. It contains superficial lymphatics and cutaneous blood vessels and nerves.
- Deep fascia is dense connective tissue.
  - It is modified to form retinacula, intermuscular septa and ligaments.
  - Retinacula hold tendons in place and act as pulleys where tendons change their direction (Fig. 1.4).

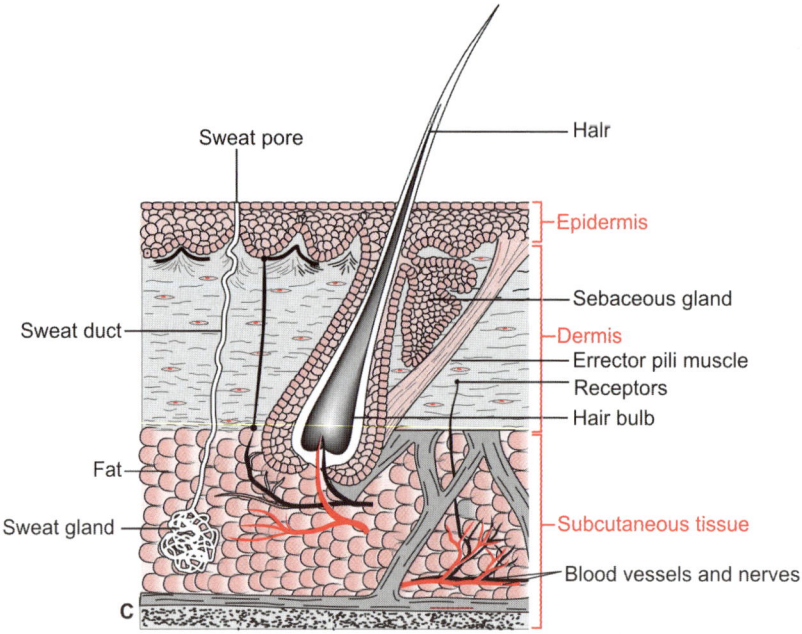

Fig. 1.3: Structure of skin

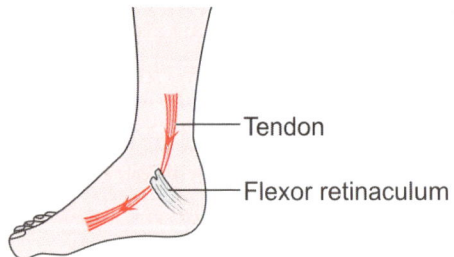

Fig. 1.4: Retinaculum at ankle

– Intermuscular septa form compartments to separate the different muscle groups. Ligaments hold bones together.
– Deep to deep fascia are the deep lymphatics, arteries and veins.
– Deep fascia helps in the venous return by forming a tight sleeve around the contracting muscles. The veins which lie between the deep fascia and muscles are thus compressed when muscles relax (milking action). Also when muscles relax blood is drawn into perforators by suction effect. This blood is pumped into deep veins by contraction of muscles. Blood in veins jumps up by this action as dictated by the direction of valves.

– The deep fascia indicates the planes along which the infection can spread from a given site.

BONES

It is a hard, living, specialized connective tissue.

Osteology

Study of bones. There are 206 bones in the body.

Functions of the Bones

• Give shape and support to the body.
• Provide surface for muscle attachments.

- Protect vital organs such as brain, heart, lung, etc.
- Bone marrow produces blood cells.
- Store house of calcium and phosphate.

The skeleton has two parts:
1. *Axial skeleton:* Skull, vertebral column, ribs, sacrum.
2. *Appendicular skeleton:* Limb bones, pectoral girdle (clavicle and scapula), pelvic girdle (hip bones).

Classification of Bones

Bones are classified according to shape, development or structure.

A. *According to Shape:*
1. *Long bones* have long shaft (diaphysis) and two ends (epiphysis), e.g. humerus, radius, ulna, femur, tibia, fibula. Meta-tarsal, metacarpals, phalanges have only one epiphysis.
2. *Short bones* are usually cuboid, cuneiform, scaphoid, etc., e.g. carpal and tarsal bones.
3. *Flat bones* resemble plates, e.g. skull bones—frontal, parietal, etc. ribs, sternum, scapula.
4. *Irregular bones,* e.g. vertebrae, hip bone.
5. *Pneumatic bones* are the irregular bones with air-filled spaces within them, e.g. maxilla, sphenoid, ethmoid.
6. *Sesamoid bones* are the bones found inside the tendons. They have no periosteum, e.g. patella, pisiform. Patella is the largest sesamoid bone.

B. *According to Development:*
1. *Membranous bones* ossify in membrane, e.g. frontal bone in the skull, clavicle.
2. *Cartilaginous bones* ossify in cartilage, e.g. bones of the limbs, vertebral column.

C. *According to Structure:*
1. *Compact bone* dense in texture, e.g. cortex of long bones (greatest in shaft region).

2. *Spongy* or *cancellous bone* made of meshwork of trabeculae and spaces, e.g. ends of long bones.

Parts of a Long Bone

A long bone has a shaft (diaphysis) and two ends (epiphysis).

- *Periosteum:* The shaft is covered by periosteum and has a cortex and a medullary (marrow) cavity. The periosteum is a fibrous membrane. It is made of outer fibrous and inner cellular layer. Periosteum has a rich nerve supply which makes it very sensitive. The muscles are attached to the periosteum. It is supplied by the periosteal arteries.
- *Endosteum* is a vascular membrane lining the marrow cavity.

Blood supply of a long bone is derived from (Fig. 1.5):
1. Nutrient artery.
2. Periosteal arteries.
3. Epiphyseal arteries.
4. Metaphyseal arteries.

Development of Bones

- Develop from either cartilaginous or membranous ossification.
- Primary centers of ossification appear before birth. Secondary centers appear after birth.
- Lower end of femur is exception and has medicolegal importance. Its lower end has the secondary center which appears just before birth and indicates viability of baby which is dead.

CLINICAL ASPECTS

1. *Osteomalacia:* Softening of bone due to lack of calcium because of vitamin D deficiency (adults).
2. Rickets is a metabolic disturbance resulting in inadequate calcification (children).

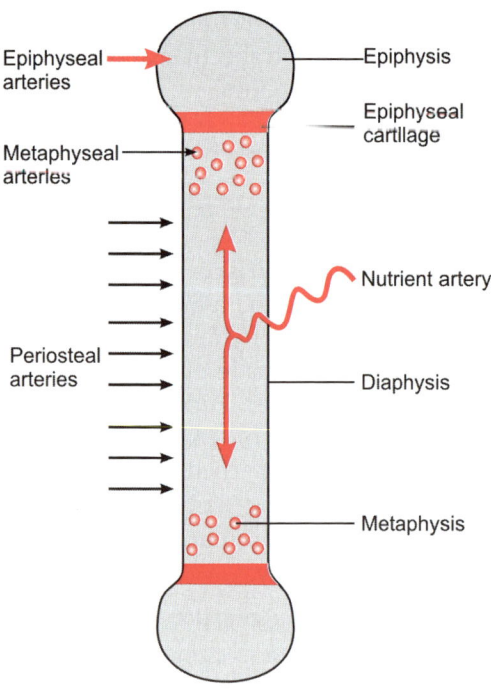

Fig. 1.5: Blood supply of a long bone

3. *Osteomyelitis:* Inflammation of bone marrow and adjacent bone.
4. Epiphyseal cartilage/plate fractures are serious as they cause shortening of the bone.
5. *Osteoporosis:* Decrease in organic and inorganic components of bone.
6. *Fracture* is a break in the continuity of bone; commonly due to an injury. It may be an open (exposed to exterior by torn skin) or closed fracture (not exposed to exterior by intact skin). Healing is by formation of a collar and callus (remember 2 Cs).

Bones of the Limbs

Upper limb

Clavicle	Collar bone
Scapula	Shoulder blade
Humerus	Arm bone
Radius/ulna	Forearm bone
Carpal bone	Wrist bone
Metacarpal	Hand bone
Phalanges	Digits

Lower limb

Hip bone	
Femur	Thigh bone
Patella	Knee caps
Tibia	Shin bone (leg)
Fibula	Leg bone
Tarsal Bones	Ankle/heel
Metatarsal	Foot
Phalanges	Digits

Terms used for describing Bony Features

1. Elevations.
   a. *Linear elevations:* Line, lip or crest.
   b. *Sharp elevations:* Spine, styloid process, etc.
   c. *Rounded elevations:* Tubercle, tuberosity, malleolus, trochanter, epicondyle.
2. Depressions—Pit, fovea, fossa, groove, notch, sulcus.
3. Openings—Foramen, canal, hiatus.
4. Cavities—Sinus, antrum.
5. Smooth articular areas—Facet, condyle, head, capitulum, or trochlea.
6. Ramus is a broad process.

Head	Enlarged part at the end, usually proximal.
Anatomical neck	Narrow part.
Surgical neck	Part of bone most likely to break.
Shaft	Long, smooth part of bone between ends.
Crest	Ridge for muscle attachment.
Condyle	Rounded part, for joints.
Fossa	Hollow or depressed area.

Epicondyle	Bump near condyle, for muscle attachment.
Tubercle	Small bump, for muscle attachment.
Tuberosity	Larger bump, for muscle attachment.
Trochanter	Large protrusion, for muscle attachment (found only in femur).
Foramen	Opening for nerves and blood vessels.

JOINTS

Site where two or more bones meet (Table 1.1). *Types:*

- *Fibrous joint:* Articular surfaces joined by fibrous tissue. Little/no movement possible (Fig. 1.6A).
- *Cartilaginous joint:* Little/no movement possible.
  - *Primary*—Bone ends are united by hyaline cartilage (Fig. 1.6B).
  - *Secondary*—Bone ends are covered by hyaline cartilage and united by fibro-cartilage (Fig. 1.6C).
- *Synovial joint:* Bone ends are covered by hyaline cartilage (articular cartilage). Have capsule, synovial membrane, synovial fluid in cavity, and are most mobile joints. They may be of the following variety: Plane, hinge, pivot, condyloid, ellipsoid, saddle, or ball and socket type (Figs 1.6D and 1.7).

CLINICAL ANATOMY

- Dislocation is disruption of the normal anatomical relationship that 2 or more articulating surfaces share at a joint.
- Subluxation is partial dislocation.
- Arthritis (inflammation).
- Arthroscopy is visualizing the interior of a synovial joint for pathology using a small telescopic device.

Ligaments

Ligaments are tough bands of connective tissue going from bone to bone. They are important factors to maintain stability of a joint, e.g. cruciate, deltoid, ligamentum flavum and nuchae.

CLINICAL ANATOMY

Sprain is an injury to a ligament as a result of undue stretch, to which it may be subjected.

BURSAE AND SYNOVIAL SHEATHS

- They contain synovial fluid which is a clear or pale yellow, viscous fluid (Fig. 1.8).
- They may become inflamed resulting in bursitis or tenosynovitis.
- Bursae prevent friction when one structure like muscle, tendon or skin slides over bone.
- Synovial sheaths envelop tendons and prevent them from being subjected to friction while sliding.

MUSCLES

Tissues endowed with the property to contract and relax. These are of three varieties

1. *Skeletal:* Strong, quick, voluntary contraction. Found attached to skeleton.
2. *Cardiac:* Strong, quick, involuntary contraction. Found in heart.
3. *Smooth:* Weak, slow, involuntary contraction. Found in wall of hollow viscus, vessels, etc.

Muscle Attachments and Terms Used

- *Origin:* The end of the muscle which is relatively fixed during contraction (on stationary bone—fixed) (Fig. 1.9).
- *Insertion:* End which moves (on bone that is moving—movable).
- *Proximal and distal attachments* (better descriptions that can be used in limbs).

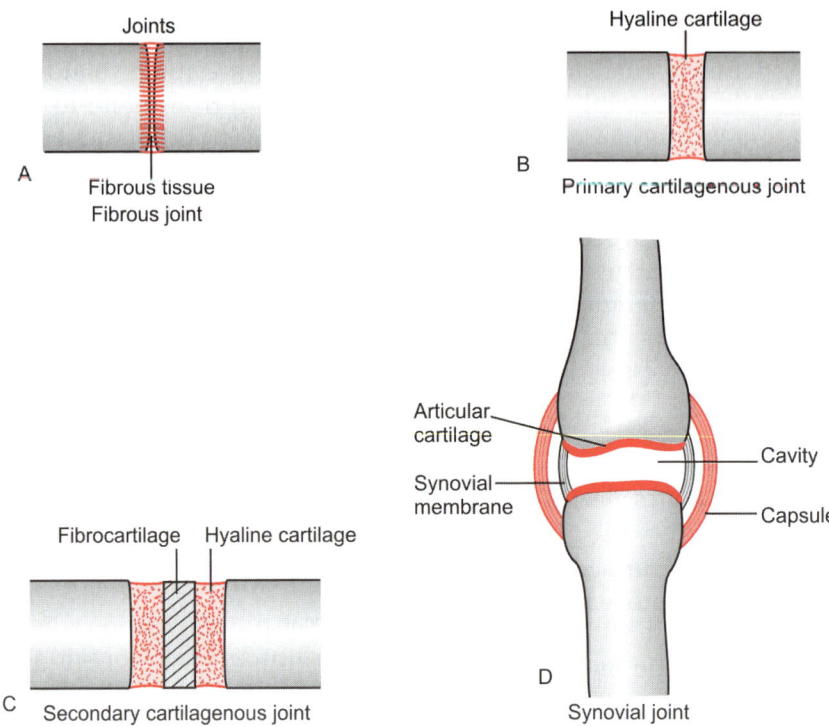

Fig. 1.6: Types of joints

Table 1.1: Examples of joint types		
Joint types	*Examples*	
Fibrous joint	Sutures	Skull
	Syndesmosis	Interosseous membrane and inferior tibiofibular joint
	Gomphosis	Between teeth and jaws
Cartilaginous joint	Primary cartilaginous joint	Epiphyseal plates of long bones, between occipital and sphenoid bones of skull
	Secondary cartilaginous joint	Intervertebral discs, symphysis pubis
Synovial joint	Plane	Acromioclavicular
	Hinge	Elbow
	Pivot	Superior radioulnar and median atlantoaxial
	Condyloid	Knee
	Ellipsoid	Wrist
	Saddle	Carpometacarpal joint of thumb
	Ball and socket	Hip and shoulder

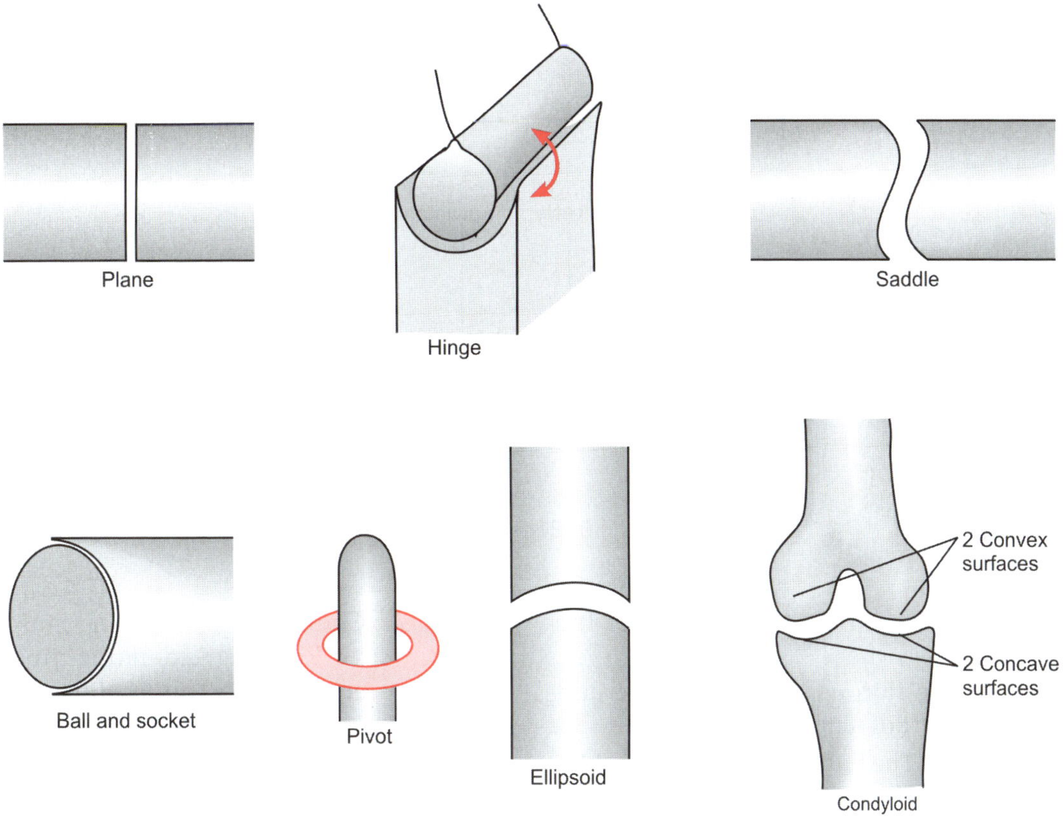

Plane

Hinge

Saddle

Ball and socket

Pivot

Ellipsoid

2 Convex surfaces

2 Concave surfaces

Condyloid

Fig. 1.7: Types of synovial joints

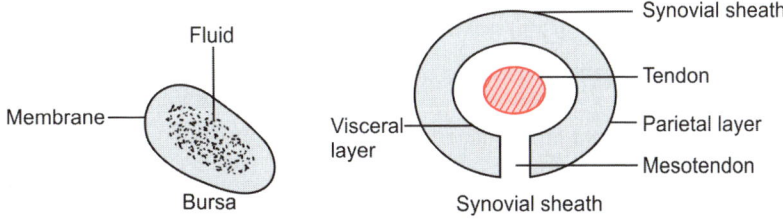

Fluid

Membrane

Bursa

Synovial sheath

Tendon

Visceral layer

Parietal layer

Mesotendon

Synovial sheath

Fig. 1.8: Bursa and synovial sheath

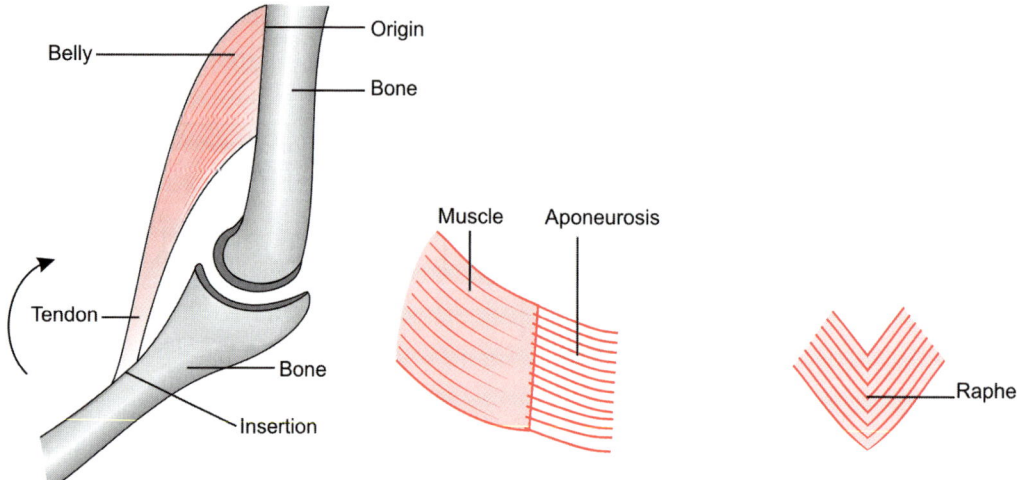

Fig. 1.9: Parts of muscle

- *Belly:* Fleshy and contractile part of the muscle.
- *Tendon:* The fibrous, non-contractile and cord-like part of a muscle.
- *Aponeurosis:* The flattened tendon (Fig. 1.9).
- *Raphe* is a fibrous band of interdigitating fibres of tendons or aponeurosis (Fig. 1.9).
- *Compartments:* Units of muscles with similar actions, blood supply, and innervations.

- *Agonists:* Contracting/shortening muscles.
- *Antagonists:* Relaxing/extending muscles usually opposite to the agonist group muscles.

Table 1.2: Classification based on arrangement of fibres (Fig. 1.10)			
Classification	*Arrangement of fibres*		*Examples*
Parallel	Muscle fibers parallel to one another	Strap-like	Sartorius
		Quadrilateral	Thyrohyoid
		Fusiform	Lumbricals
Triangular	Muscle fibers converge into a tendon		Temporalis
Pennate	Muscle fibers present on one side of tendon	Unipennate	Peroneus tertius
	Muscle fibers present on two sides of tendon	Bipennate	Dorsal interossei
		Multipennate	Deltoid
	Muscle fibers converge on tendon which is in the central axis of the muscle	Circumpennate	Tibialis anterior

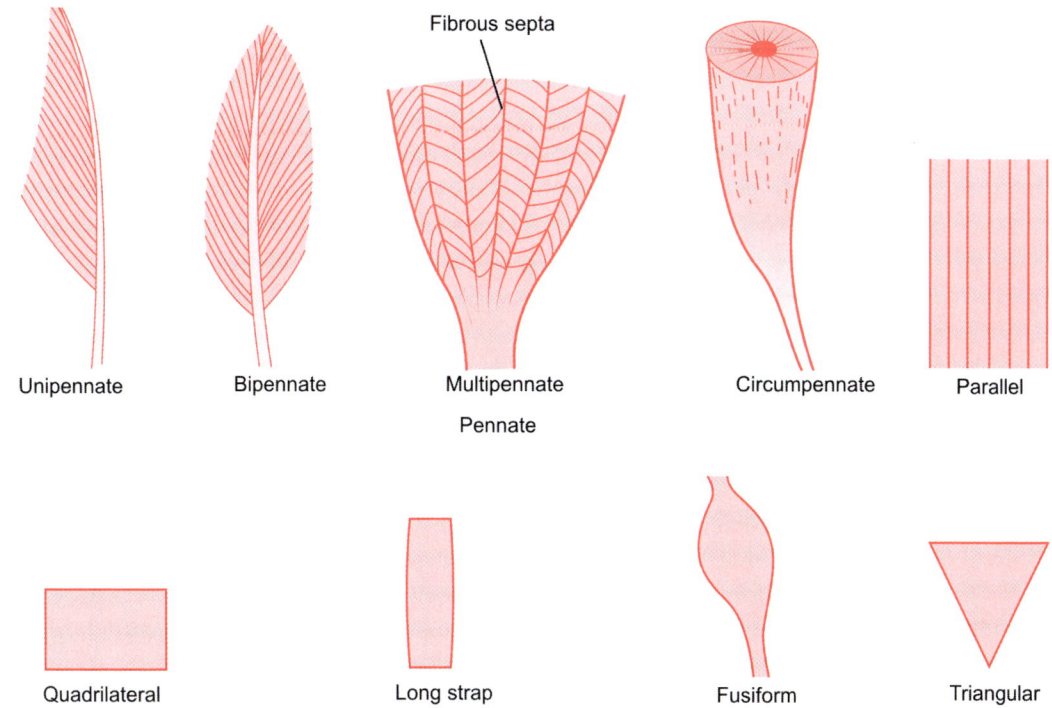

Fig. 1.10: Arrangement of fibers in skeletal muscle

Unipennate Bipennate Multipennate Circumpennate Parallel

Pennate

Fibrous septa

Quadrilateral Long strap Fusiform Triangular

CIRCULATORY SYSTEM

Includes:

- *Systemic circulation* from left ventricle of heart to tissues of body and back to right atrium of heart.
- *Pulmonary circulation* from right ventricle of heart to lungs and back to left atrium of heart.
- *Portal circulation* from one capillary bed to another before reaching the heart. They are uncommon as the capillary beds normally drain into the heart and not into another capillary bed (Fig. 1.11).
- *Lymphatic system* includes lymphoid organs and lymphatic vessels. Functions to protect the body from invasion and damage by microorganisms and foreign substances. Lymphoid organs or tissues include:
  - Lymph nodes.
  - Thymus.
  - Spleen.
  - Tonsils.
  - Bone marrow.

Terms used for describing vessels:

1. *Arteries:* Carry oxygenated blood away from heart. Exceptions are pulmonary and umbilical arteries which carry deoxygenated blood. Arteries are like trees. They have branches. No valves are present.

2. *Veins:* Carry deoxygenated blood from the heart. Exceptions are pulmonary and umbilical veins. Veins are like rivers. They receive tributaries. Venous plexus is communication between veins. Valves are seen.

3. *Capillaries:* These are network of microscopic vessels (Fig. 1.12).

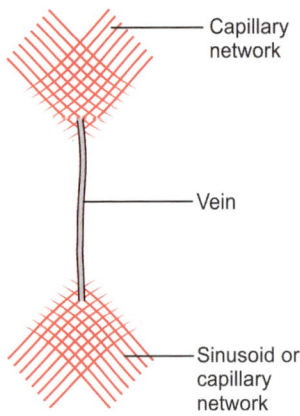

Fig. 1.11: Portal circulation

4. *Anastomosis* is a communication between neighboring arteries which helps in collateral circulation (Fig. 1.12).
5. *Arteriovenous shunts* provide direct routes between arteries and veins bypassing capillaries.

6. *Lymphatics* carry tissue fluid. Lymphatic vessels include lymph capillaries, smaller and larger lymphatic vessels and terminal collecting ducts [right lymphatic duct and left lymphatic duct (thoracic duct)]. The bigger lymph vessels [right lymphatic duct and left lymphatic duct (thoracic duct)] drain into the veins at the root of the neck. Lymph vessels have valves to prevent backflow of lymph.

Note
1. *End arteries:* These arteries do not have anastomoses with neighbouring arteries. Their blockade results in death of tissue supplied by them, e.g. arteries in kidney and spleen, coronary arteries, central artery of retina, central arteries of brain. They may be anatomical or functional end arteries.

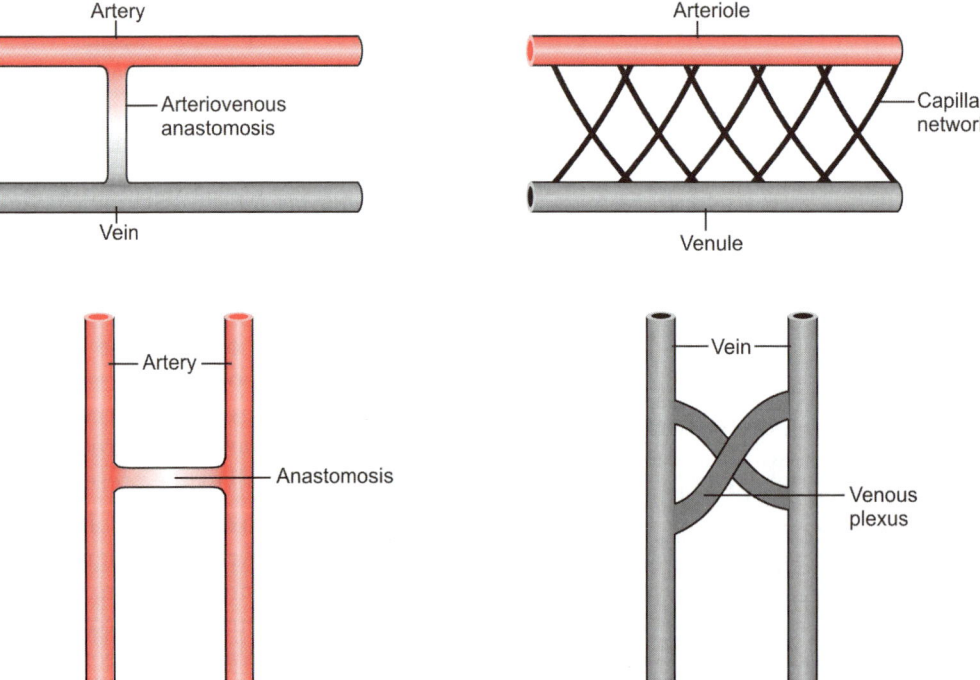

Fig. 1.12: Connections between arteries and veins

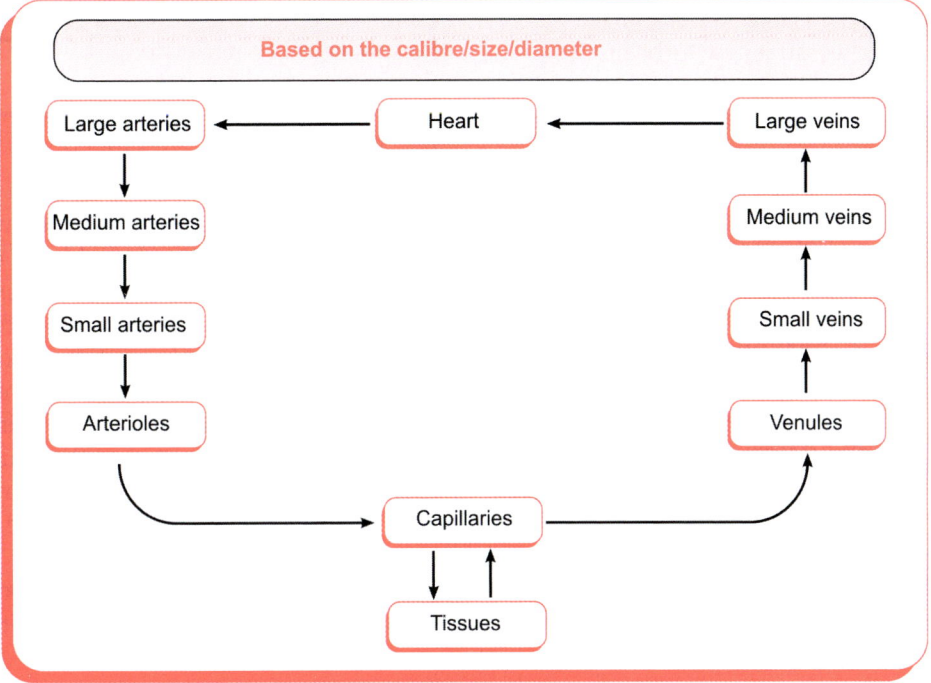

Fig. 1.13: Direction of blood flow in circulatory system

2. *Tortuous or wavy arteries:* They run a wavy course to allow for their elongation; in times of:
   a. The area of their location being subjected to movement [facial artery (face), lingual artery (tongue)]; or
   b. Movements of the organ which they supply [splenic artery (spleen), uterine artery (allow for increased size of uterus in pregnancy)].

CLINICAL ANATOMY

- *Atherosclerosis* is accumulation of fat in walls of the arteries, leading to the narrowing of their lumen.
- *Varicose veins* is abnormally dilated and tortuous veins.

- *Lymphangitis* and *lymphedema* refer to inflammation of lymph vessels and lymph nodes respectively.

NERVOUS SYSTEM

The nervous system is divided structurally into:
1. Central nervous system.
2. Peripheral nervous system.

Central nervous system is made up of:
1. Brain.
2. Spinal cord.
   - The brain is safely preserved in the cranial cavity and is surrounded by the meninges of the brain (cranial).
   - The spinal cord is present inside the vertebral canal and is covered by the spinal meninges.

Peripheral nervous system is made up of:
1. Cranial nerves attached to brain.
2. Spinal nerves attached to spinal cord.
The nervous system is divided functionally into:

1. *Somatic nervous system* (under will)—somatic parts of central and peripheral nervous system.
2. *Autonomic nervous system* (not under will)—autonomous parts of central and peripheral nervous system.

Autonomic nervous system is self-regulating. Higher centers are in brainstem and hypothalamus. Two components: Sympathetic and parasympathetic.
- Sympathetic mobilizes body energy to deal with stress and emergency.
- Parasympathetic conserves body energy.

Both comprise preganglionic and post-ganglionic neurons with ganglion intervening.

Ganglia are groups of neuronal cell bodies in Peripheral nervous system.

Typical Spinal Nerve

It is formed as follows: (Fig. 1.14)
1. Ventral rootlets from ventral horn of spinal cord join to form ventral root (motor).
2. Dorsal rootlets from dorsal horn of spinal cord join to form dorsal root (sensory).
3. Ventral and dorsal root join to form spinal nerve. Close to this formation, a dorsal root or spinal ganglion is present on dorsal root.
4. Immediately after formation of spinal nerve (in intervertebral foramen) the spinal nerve divides into ventral and dorsal rami. Each of these rami contains autonomic, sensory and motor fibres.
5. The ventral ramus is connected to sympathetic ganglion by a lateral white ramus

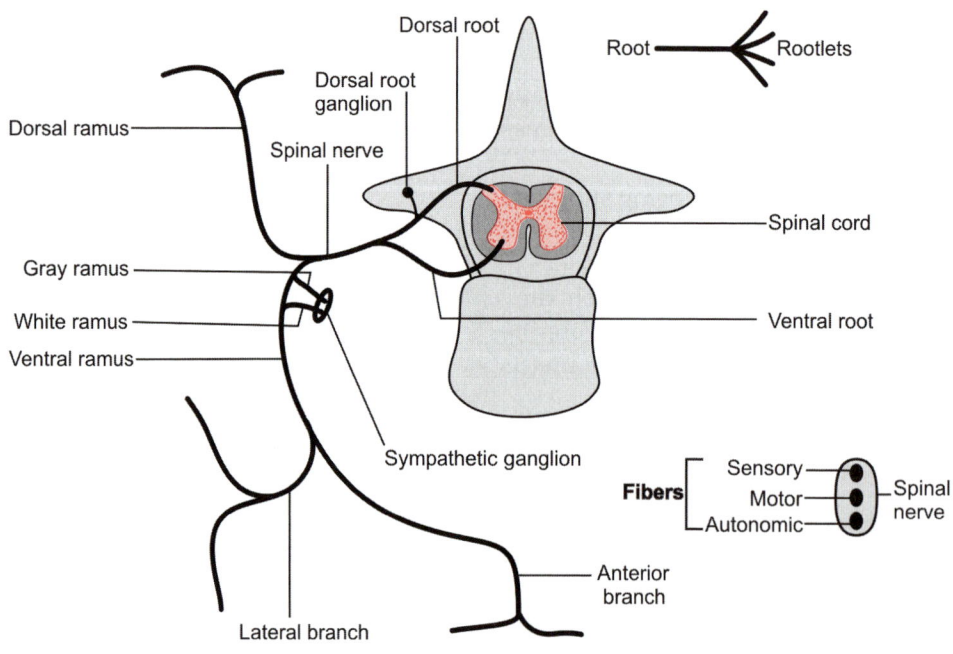

Fig. 1.14: Typical spinal nerve

communicans (contains myelinated fibers, myelin gives white colour hence called so) and a medial grey ramus communicans (contains unmyelinated fibers giving greyish colour hence called so).

IMAGING TECHNIQUES

These are employed to study the different structures of the body in a noninvasive manner (without cutting the body) to detect any abnormalities. These include:
- Conventional radiography (uses X-rays).
  - Cheap.
  - Risks exposure to X-rays.
- CT (computerized tomography) scan (uses X-rays).
  - Reliable.
  - Risks exposure to X-rays.
- MRI (magnetic resonance imaging) scan (uses magnetic field and radio waves).
  - Reliable.
  - No risk of exposure to X-rays.
  - Expensive.
- Ultrasound scan (uses sound waves).
  - Safe.
  - Fails to visualize structures hidden by bone as ultrasound has difficulty in penetrating the bone.

Upper Limb

2

Upper limb is a specialized part designed to hold, handle and manipulate. All the joints of the upper limb are very freely mobile. Clavicle holds the upper limb clear off the trunk. Fingers are long and freely movable. The thumb is set at right angles to other digits. This helps to oppose the thumb to other digits. This is the main event which makes man an advanced individual. Otherwise we would not have written or cooked food or buttoned our shirts. Just try and it is impossible to button without the help of the thumb.

That is the reason why even a small injury to the hand renders the individual more disabled.

Shoulder Girdle

A girdle is used as a beam to transmit the weight between the columns. The skeleton of the upper limb is one column and the skeleton of the vertebral column is another column. These two columns are connected by a girdle at the shoulder and this is called the shoulder girdle. Its main purpose is to transmit the weight of the upper limb to the axial skeleton.

- The clavicle and scapula together form the shoulder girdle.
- The clavicle is the bone which is exclusively designed to transmit the weight of the upper limb while the scapula is designed to support the clavicle by giving extensive attachments to muscles and

helps increase the range of movements at the so-called scapulothoracic joint. Now let us study the clavicle.

CLAVICLE

- It is colloquially known as the collar bone and is easily visible and palpable. It is called clavicle as it resembles a curved window fastener.
- It is curved like letter "S" (Fig. 2.1).
- The curve gives resilience to the bone otherwise it would not have been suitable to transmit the weight of the upper limb.
- The curve allows space for the neurovascular bundle to go to the upper limb under its protection.
- Medullary cavity is formed in a cartilaginous bone. The clavicle is a membranous bone and, therefore, there is no chance of a medullary cavity.
- Once bone is formed whether it is cartilaginous or membranous, it has the same property. The clavicle is precautiously membranous as the formation of bone is quite early and quick and that is indeed suitable for weight transmission.
- It is a long bone. It transmits the weight of the upper limb to the axial skeleton.
- It does not agree with many of the specifications of long bones. Look at the

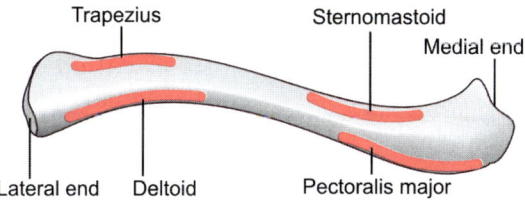

Fig. 2.1A: Right clavicle (superior aspect)

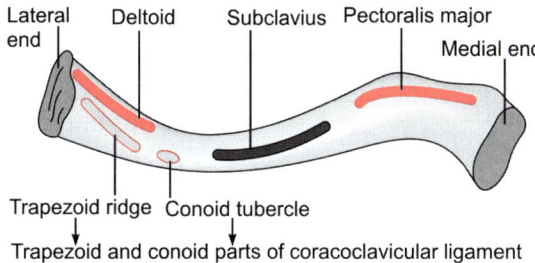

Fig. 2.1B: Right clavicle (inferior aspect)

following and compare the long bone characteristics with that of the clavicle.

Side Determination

- The lateral end is flat.
- The medial two-thirds of the shaft is convex anteriorly.
- There is a subclavian groove on the inferior surface.

These three points are sufficient to assign the clavicle to its correct side.

Joints of the Clavicle

- Medially, it joins the manubrium sternum to form a sternoclavicular joint.
- Laterally, it joins the acromion of the scapula to form the acromioclavicular joint.
- They must be freely movable joints. Therefore, the sternoclavicular joint is a saddle type of synovial joint. Keep your

Long bones	Clavicle
They are vertically placed. They have medullary cavity.	It is placed horizontally. No medullary cavity.
Ossified in cartilage.	Ossified in membrane.
They have one primary center for the body.	There are two primary centers.
Not pierced by any cutaneous nerve.	It is often pierced by cutaneous (supraclavicular) nerve.

fingers over the medial end of the clavicle and move the arm backward, you will see the sternal end moving forward. Similarly, when the shoulder is elevated the clavicle is depressed at its medial end.

What is Shoulder Separation?

- When a person falls very heavily on the side of the shoulder, the acromion may get dislocated under the lateral end of the clavicle. This is called shoulder separation.

Symptoms of shoulder separation:
1. Shoulder pain.
2. Shoulder tenderness.
3. A bump over the lateral end of the clavicle.

Ligaments attached to the Clavicle

- *Medial end:* Sternoclavicular and costo-clavicular.
- *Lateral end:* Acromioclavicular and coraco-clavicular.

Muscles attached to the Clavicle

1. Sternocleidomastoid.
2. Pectoralis major.
3. Deltoid.
4. Trapezius (inserts to the lateral 1/3rd).
5. Subclavius (inserts to the inferior surface).

Subclavius

- The subclavius is attached to the groove on the inferior surface of the clavicle. It holds the clavicle to the first rib around which it can rotate. It helps to hold the SC (sterno-clavicular joint) intact. Otherwise the SC joint would have given way in a tug of war competition. Subclavius also protects the underlying vessels from the broken pieces of clavicle.

CLINICAL ANATOMY

- Fracture of clavicle:
  1. Common.
  2. Junction of medial 2/3rd and lateral 1/3rd is weakest part in children. Greenstick fracture may ensue.

SCAPULA

- It is called scapula as it resembles a triangular-shaped digging tool.
- It is designed to give attachment to scapulo-thoracic muscles.
- It floats in a sea of muscles.
- It has three borders, three angles, three fossae, three important bony projections.
- *Three borders are:* Lateral, medial and superior.
- *Three angles are:* Superior, inferior and lateral. Lateral angle carries the glenoid cavity.
- *Three fossae are:* Subscapularis, supra-spinous and infraspinous.
- *Thee important bony projections are:* Coracoid process (it resembles a crow's beak); acromion (the top) and the spine of the scapula.
- Its lateral border is thick otherwise it would have buckled or bent by the shearing forces that the scapula is subjected to. Its lateral border gives attachment to the following muscles: Teres minor above and teres major below. The upper end of the lateral border has the infraglenoid tubercle just below the glenoid cavity and this tubercle gives origin to the long head of the triceps. Lateral border ends inferiorly at the inferior angle which gives origin to the latissimus dorsi muscle. Note that all these four muscles of the lateral border are supplied by the branches of the posterior cord of the brachial plexus.
  1. Long head of triceps—radial nerve.
  2. Teres minor—axillary nerve.
  3. Teres major—lower subscapular nerve.
  4. Latissimus dorsi—thoracodorsal nerve or nerve to latissimus dorsi.
- Medial border of scapula is thin and it gives attachment to three muscles on its dorsal aspect and one muscle along its costal surface. Totally you have to remember four muscles along the medial border like the lateral border.

The three muscles which are attached to the dorsal aspect of the medial border are (Fig. 2.2):

1. Levator scapulae—from the superior angle to the root of the spine.
2. Rhomboideus minor—opposite the root of the spine of the scapula
3. Rhomboideus major—from the root of the spine till the lower end of the medial border.

Serratus anterior is inserted into the costal surface of the medial border. But it is denser at the lower end.

Note: All these four muscles of the medial border are supplied by the roots of the brachial plexus.

- C5 root supplies the levator scapulae and rhomboids through the dorsal scapular nerve.
- Serratus anterior is supplied by the long thoracic nerve which derives its fibers from the root of C5, 6 and 7.

Supraspinous fossa gives origin to the supraspinatus (Fig. 2.2).

Infraspinous fossa gives origin to infraspinatus while subscapularis arises from the subscapular fossa (Fig. 2.3). Note that these muscles arise only from the medial two-thirds of the fossa. This allows space for the contraction of these muscles.

The two muscles of the dorsal surface, the supraspinatus and infraspinatus, are supplied by the suprascapular nerve. The subscapularis is supplied by the branches of the posterior cord of the brachial plexus, the upper and lower subscapular nerves.

- Spine and acromion are so prominent because they give attachment to two large muscles.

- They are trapezius coming from above and deltoid going down to insert into the arm.

Note that the long head of the biceps arises from the supraglenoid tubercle.

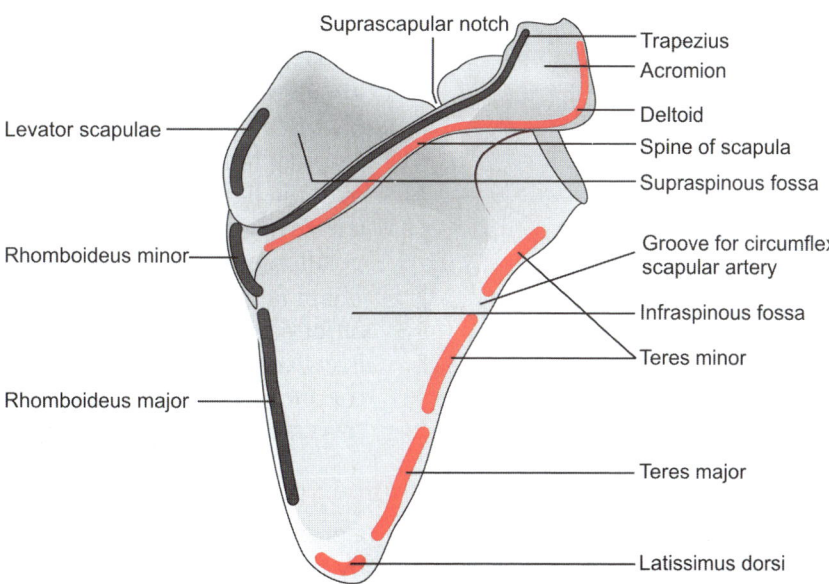

Fig. 2.2: Right scapula (posterior aspect)

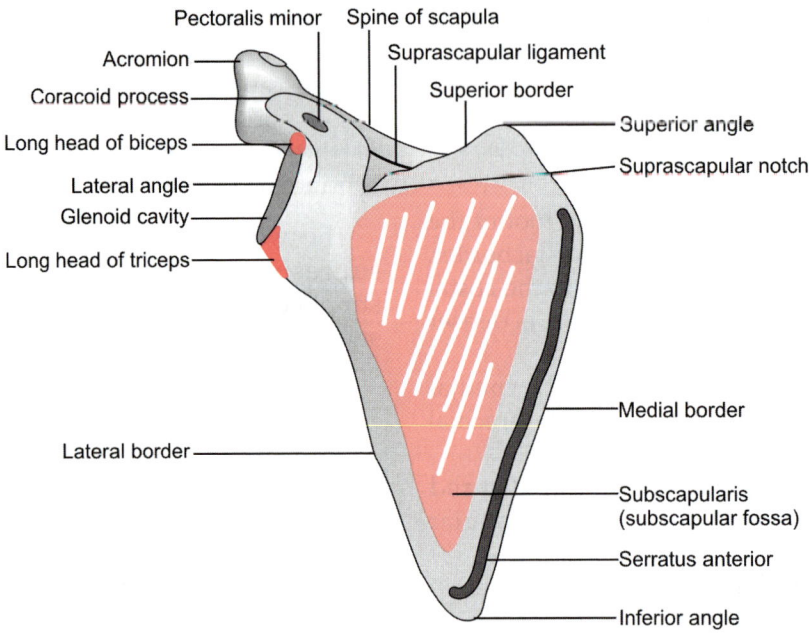

Fig. 2.3: Right scapula (anterior aspect)

The following muscles and ligaments are attached to the *coracoid process*. Three muscles are:

1. Pectoralis minor (insertion).
2. Short head of biceps (origin).
3. Coracobrachialis (origin).

Three ligaments are:
1. Coracoclavicular.
2. Coracoacromial.
3. Coracohumeral.

The Joints of Scapula

- In fact, only one joint is really associated with this bone and that is acromioclavicular joint. The other is only a conceptual joint called scapulothoracic between scapula and thorax separated by the serratus anterior and subscapularis.

The Two Notches of the Scapula

- At the lateral end of the superior border of the scapula, there is a suprascapular notch which allows the suprascapular nerve to pass through it. It is covered by the suprascapular ligament. Suprascapular vessels lie over the ligament (Mnemonic "**n**avy under the bridge" is useful to remember the position of nerve under the ligament).
- There is another notch between the spine of the scapula and the glenoid cavity and it is called the spinoglenoid notch. It allows the suprascapular vessels and nerve to traverse it to reach the infraspinous fossa.

The Ligaments of the Scapula

- Coracoid process is connected to the clavicle by the coracoclavicular ligament and it has two parts: The conoid and trapezoid part.

This ligament is very important as it transmits the weight of the upper limb to the clavicle.

- Coracoacromial ligament is a strong ligament of the scapula which forms the coracoacromial arch along with the acromion and the coracoid process. It is the protective hood of the shoulder joint.

HUMERUS

- This is a funny bone as it gives a peculiar funny sensation when posterior part of the medial epicondyle is hit accidentally.
- It is a long bone having an upper end, lower end and a shaft (Figs 2.4 and 2.5).
- Upper end has a head and two tubercles.
- Head of the humerus forms the shoulder joint with the glenoid cavity of the scapula.

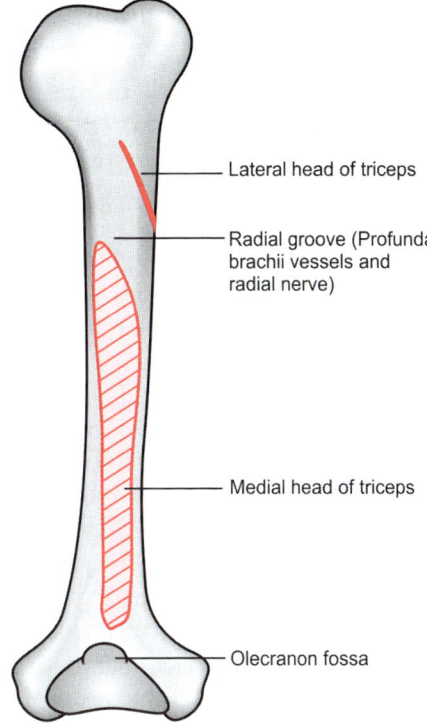

Fig. 2.5: Right humerus (posterior aspect)

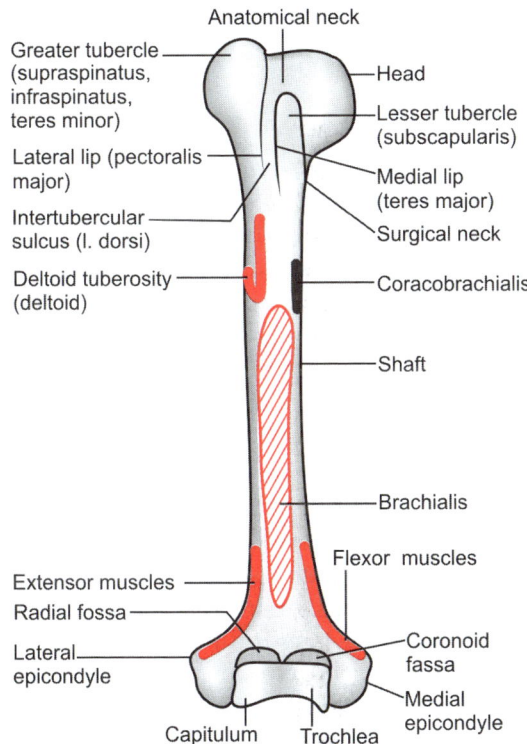

Fig. 2.4: Right humerus (anterior aspect)

- Greater tubercle is larger because it gives attachment to three muscles. Lesser tubercle is apparently small because it gives attachment to only one muscle.
- It is interesting to note that all the muscles attached to the upper end are insertions and they are designed to protect the shoulder joint and also allow the movements in the bargain.
- The muscles attached to the greater and lesser tubercles are called the muscles of muscular rotator cuff of shoulder joint.

SIT muscles are inserted into the greater tubercle.

They are:

S—Supraspinatus

I—Infraspinatus

T—Teres minor

Subscapularis is Inserted into the Lesser Tubercle

- Tendon of long head of biceps passes through the shoulder joint and emerges between the two tubercles of the upper end. Therefore, this intertubercular groove is also called the bicipital groove.
- Note that the tendon of long head of biceps arises from the supraglenoid tubercle and it is intracapsular and extrasynovial.
- The groove around the head of the humerus which excludes the tubercles is called the anatomical neck of the humerus. Capsule of the shoulder joint is attached to the anatomical neck which extends slightly inferiorly on the medial side to allow abduction.
- The lower end has two nonarticular epicondyles, articular capitulum and trochlea.
- Medial epicondyle gives attachment to the common flexor tendon of the flexor muscles of the forearm (epicondylitis results in golfers' elbow).
- Lateral epicondyle gives attachment to the common extensor tendon of the extensor muscles of the forearm (epicondylitis results in tennis elbow).
- Posterior part of the shaft gives origin to the lateral and medial heads of triceps. The groove between the origins of these two muscles is called the spiral or radial groove.
- The front of the shaft of the humerus gives insertion to the deltoid at the anterolateral part of its middle.
- Coracobrachialis is inserted into the middle of the medial border of the shaft of the humerus.
- The lower part of the front of the humerus gives origin to the brachialis muscle.
- Lateral supracondylar ridge gives origin to the brachioradialis, extensor carpi radialis longus. While the medial supracondylar ridge gives origin to the pronator teres.

What are the Nerves which are likely to be Injured in the Fractures of Humerus?

- Axillary nerve as it lies along the surgical neck of the humerus going around it from medial and posterior aspects towards the front.
- Radial nerve as it runs along with the deep artery of the arm in the spiral groove.
- Ulnar nerve as it lies behind the medial epicondyle of the humerus.
- Median nerve is likely to be injured when the lower end of the shaft of the humerus is fractured as it lies very close to it though separated from it by the brachialis muscle.

MAMMARY GLAND

Introduction:
- Position—lies in superficial fascia.
- In males, rudimentary. In females, well developed during puberty and pregnancy.

Parts:
1. Base.
2. Apex.
3. Tail of Spence.

1. *Base* extends from sternum to mid axillary line and vertically from 2nd to 6th rib.
   Deep relations (base) are 3 muscles (Fig. 2.6):
   - Pectoralis major mainly; serratus anterior and external oblique.
   - Between breast and pectoral fascia covering pectoralis major muscle is loose connective tissue called retromammary space.

2. *Apex* is formed by nipple which lies at level of 4th intercostal space (variable in pendulous breasts). It is surrounded by an area of pigmented skin called areola. No subcutaneous fat in nipple and areola. Circular and longitudinal smooth muscle fibers are seen which cause erection or flattening of nipple respectively.

3. *Tail of Spence* is an extension of the base towards the axilla.

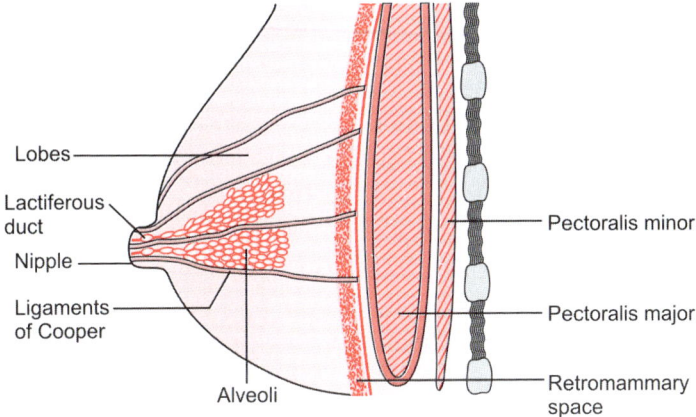

Lobes

Lactiferous duct

Nipple

Ligaments of Cooper

Alveoli

Pectoralis minor

Pectoralis major

Retromammary space

Fig. 2.6: Structure and relations of breast

Internal Structure

- Lobes—15–20 (Fig. 2.6).
- No capsule.
- Suspensory ligaments (Cooper) are fibrous condensations that support the breast tissue. The fibrous ligaments of Cooper separate the lobes and anchor the gland to both skin and deep fascia.
- Each lobe is drained by a lactiferous duct which has a lactiferous sinus (dilated portion) close to the areola.
- 15–20 lactiferous ducts converge onto the nipple like the spokes of a wheel and open here.
- The secretory element of the gland is seen as grape-like clusters within lobes.
- Suckling by the infant causes release of milk by suckling reflex or milk let down reflex or milk ejection reflex.

Breast Quadrants

The breast is divided into quadrants. It is helpful for purposes like describing the position of breast tumors and explaining the lymphatic drainage.

Blood supply:
- Branches of internal thoracic, lateral thoracic, superior thoracic and posterior intercostal.
- Veins accompany corresponding arteries.

Lymphatic Drainage

Mainly into:
- Axillary (Fig. 2.9)
- Parasternal.

Some lymph also drains into posterior intercostal nodes and communicates with other breast and rectus sheath.

- Lymph vessels—superficial and deep.
- Superficial drain skin of breast except nipple and areola into axillary, supra-clavicular group of lower deep cervical LN and parasternal in a radial manner.
- Deep lymphatics—75% of breast paren-chyma especially lateral quadrant and skin of nipple and areola (subareolar plexus of Sappey) drains into axillary (mainly anterior). Medial quadrant drains into parasternal. Lymphatics from deep surface drain into apical group after passing through pectoralis major and clavipectoral fascia.

Colostrum or first milk is produced by the female breast for the first few days following delivery or in late pregnancy.
- It is creamy white to yellow in color.
- Colostrum is rich in protein and antibodies (immunoglobulins) which is supposed to have a protective role.

Brief Development

Milk line or ridge extends from axilla to groin. All along this, breasts are developed in some animals like dogs, pigs. But in humans it develops only in pectoral regions and disappears in other areas. So humans have breast only in pectoral region.

Congenital Anomalies

- Micromastia—abnormally small.
- Macromastia—abnormally large.
- Polythelia—many nipples.
- Athelia—nipple absent.
- Polymastia—many breasts.
- Amastia—breasts absent.

Clinical Anatomy

- Cancer—lymphatic spread to other breast and distant sites (metastasis)
- Peau d'orange—blockage of superficial lymphatics results in edema of skin which gives an orange skin appearance.
- Surgical incision for drainage of breast abscess done radially to avoid damage to lactiferous ducts.
- Mammography is an imaging technique to distinguish certain breast disorders.
- Gynecomastia—males have enlarged breasts as in females.
- Treatment of breast cancer—surgery, chemotherapy and radiotherapy.

Surgery	Structures removed
Radical mastectomy—rarely performed	Breast, axillary nodes, pectoralis major, pectoralis minor
Modified radical mastectomy—widely used.	Tissues mentioned above but leaves pectoral muscles intact. Breast reconstruction can be attempted.
Simple mastectomy	Breast is removed till the retromammary space. All other structures mentioned above are spared.
Lumpectomy	Only tumor and surrounding tissue removed.

Chemotherapy is use of anticancer drugs.
Radiotherapy is use of radiation to destroy cancer cells.

Cosmetic Breast Surgeries

1. Breast reconstruction is reconstructing a patient's breast following mastectomy. Patient's own tissue flaps (latissimus dorsi) or prosthetic implants are used.
2. Breast lift surgery or mastopexy lifts the breast on the chest wall when flaccidity and loss of volume causes drooping of breast (seen in weight loss and aging).
3. Breast augmentation is enhancement of breast size or volume in patients who opt for it.
4. Breast reduction—reducing the size of breasts.

Pectoralis Major

- This is a massive muscle which arises from the anterior surface of the medial part of the clavicle, sternum and 2nd–6th costal cartilages.

- It is inserted into the lateral lip of the bicipital groove.
- *Nerve supply:* Lateral and medial pectoral nerves.
- It crosses the shoulder joint in front from medial to lateral side and, therefore, it has the following actions:
    1. Flexion.
    2. Adduction.
    3. Medial rotation

DELTOPECTORAL TRIANGLE (GROOVE)

This lies between the deltoid and pectoralis major muscles. It contains the following:

1. Cephalic vein and accompanying lymph vessels.
2. Deltopectoral lymph node.

AXILLA

- It is a pyramidal space which lies on the side of the upper part of thorax and medial side of the upper part of the arm (Fig. 2.7).
- It has an apex, base, anterior, posterior, medial and lateral walls (Fig. 2.8).

Apex is formed by three bony structures:
1. The clavicle.
2. Outer border of the first rib.
3. Superior border of the scapula.

Base is formed by three structures:
1. Skin.

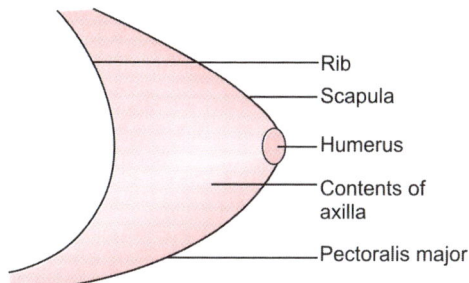

Fig. 2.7: Left axilla: Boundaries (seen from above)

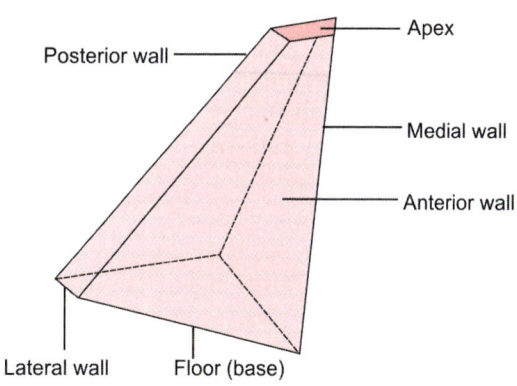

Fig. 2.8: Right axilla: Walls

2. Superficial fascia.
3. Deep fascia.

Anterior wall is formed by three structures:
1. Pectoralis major.
2. Pectoralis minor.
3. Clavipectoral fascia.

Posterior wall is formed by three structures:
1. Subscapularis.
2. Teres major.
3. Latissimus dorsi.

Medial wall is formed by three structures:
1. Upper three or four ribs.
2. Intervening intercostal spaces and inter-costal muscles.
3. Upper digitations of serratus anterior.

Lateral wall is formed by three structures:
1. Intertubercular groove.
2. Long head of biceps.
3. Common tendon of short head of biceps and coracobrachialis lying medial to it.

Contents of Axilla

1. Vessels.
2. Nerves—cords of brachial plexus and its branches.
3. Lymph nodes and lymph vessels.

Vessels

- The artery present in the axilla is the axillary artery (its branches).
- The vein present in the axilla is the axillary vein (its tributaries).

Pectoralis Minor

- It arises from the 3rd, 4th and 5th costochondral junctions and is inserted into the coracoid process.
- It does not cross a joint. Therefore, it depresses the scapula and pulls it forwards when we try to reach forward.
- *Nerve supply:* Medial and lateral pectoral nerves. Medial pectoral nerve is its main nerve supply as it pierces it.

Clavipectoral Fascia

It is a triangular-shaped fascia which bridges the gap between the clavicle and upper border of the pectoralis minor.

It is pierced by the following structures:
1. Cephalic vein.
2. Lateral pectoral nerve.
3. Acromiothoracic artery.
4. Vessels (lymph) (remember the first four letters of clavipectoral **CLAV** for mnemonic).

Axillary Group of Lymph Nodes

There are five groups of axillary lymph nodes. They are (Fig. 2.9):
1. Anterior (pectoral).
2. Posterior (subscapular).
3. Lateral.
4. Central.
5. Apical.
- Anterior group lies along the lateral border of the pectoralis minor and accompanies the lateral thoracic vessels.
- Posterior group lies along the posterior wall of thorax and accompanies the subscapular vessels.

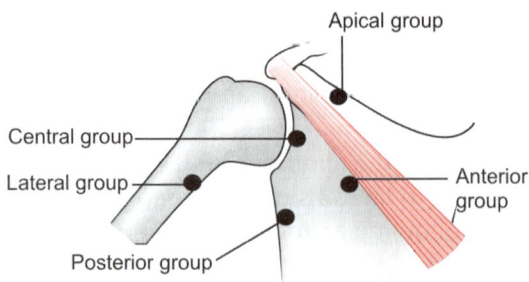

Fig. 2.9: Axillary lymph nodes (right)

- Lateral group lies along the axillary vessels in the lateral wall of the axilla.
- Central group lies in the middle of the axilla amidst the fat.
- Apical group lies at the apex of the axilla.

Axillary Artery

This is the continuation of subclavian artery (Fig. 2.10).
- Axillary artery begins at the outer border of the first rib and continues as the brachial artery at the lower border of the teres major muscle.
- It is divided into three parts by the pectoralis minor muscle.

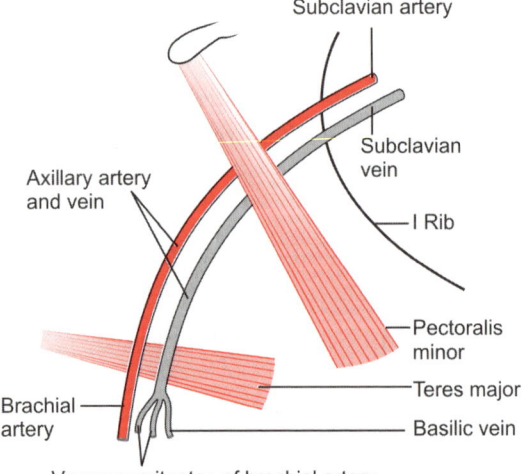

Fig. 2.10: Right axillary vessels

I part: It lies superior and medial to the pectoralis minor. It gives one branch and that is: superior thoracic artery

II part: It lies behind the pectoralis minor muscle. It gives two branches:
1. Thoracoacromial.
2. Lateral thoracic.

III part: It lies below the level of pectoralis minor: It gives three branches:
1. Subscapular.
2. Anterior circumflex humeral.
3. Posterior circumflex humeral.
- Axillary artery is related to the cords and branches of the brachial plexus.
- The first part of the axillary artery has lateral pectoral nerve and lateral cord of the brachial plexus lying lateral to it.
- Medial pectoral nerve and other cords lie behind the first part of the artery.
- The cords of the brachial plexus are named as lateral, medial and posterior depending on their relationship to the second part of the axillary artery.
- Therefore, second part of the axillary artery has lateral cord lateral to it, medial cord medial to it and posterior cord posterior to it.
- The third part of the axillary artery is related to the branches of the brachial plexus.
- Musculocutaneous nerve, lateral root of median nerve and median nerve lie lateral to the third part of the axillary artery.
- Medial root of median nerve lies anterior to it.
- Ulnar nerve and medial cutaneous nerve of forearm lie between the third part of axillary artery and axillary vein.
- Medial cutaneous nerve of arm lies medial to the axillary vein.
- All the branches of posterior cord lie behind the 3rd part of axillary artery.
- Axillary vein lies medial to all 3 parts of axillary artery.

Axillary Vein
- It lies medial to the axillary artery (Fig. 2.10).
- It is formed by the union of basilic vein with the venae comitantes of the brachial artery at the inferior border of the teres major muscle.
- It becomes the subclavian vein at the outer border of the first rib.
- It receives tributaries that correspond to branches of axillary artery.
- Ulnar nerve and medial cutaneous nerve of forearm lie between the axillary vein and third part of the axillary artery.
- Medial cutaneous nerve of arm lies medial to the axillary vein.

- Cephalic vein is the important tributary of the axillary vein. Cephalic vein pierces the clavipectoral fascia and then opens into the axillary vein at an angle. Therefore, cephalic vein is not preferred for cardiac catheterization. Basilic vein which is relatively straight is preferred.
- A collateral route is established between the tributaries of the inferior vena cava and axillary vein when thoracoepigastric veins open up in the event of obstruction to the major veins superior and inferior vena cavae.
- Wound to the axillary vein may result in air embolism and subsequent fatal pulmonary embolism.

BRACHIAL PLEXUS

- It is formed by the ventral rami of lower four cervical nerves and first thoracic nerve (Fig. 2.11).
- All plexuses are always formed by the ventral rami (Dorsal rami do not supply the skin or muscles of the upper limb).
- The roots of the brachial plexus are five in number and they are C5, 6, 7, 8 and T1.

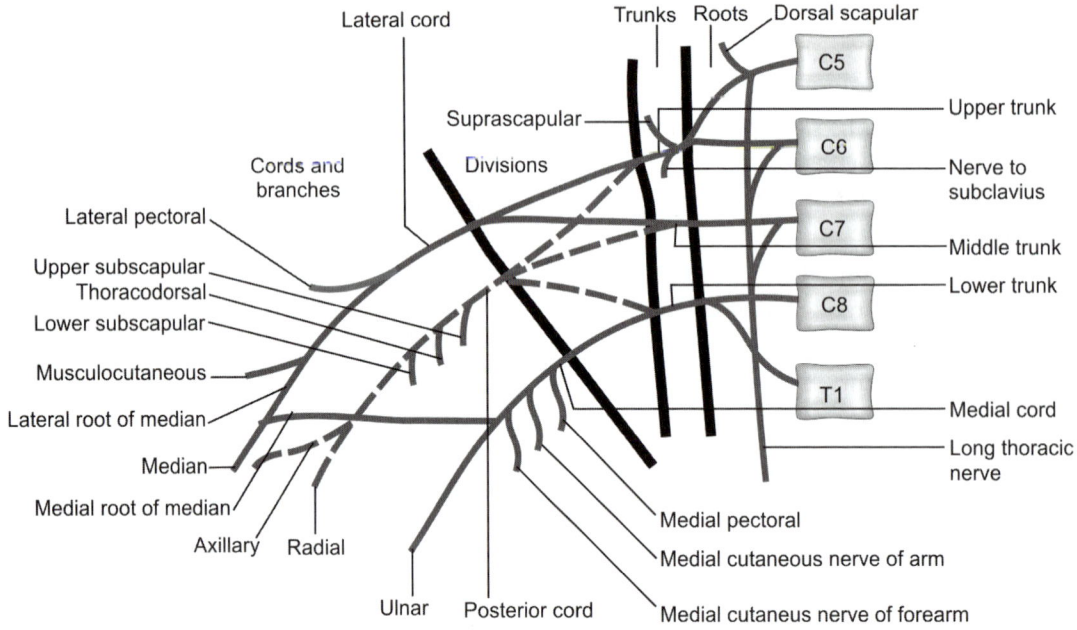

Fig. 2.11: Brachial plexus

- The roots lie between the scalenus anterior and scalenus medius.
- Upper two roots, C5 and C6, join together to form the upper trunk.
- Lower two roots, C8 and T1, join together to form the lower trunk.
- The remaining root C7 forms the middle trunk.
- Trunks lie in the posterior **T**riangle of the neck (remember **T** in **T**).
- Infraclavicular part of the brachial plexus lies in the axilla.
- Infraclavicular part includes the cords and the branches.

Note: Each trunk divides into anterior and posterior divisions. The anterior divisions of upper and middle trunks unite to form the lateral cord. The anterior division of the lower trunk continues as the medial cord. All the posterior divisions join to form the posterior cord of the brachial plexus.

Lateral Cord

It lies lateral to the second part of the axillary artery. It gives following branches:

1. Lateral pectoral.
2. Lateral root of median nerve.
3. Musculocutaneous nerve (mnemonic: **L**ady **L**oves **Me**).

Medial Cord

It lies medial to the second part of the axillary artery and lies lateral to the axillary vein. It gives the following branches:

1. Medial pectoral nerve.
2. Medial cutaneous nerve of arm.
3. Medial cutaneous nerve of forearm.
4. Ulnar nerve.
5. Medial root of median nerve (mnemonic: **M**ost **M**edical **M**en **U**se **M**orphine).

Posterior Cord

It lies behind the second part of the axillary artery. It gives the following branches:

- Upper subscapular.
- Lower subscapular.
- Nerve to latissimus dorsi.
- Axillary.
- Radial (remember ULNAR as mnemonic but ulnar nerve is not a branch of the posterior cord of the brachial plexus).

Branches from the Roots

1. To scalene muscles (these muscles have to be given branches as the roots lie between scalenus anterior and medius).
2. Nerve to longus colli (a neck muscle).
3. Dorsal scapular nerve (C5).
4. Long thoracic nerve (C5, 6 and 7).

Note: Dorsal scapular nerve supplies the muscles attached to the dorsal aspect of the medial border of the scapula and they are three in number:

1. Levator scapulae.
2. Rhomboid minor.
3. Rhomboid major.

   - Long thoracic nerve lies posterior to the brachial plexus but superficial to the serratus anterior muscle which it innervates.

It is more prone to be injured during the removal of the axillary lymph nodes. When it is injured, it results in winging of the scapula.

Branches from the Trunks

- Only upper trunk gives two branches and other trunks do not give branches. Two branches of the upper trunk are:

1. Suprascapular.
2. Nerve to subclavius.

CLINICAL ANATOMY

- When upper trunk is severed it results in *Erb-Duchenne palsy*. In this palsy, the free upper limb is pronated, adducted and medially rotated. The palm is in the semiflexed state. All this resembles to a clandestine seeking of tips either from a traffic policeman or a porter. Therefore, it is called *policeman's* or *porter's tip hand*. This accident occurs when a motorcycle rider falls on the side of the head which stretches the angle between the shoulder and head or during shoulder presentation of the fetus and associated difficult delivery.
- When lower trunk is injured it results in *Klumpke's palsy*. This occurs when a falling man holds on to a branch of a tree or something in a reflex.
- Brachial plexus block involves injecting anesthetic into angle between posterior border of sternomastoid and clavicle.

Serratus Anterior

- This muscle arises from upper eight ribs by eight digitations and is inserted into the costal surface of the medial border of the scapula.
- It helps in dragging the scapula forwards which is called protraction.
- Its nerve lies superficial to it.
- Long thoracic nerve supplies it.

TRAPEZIUS

This muscle is called trapezius because it resembles a trapezium when muscles of both sides are seen together (Fig. 2.12).

- *Origin*
   1. Medial part of the superior nuchal line.
   2. Ligamentum nuchae.
   3. Spines of all thoracic vertebrae.

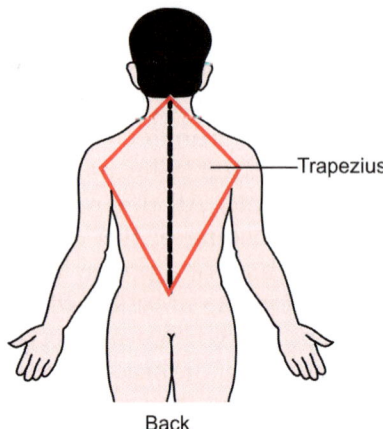

Back

Fig. 2.12: Trapezius

Remember: Whenever a muscle arises from more than one bone, the origin is always continuous. Now appreciate the continuous origin of the trapezius. If the origin were to be discontinuous, we would have given different names to it.

- *Insertion:* It is inserted in one continuous line into the following structures in the shape of letter "U".
  1. Lateral part of the posterior aspect of the clavicle.
  2. Medial border of the acromion.
  3. Upper lip of the crest of the spine of the scapula.

Direction of the Fibers

- Upper fibers are directed downwards and laterally.
- Middle fibers run horizontally.
- Lower fibers are directed upwards and laterally.

Note: Its action is mainly on the movement of the scapula.

Action

- Upper fibers elevate the scapula as in shrugging (when you say, "I don't know").

- Middle fibers retract and move the scapula towards the median plane. This is a movement through which the two scapulae come near to each other (imagine an old guy lazily walking with his hands clasped on the back of the hip).

Nerve Supply

- Its motor nerve supply is from the spinal part of accessory nerve. Its sensory innervation comes from C3 and C4 fibers.
- When the muscle is paralyzed it results in the bottle neck paralysis. Head, neck and trunk resemble a bottle neck.

Structures that Lie deep to Trapezius

- The nerve supplying a muscle lies deep to the said muscle. Similarly, spinal part of accessory nerve and branches of C3 and C4 lie deep to trapezius.
- Superficial branch of transverse cervical artery lies deep to the muscle.
- There are three muscles which lie deep to it in the scapular region:
  - Levator scapulae.
  - Rhomboid minor.
  - Rhomboid major.

Movements of the Scapula

- Elevation of the scapula as in shrugging of the shoulder. This movement is carried out by the upper fibers of trapezius and levator scapulae.
- Depression is carried out by the gravity assisted by the lower fibers of trapezius.
- *Protraction:* Serratus anterior and pectoralis minor.
- *Retraction:* Rhomboid muscles and middle fibers of trapezius.
- *Lateral rotation:* This is called lateral rotation because the inferior angle of the scapula moves laterally. This movement is observed

when hand is raised above the level of the head. Two muscles that help in this movement are trapezius and serratus anterior.

- *Medial rotation:* It is opposite of the lateral rotation. Muscles attached to the dorsal aspect of medial border namely levator scapulae, rhomboid muscles assisted by the pectoralis minor help bring about this movement.

Latissimus Dorsi

- This is another massive muscle seen on the back. It is called latissimus because it is very wide.
- It arises from the iliac crest, lumbar fascia and the spines of lower thoracic vertebrae and inferior angle of the scapula.

Note: Appreciate the continuous origin of this muscle from the bony points given above.

- The muscle goes around the teres major and moves anterior to it. Therefore, the two muscles, teres major and latissimus dorsi, form the posterior fold of the axilla.
- It is inserted into the floor of the intertubercular sulcus which is also called the bicipital groove.

Action

- It helps to draw the arm backwards and medially. Therefore, it has three actions: (1) extension (2) adduction (3) medial rotation.
- (If you ever forget the action of this muscle just scratch the back of the opposite scapula with the arm over the back.) It is also known as swimmer's muscle as it is very evident in the back stroke swimming. It is well developed in boat rovers and canoers.

- When the muscle is paralyzed one cannot take the pull ups over a horizontal exercise bar. But for weakness in extension and adduction at shoulder, there is no other appreciable disability following the paralysis of the muscle. Therefore, they may sacrifice the nerve to latissimus dorsi, if need be, while removing the cancerous axillary lymph nodes but not nerve to serratus anterior.

Remember that a patient with latissimus dorsi paralysis cannot use crutch.

Nerve supply: It is supplied by the nerve to latissimus dorsi (thoracodorsal nerve) which arises from the posterior cord of the brachial plexus.

Triangle of Auscultation

- It is a triangular gap between the trapezius and latissimus dorsi muscle near the inferior angle of the scapula.
- Superiorly it is bounded by the inferolateral border of the trapezius.
- Inferiorly it is bounded by the superior horizontal border of the latissimus dorsi muscle.
- Laterally it is bounded by the lower part of the medial border of the scapula.

When the arms are folded across the front of the chest and the trunk is flexed, the scapulae are drawn anteriorly so that triangle of auscultation enlarges. It is through this triangle that posterior segments of the lung are examined using a stethoscope.

Do you know? Before the advent of stethoscope, physicians used to listen to the sound of spurting of fluid into the stomach by applying their ears to this triangle on the left side.

DELTOID

- It is called deltoid because it is shaped like inverted Greek letter "delta".
- It is responsible for the smooth contour of the shoulder.
- It is the principal abductor of the shoulder.

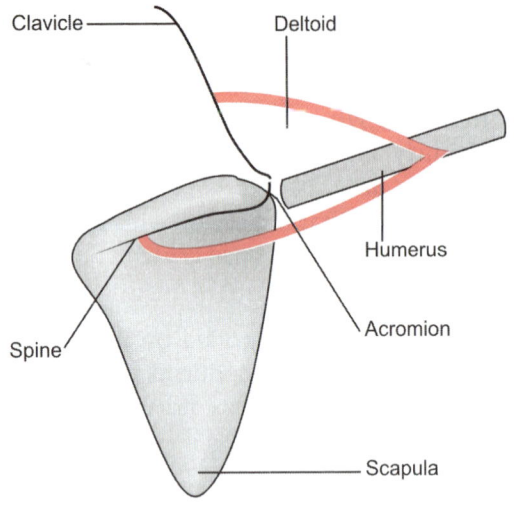

Fig. 2.13: Deltoid

Origin

It has a continuous origin from:
- Anterior aspect of the lateral part of the clavicle.
- Lateral margin of the acromion.
- Lower lip of the crest of the spine of the scapula.
- The origin is shaped like letter "U" placed sideward.

Insertion

Deltoid tuberosity on the lateral part of the middle of the humerus.
Nerve supply: Axillary nerve.

Action

- Anterior fibers help in the flexion and medial rotation of the shoulder.
- Posterior fibers help in the extension and lateral rotation of the shoulder.
- Anterior and posterior fibers alternately contract while walking.
- Middle fibers are multipennate and abduct the shoulder joint.

Structures that lie deep to deltoid (Fig. 2.14):
1. Shoulder joint.
2. Subacromial bursa.
3. Axillary nerve.
4. Anterior and posterior circumflex humeral vessels.
5. Supraspinatus.
6. Coracoid process and origin of coraco-brachialis and short head of biceps from it.
7. Insertion of pectoralis minor into the coracoid process. Coracoclavicular and coracoacromial ligaments.
8. Origin of long head of triceps.
9. Upper end of humerus.
10. Triangular and quadrangular muscular spaces.

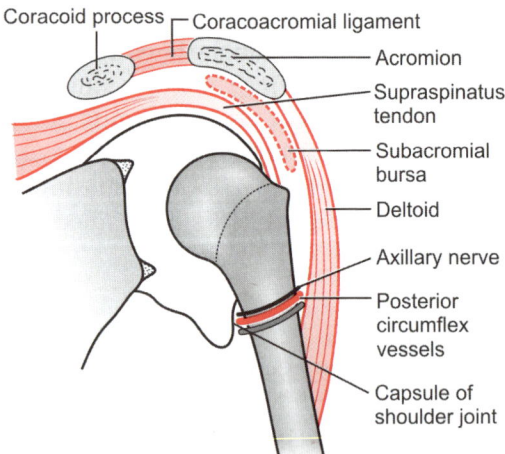

Fig. 2.14: Structures under cover of deltoid

Quadrangular Space

It is a muscular space which lies inferior to the lateral border of the scapula (Fig. 2.15).

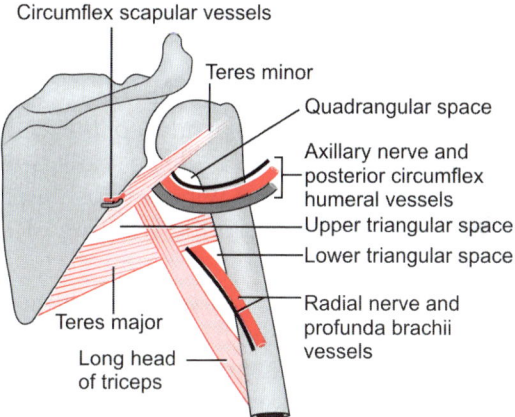

Fig. 2.15: Triangular and quadrangular spaces

Boundaries

- *Medially:* Long head of triceps.
- *Laterally:* Upper end of the humerus.
- *Superiorly:* Subscapularis in front and teres minor behind.
- *Inferiorly:* Teres major.
- *Contents:* Axillary nerve and posterior circumflex humeral artery.

Upper Triangular Space

- It lies medial to the long head of triceps (Fig. 2.15).
- *Superomedially:* Subscapularis in front and teres minor behind.
- *Inferiorly:* Teres major.
- *Laterally:* Long head of triceps.
- *Contents:* Circumflex scapular artery, a branch of subscapular artery lies in it (not ideally a content).

Lower Triangular Space

- There is a lower triangular space below the teres major (Fig. 2.15).
  The boundaries are:
  - *Superiorly:* Teres major.
  - *Laterally:* Shaft of the humerus.

- *Medially:* Long head of the triceps.
- *Contents:* Radial nerve and deep artery of the arm.

Muscular Rotator Cuff of the Shoulder Joint

These are the muscles which immediately surround the capsule of the shoulder joint. Following are the rotator cuff muscles:

1. Subscapularis.
2. Supraspinatus.
3. Infraspinatus.
4. Teres minor.
   These muscles are inserted into the greater and lesser tubercles.
- Three muscles are inserted into the greater tubercle.
  1. Supraspinatus.
  2. Infraspinatus.
  3. Teres minor (SIT muscles).
  Subscapularis is inserted into the lesser tubercle.
- They act like expansile ligaments and protect the shoulder joint. The tonic contraction of the muscles helps keep the head of the humerus opposed to the glenoid cavity.

Nerve Supply of the Muscles of Rotator Cuff

- Supraspinatus and infraspinatus—supras-capular nerve.
- Teres minor—axillary nerve.
- Subscapularis—upper and lower sub-scapular nerves.

AXILLARY NERVE

- It arises from the posterior cord of the brachial plexus (Fig. 2.16).
- Its root value is C5 and C6.
- It lies anterior to the subscapularis muscle.
- It passes through the quadrangular space.

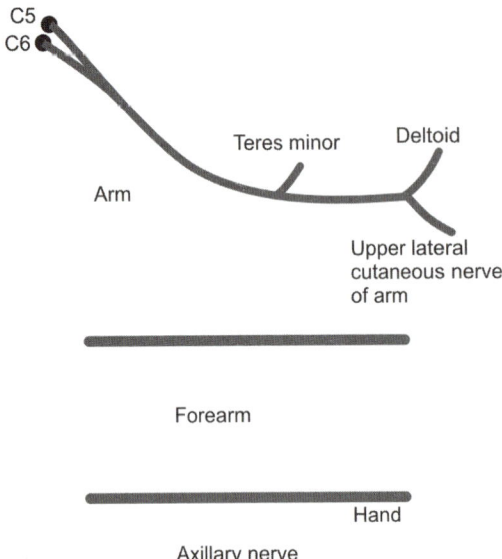

Fig. 2.16: Muscular branches of axillary nerve

- It divides into anterior and posterior branches.
- Posterior branch supplies the teres minor and deltoid and becomes the superior lateral cutaneous nerve of arm.
- Anterior branch supplies the anterior part of the deltoid and winds around the surgical neck of the humerus. Anterior branch accompanies the posterior circumflex humeral artery.
- It is commonly injured in the fractures of surgical neck of the humerus.
- It supplies the shoulder joint from main trunk.

- It might be injured in the inferior dislocation of the shoulder joint.
- It is usually involved in the fracture of the surgical neck of the humerus.
- Following injury to the axillary nerve the rounded contour of the shoulder is lost and and abduction is not possible in 15 to 90 degrees range.

Testing of Muscles

- *Serratus anterior:* Patient is asked to push the wall or asked to abduct the arm over his head. If this muscle is paralyzed, the medial border and inferior angle of the scapula protrudes back like a wing on pushing the wall and this is called the **winging of the scapula.**
- *Latissimus dorsi:* It is tested by asking the patient to touch the back of the opposite scapula. When this muscle is paralyzed, it is not possible to take pull ups on a horizontal bar. It is also not possible to use axillary crutch when this muscle is paralyzed.
- Upper fibers of trapezius are tested by asking the patient to shrug against the resistance.
- *Deltoid:* It is tested by asking the patient to abduct against resistance beyond 15 degrees.
- *Supraspinatus:* Tested by asking the patient to abduct for initial 15 degrees against resistance.
- *Infraspinatus:* Tested by asking the patient to laterally rotate the adducted arm against resistance.
- *Clavicular fibers of pectoralis major:* Patient is asked to flex the arm against resistance.
- *Sternoclavicular fibers of pectoralis major:* Patient is asked to adduct and medially rotate the arm against the resistance.

Anastomoses around the Scapula

- There are three arteries which take part in the anastomosis around the scapula (Fig. 2.17).
  1. Suprascapular artery.
  2. Deep branch of the transverse cervical artery which is also called the dorsal scapular artery.
  3. Circumflex scapular artery, a branch of subscapular artery.

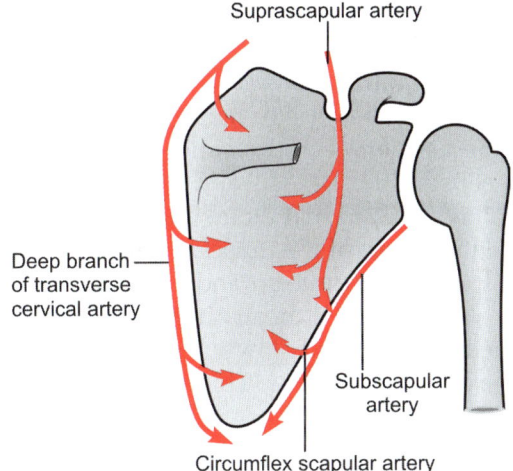

Fig. 2.17: Anastomoses around the scapula

In the event of block or ligation of first or second part of axillary artery, blood reaches the scapular region through the suprascapular artery and the deep branch of transverse cervical artery and from there it goes in reverse direction to the third part of the axillary artery through the circumflex artery and its parent trunk the subscapular artery.

Anterior Compartment of the Arm

- Identify the cephalic vein on the lateral side and basilic vein in the lower part of the medial side of the arm superficial to the deep fascia.
- Basilic vein pierces the deep fascia at the middle of the medial side of the arm.

Muscles of the anterior compartment of the arm are (Fig. 2.18):

1. Biceps brachii.
2. Coracobrachialis.
3. Brachialis.

Note: All these three muscles are supplied by the musculocutaneous nerve (mnemonic BBC).

Biceps Brachii

- *It has two heads:* A short and a long head.
- Short head arises from the coracoid process along with the coracobrachialis.
- Long head arises from the supraglenoid tubercle and lies inside the capsule of the shoulder joint.
- The tendon of long head of biceps is intracapsular and extrasynovial.

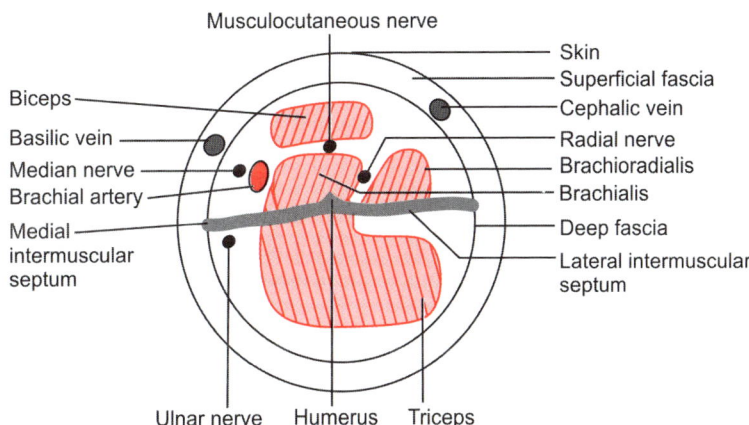

Fig. 2.18: Transverse section through the lower third of the arm

- It emerges through the intertubercular groove and joins the short head.
- It is inserted into the posterior part of the radial tuberosity.
- It crosses the shoulder, elbow and superior radioulnar joints. Therefore, it has actions on all these three joints.

Action on the shoulder joint: Long head prevents upwards dislocation of the head of the humerus and acts like a protective expansible ligament. Short head assists coracobrachialis in the flexion of the shoulder joint.

Action on the elbow joint: It flexes the elbow joint as it crosses anterior to the joint.

Action on the superior radioulnar joint: It supinates the forearm as it crosses the vertical axis of supination and pronation. It is a powerful supinator and that is the reason why all screws are tightened by supination action and loosened by pronation.

Nerve supply: Musculocutaneous nerve.

Coracobrachialis

- It arises from the coracoid process along with the short head of the biceps. It is inserted into the middle of the medial side of the humerus.
- It crosses the shoulder joint anteromedially, therefore, it serves as the flexor of the shoulder joint.

Note: It is pierced by the musculocutaneous nerve and musculocutaneous nerve supplies this muscle before it passes through it.

Brachialis

- It arises from the lower part of the front of the humerus.
- It is inserted into the ulnar tuberosity of ulna.

- It protects the elbow joint in front. It lies immediately outside the capsule of the elbow joint.
- *It is supplied by two nerves:* Musculo-cutaneous nerve—motor and radial nerve—sensory.
- It is also said that radial nerve supplies the lateral part of the muscle.
- It lifts the drink up and keeps the empty glass down. It means it helps to flex the elbow joint and slowly relaxes during the extension of elbow. This slow relaxation is called the paying out rope action. That results in a smooth extension.

BRACHIAL ARTERY

- It is the continuation of the axillary artery.
- It begins at the level of the lower border of the teres major.
- It terminates opposite the neck of the radius by dividing into two terminal branches, radial and ulnar.
- Its pulsations are readily felt in the middle of the arm medial to the biceps.

- This artery is used to measure the blood pressure.
- It may be compressed near the middle of the arm.

Branches

1. Arteria profunda brachii (deep artery of the arm).
2. Nutrient artery to humerus.
3. Superior ulnar collateral artery.
4. Inferior ulnar collateral artery.
5. Muscular branches.
6. Two terminal branches: Radial and ulnar.

Anastomoses around the Elbow

It exists between branches of brachial artery, profunda brachii artery, radial artery, ulnar artery and posterior interosseous artery (Fig. 2.19).

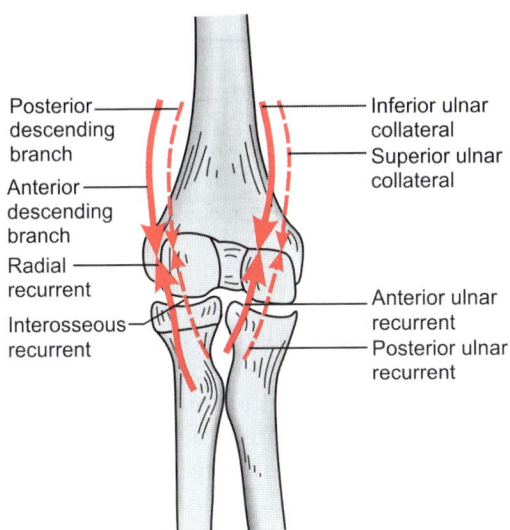

Fig. 2.19: Anastomoses around the elbow

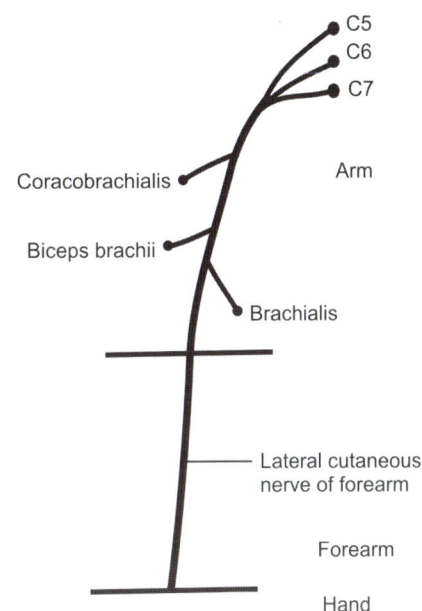

Fig. 2.20: Muscular branches of musculocutaneous nerve

It occurs around the elbow as follows:

1. In front of medial epicondyle between inferior ulnar collateral branch of brachial and anterior ulnar recurrent branch of ulnar.
2. Behind medial epicondyle between superior ulnar collateral branch of brachial and posterior ulnar recurrent branch of ulnar.
3. In front of lateral epicondyle between anterior descending branch of profunda brachii and radial recurrent branch of radial.
4. Behind lateral epicondyle between posterior descending branch of profunda brachii and interosseous recurrent branch of posterior interosseous artery.

It helps in collateral circulation when terminal part of brachial artery is compressed in flexion of elbow.

MUSCULOCUTANEOUS NERVE

- This nerve arises from the lateral cord of the brachial plexus (Fig. 2.20).
- It pierces the coracobrachialis.

- It becomes the lateral cutaneous nerve of forearm.
- *It supplies:* Biceps brachii, coracobrachialis and brachialis muscles.

Median Nerve in the Arm

- It lies on the lateral side of the brachial artery as far as the insertion of the coracobrachialis and later it crosses the artery anteriorly and goes medial to it.
- It does not give any muscular branch or any other named branch in the arm. It may give unnamed vascular branches and sometimes nerve to pronator teres in the lower part of the arm.

Ulnar Nerve in the Arm

- It lies medial to the brachial artery as far as the insertion of coracobrachialis. Later it goes far more medial and pierces the medial intermuscular septum. Later it lies posterior to the medial epicondyle of the humerus.

Name the different relations at the level of insertion of coracobrachialis in the arm:

- Median nerve crosses from lateral to medial side.
- Ulnar nerve goes far more medial at this level.
- Nutrient artery to humerus is given.
- Basilic vein pierces the deep fascia.
- The brachial artery passes from the medial side of the arm to its anterior aspect.

Cubital Fossa

- Triangular fossa at the junction of arm and forearm (Fig. 2.21).
- Base is formed by the imaginary line connecting the two epicondyles of the humerus.
- Medial boundary is formed by the pronator teres.
- Lateral boundary is formed by the brachioradialis.
- Floor is formed by brachialis and supinator muscles.

The roof of the cubital fossa which is formed by skin and fasciae contains the following:
1. Median cubital vein.
2. Bicipital aponeurosis.

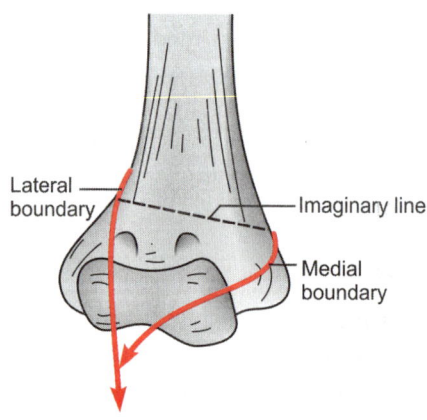

Fig. 2.21: Cubital fossa: Boundaries

3. Medial cutaneous nerve of forearm.
4. Lateral cutaneous nerve of forearm.

Following are the contents:
1. Median nerve.
2. Brachial artery.
3. Tendon of biceps.
4. Radial nerve.

For structures 3, 2, 1 the mnemonic is **TAN** from lateral to medial.

Logic: The median nerve has already crossed the brachial artery from the lateral to medial side at the insertion of the coracobrachialis in the mid-arm. Therefore, the median nerve must lie most medially followed by the brachial artery. The radial nerve should be the most lateral structure. Palpate the tendon of biceps in the cubital fossa.

Back of the Arm

Triceps

Large triceps muscle lies deep to the deep fascia. It has three heads:

- *Long head:* It arises from the infraglenoid tubercle which lies outside the capsule of the shoulder joint.
- *Lateral head:* It arises from the posterior surface of the shaft superior to the spiral line.
- *Medial head:* It arises from the lower part of the posterior surface of the humerus.
- *Insertion:* All three heads join to form the belly of triceps and its tendon is inserted into the olecranon process of ulna.
- *Nerve supply:* Radial nerve.
- *Action:* Extends elbow.

Radial Groove

- It is a spiral groove which lies between the medial and lateral heads of triceps muscle.
- It contains the radial nerve, its branches and profunda brachii artery.

The following branches of radial nerve lie in the radial groove:
1. Branch to lateral head of triceps.
2. Branch to medial head of triceps.
3. Nerve to anconeus.
4. Lower lateral cutaneous nerve of arm.
5. Posterior cutaneous nerve of forearm.

Identify the following bony landmarks on humerus:
- Lateral epicondyle of the humerus.
- Medial epicondyle of the humerus.
- Capitulum.
- Trochlea.
- Medial flange of trochlea is more prominent than the lateral flange and this causes the carrying angle.

The carrying angle is the angle described laterally between the long axis of arm and forearm. The angle is less and forearm is more bent in the case of female. In the case of male, the bend is less.

Identify the following fossae in the lower end of the humerus:
1. Olecranon fossa.
2. Radial fossa.
3. Coronoid fossa.

The radius presents the following landmarks:
- The head.
- The neck.
- The tuberosity of radius.
- Styloid process of radius.
- Dorsal tubercle of radius.
- Interosseous border of radius.

CLINICAL ANATOMY

- Lower end of the radius is usually fractured when a person falls on the outstretched hand. The broken distal segment of radius

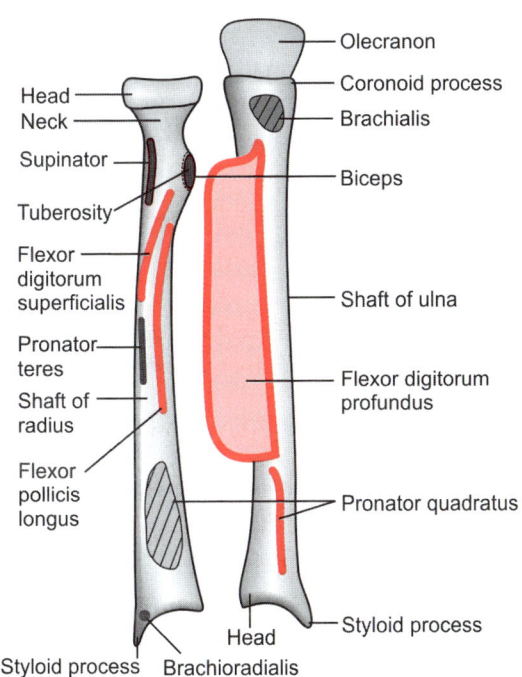

Fig. 2.22: Right radius and ulna (anterior aspect)

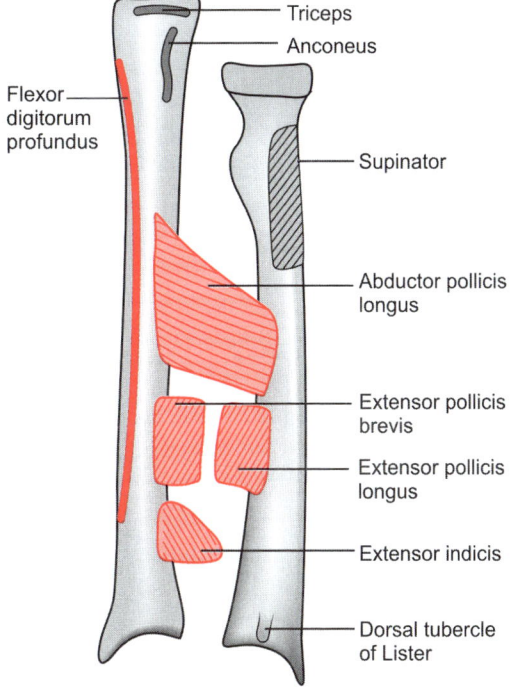

Fig. 2.23: Right radius and ulna (posterior aspect)

is displaced dorsally and it is called **Colle's fracture.**

- If a person falls on the back of the hand and if the fractured radius is displaced ventrally then it is called **Smith's fracture.**

The ulna presents the following landmarks:
- Coronoid process.
- Olecranon process.
- Trochlear notch.
- Ulnar tuberosity.
- Head of ulna.
- Styloid process of ulna.
- The posterior border of ulna presents a groove on the back of the forearm in the living. This can be easily seen on the back of the flexed forearm. You can trace this groove to the head of ulna inferiorly.
- The styloid process of radius is at a lower level when compared to the styloid process of ulna. The radial styloid process lies in the anatomical snuff box.

(Palpate the ulnar and radial styloid processes).

Following parts of the ulna can be palpated:
- Head of ulna.
- Styloid process of ulna.

- Olecranon.
- Posterior border of ulna.

Anterior Compartment of the Forearm

There are four superficial muscles of the forearm which arise from the medial epicondyle of the humerus. They are:

1. Pronator teres.
2. Flexor carpi radialis.
3. Palmaris longus.
4. Flexor carpi ulnaris.

Pronator Teres

- It arises from the medial epicondyle of the humerus.
- It also arises from the medial border of olecranon process of ulna.
- Therefore, it has two heads: the humeral (superficial) and ulnar (deep) heads.
- Median nerve runs between its two heads and it is the site of compression of median nerve.
- Deep head of pronator teres separates the median nerve from the ulnar artery.
- Ulnar artery lies deep to the deep head of pronator teres.

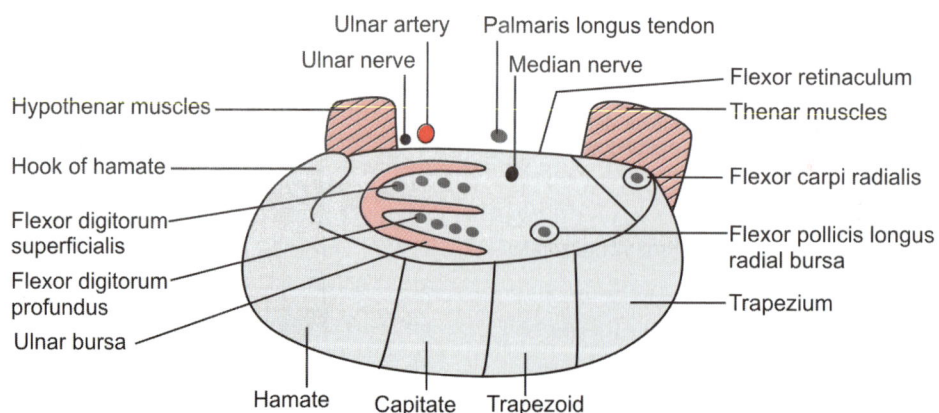

Fig. 2.24: Flexor retinaculum and carpal tunnel

- Pronator teres is inserted into the maximum convexity on the shaft of the radius.
- It is supplied by the median nerve.
- It acts as a pronator of the forearm.
- It forms the medial boundary of the cubital fossa.

Flexor Carpi Radialis

- It arises from the medial epicondyle of the humerus.
- It lies within a separate compartment deep to the flexor retinaculum (Fig. 2.24).
- It is inserted into the bases of second and third metacarpal bones.
- Why is it inserted into both second and third metacarpals? It is because it has to counteract the extensor muscles; extensor carpi radialis longus and brevis.
- It is supplied by the median nerve.
- It flexes the wrist. It abducts the wrist joint when it acts with the extensor carpi radialis longus and brevis.

Palmaris Longus

- It arises from the medial epicondyle of the humerus.
- It lies superficial to the flexor retinaculum and is inserted into the palmar aponeurosis (Fig. 2.24).
- It is often absent and it is supplied by the median nerve.

  You know this interesting point!! Some of the muscles which begin with the letter "P" are often absent (considered vestigial) and they are:
1. Palmaris longus.
2. Palmaris brevis.
3. Psoas minor.
4. Plantaris.
5. Pyramidalis.

Flexor Carpi Ulnaris

- It arises from the medial epicondyle of the humerus.

- It also arises from the posterior border of the ulna and olecranon.
- Ulnar nerve passes between the two heads of the flexor carpi ulnaris and supplies the flexor carpi ulnaris before it passes between its two heads.
- It is the site where compression of ulnar nerve can occur.
- It is inserted into the pisiform bone.
- It flexes the wrist joint and it adducts the wrist joint along with the extensor carpi ulnaris.

Flexor Digitorum Superficialis

- It arises from three bones:
  1. Medial epicondyle of humerus.
  2. Coronoid process of ulna.
  3. Oblique line of radius.
- It runs deep to the flexor retinaculum and divides into four tendons (Fig. 2.24).
- The four tendons go to the medial four digits of the hand.

  Each tendon splits into two (perforated by flexor digitorum profundus) and is attached to the sides of the middle phalanx (Fig. 2.25).
- It is supplied by the median nerve.
- It flexes the proximal interphalangeal joint.
- It also assists in the flexion of the meta-carpophalangeal and wrist joints.

Deep muscles of the front of the forearm:
There are three deep muscles:
1. The flexor digitorum profundus.
2. The flexor pollicis longus.
3. Pronator quadratus.

Flexor Digitorum Profundus

- It arises from ulna (upper 3/4th of anterior and medial surface and posterior border). It also arises from the adjoining intero-sseous membrane.

- It passes deep to the flexor retinaculum and divides into four tendons for the medial four digits (Fig. 2.24).
- The tendons give origin to four lumbricals.
- The tendon of flexor digitorum profundus is inserted into the base of the distal phalanx.
- *It is supplied by two nerves:* The medial half is supplied by the ulnar nerve while the lateral half is supplied by the anterior interosseous branch of median nerve.
- It flexes the distal interphalangeal joint.
- It also assists in the flexion of the proximal interphalangeal, metacarpophalangeal and wrist joints.

Flexor Pollicis Longus

- It arises from the anterior surface of radius between anterior oblique line and pronator quadratus. It also arises from the adjoining interosseous membrane.
- It passes deep to the flexor retinaculum and is inserted into the base of the distal phalanx of thumb (Fig. 2.24).
- It flexes the interphalangeal joint of thumb.
- It is supplied by the anterior interosseous branch of median nerve.

Pronator Quadratus

- It is a quadrilateral muscle.
- It arises from the distal 1/4th of anterior surface of ulna and is inserted into the distal 1/4th of anterior surface of radius.
- Its action is pronation.
- It is supplied by the anterior interosseous nerve of forearm.

Note: All supinators and pronators are inserted into the radius. Why? It is the radius which moves in all excursions of forearm. That is the reason why the bone is come to be called as radius. It means it moves like the radius of a circle in all rotatory movements of the forearm. Therefore, all supinators and pronators are inserted into the radius. (By this you can easily remember that biceps, supinator, pronator teres and pronator quadratus are inserted into radius).

Medial epicondylitis:
- It is also called golfer's elbow.
- It is due to the inflammation of tendon of origin of flexor muscles from the medial epicondyle of the humerus.

Flexor retinaculum of wrist:
- It is thickened band of deep fascia which bridges the concavity of carpal bones (Fig. 2.24).
- It is attached medially to the pisiform and hook of the hamate bones.
- It is attached laterally to the scaphoid and trapezium bones.

The following structures lie superficial to the flexor retinaculum of the wrist:
1. Ulnar nerve.
2. Ulnar artery.
3. Palmar cutaneous branch of ulnar nerve.
4. Palmaris longus tendon.
5. Palmar cutaneous branch of median nerve.
6. Superficial palmar branch of radial artery.

The following structures lie deep to the flexor retinaculum of wrist:
1. The median nerve.
2. Four tendons of flexor digitorum superficialis.
3. Four tendons of flexor digitorum profundus.
4. Tendon of flexor pollicis longus.
5. Tendon of flexor carpi radialis that lies in a separate compartment.

From superficial to deep, you find structures in the following order in the palm of the hand:
- The skin fibrous loculated superficial fascia.
- Palmar aponeurosis.
- Superficial palmar arch and its common digital branches.

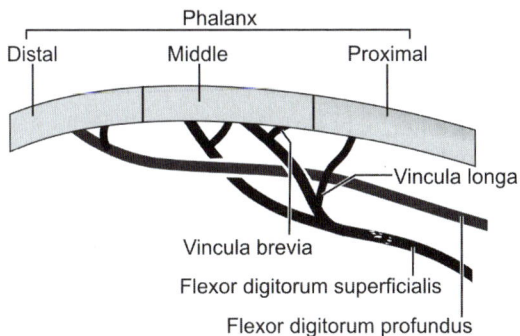

Fig. 2.25: Flexor digitorum superficialis and profundus tendons in digits

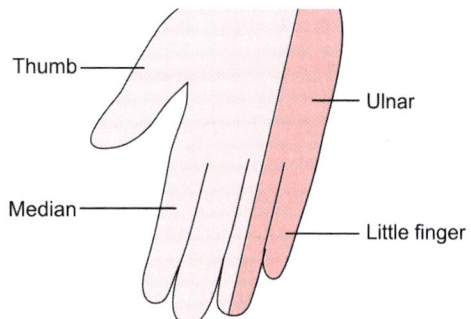

Fig. 2.26: Cutaneous innervation of front of hand (right)

- Digital branches of ulnar and median nerves.
- Tendons of flexor digitorum superficialis and profundus.
- Lumbricals arise from the tendons of the flexor digitorum profundus.
- Deep palmar arch and the deep branch of ulnar nerve lie deep to the tendons.
- Interossei muscles.

The skin is firmly attached to the underlying fascia. By this, skin does not slip and thereby enhances the grip.

Try this: You can lift the skin of the dorsum of the hand while it is not possible to pinch the skin of the palm of the hand.

Ulnar nerve supplies the medial part of the palm of the hand and medial one and half digits while the median nerve supplies the lateral part of the palm of the hand and lateral three and half digits (Fig. 2.26).

Palmar Aponeurosis

- It is a triangular, strong and well defined part of the deep fascia of the palm (Fig. 2.27).
- It covers the soft tissue and overlies the tendons of the palm of the hand.
- The proximal end is apex and is continuous with the flexor retinaculum.

- Distally it forms the four digital bands for the medial four digits.

- *Dupuytren's contracture:* It is the progressive shortening, thickening and fibrosis of the palmar aponeurosis. Little and ring fingers are partially flexed. Surgical excision of fibrotic part is curative.

Note:
- Palmar aponeurosis sends in a medial vertical septum which is attached to the fifth metacarpal bone.

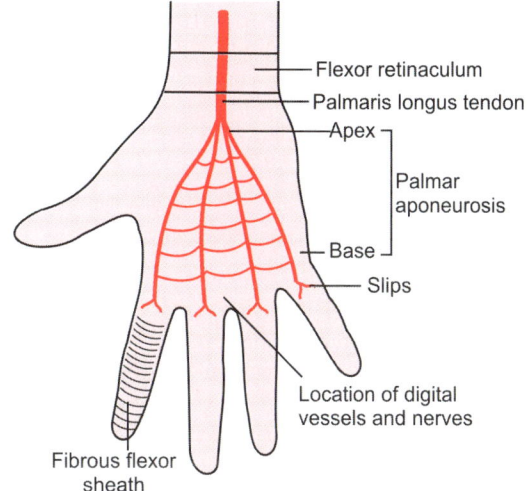

Fig. 2.27: Palmar aponeurosis and fibrous flexor sheaths

- The lateral vertical septum is attached to the first metacarpal bone.
- An intermediate septum is attached obliquely to the third metacarpal bone.
- These three septae and fascial lining divide the palm into the following compartments:
  1. Lateral thenar compartment which contains three muscles of thumb.
  2. Medial hypothenar compartment which contains three muscles of little finger.
  3. Central compartment which contains long flexor tendons and lumbricals.
  4. Adductor compartment which contains adductor pollicis muscle.
  5. Interosseous compartment containing palmar and dorsal interossei.
- In between the above said compartments, there are two spaces.
  1. Medial large midpalmar space (lies between the medial and intermediate septae).
  2. Lateral small thenar space (lies between the intermediate and lateral septae).

Facial Spaces in Palm

- Three are important.
- They are thenar, midpalmar and pulp spaces (Figs 2.28 and 2.29).

- *Thenar space:*
  - Bounded anteriorly by muscles of thenar eminence.
  - Posteriorly by adductor pollicis.
  - Medially by midpalmar space.
  - *Proximal limit:* Flexor retinaculum but may be continuous with forearm space of parona.
  - *Distally:* Continuous with I and II lumbrical canal (fascial sheath of lumbricals).
- *Midpalmar space:*
  - Bounded anteriorly by III and IV lumbricals, palmar aponeurosis.
  - Posteriorly by metacarpals 3–5 and associated interosseous muscles.
  - Medially by medial palmar septum.
  - Laterally intermediate septum and thenar space.
  - *Proximal limit:* Flexor retinaculum but may be continuous with forearm space of parona.
  - *Distally:* Continuous with III and IV lumbrical canal (fascial sheath of lumbricals).

- These are the potential spaces which may allow pus or other pathologic material to be collected in them. They can be drained

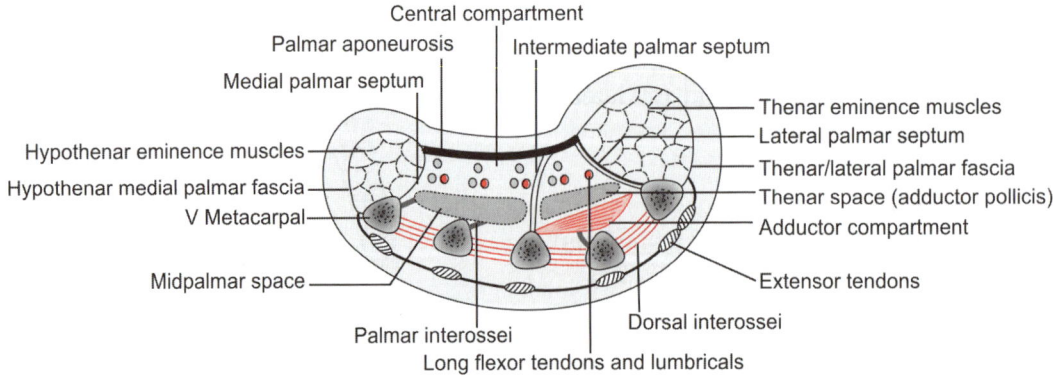

Fig. 2.28: Cross-section through the hand

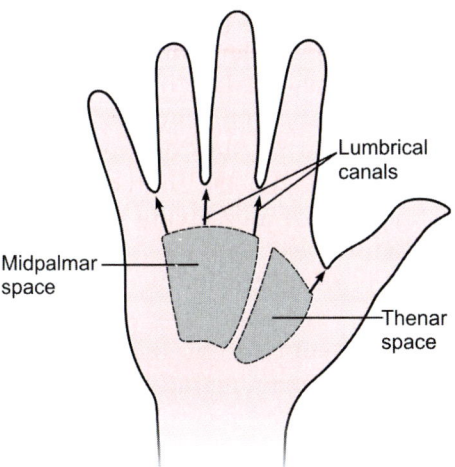

Fig. 2.29: Fascial spaces of the palm

by inserting a needle through the webs of the fingers. With the advent of antibiotics, the importance of spaces is lessened.

- *Pulp space:*
  - Seen in the pulp of the finger (Fig. 2.30).
  - Divided into many small fatty compartments by fibrous septa running from skin to the bone (terminal phalanx).

Synovial Sheaths

- *In the palm:* Ulnar and radial bursa (Fig. 2.31).
- *In the finger:* Digital synovial sheaths (Fig. 2.31).
- *Ulnar bursa:* Common flexor synovial sheath that envelopes tendons of FDS and FDP.
- *Radial bursa* is the synovial sheath of FPL tendon in the palm.
- *Digital synovial sheaths:* Envelope the long flexor tendons of the fingers within the fibrous flexor sheaths. The digital synovial sheath of little finger is continuous with ulnar bursa while that of thumb is continuous with that of radial bursa.

Hence, infections of little finger and thumb can spread proximally into hand easily unlike infections of other digits.

Thenar Muscles

- The thenar eminence has three thenar muscles.

They are:
1. Abductor pollicis brevis.
2. Flexor pollicis brevis.
3. Opponens pollicis.

All these three muscles are supplied by the median nerve.

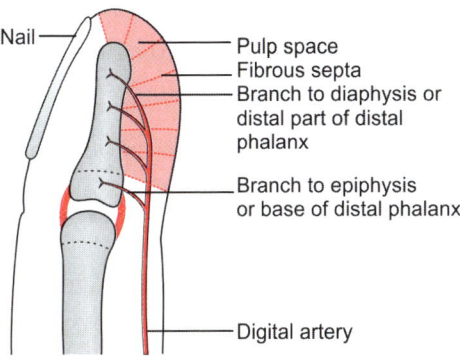

Fig. 2.30: Pulp spaces of the digits

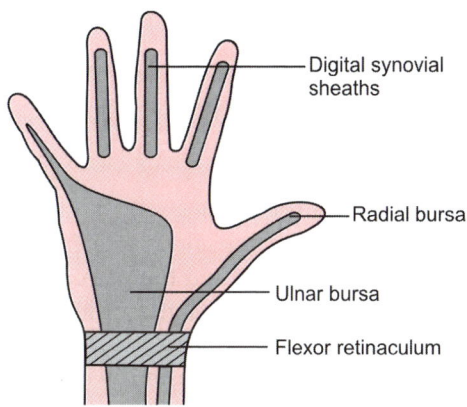

Fig. 2.31: Synovial sheaths of the hand

Abductor Pollicis Brevis

• It arises from the trapezium and flexor retinaculum. It is inserted into the lateral side of the base of the proximal phalanx of the thumb.

Flexor Pollicis Brevis

• It arises from the flexor retinaculum and trapezium and it is inserted into the lateral side of the base of the proximal phalanx of the thumb. Superficial head is supplied by median nerve and deep head is supplied by deep branch of ulnar nerve.

Opponens Pollicis

• It arises from the flexor retinaculum and trapezium and is inserted into the shaft of the first metacarpal bone.

Adductor Pollicis

• It is a thenar muscle but not a muscle of thenar eminence. It has 2 heads—oblique and transverse. Oblique arises from bases of 2nd and 3rd metacarpal and capitate. Transverse arises from palmar aspect of shaft of 3rd metacarpal. Inserted into medial side of base of proximal phalanx of thumb.

Action: The name of the muscles suggests its action. For example: The opponens pollicis opposes the thumb with other digits.

Hypothenar Muscles

They are three in number:
1. Abductor digiti minimi.
2. Flexor digiti minimi.
3. Opponens digiti minimi.
   • All these three muscles arise from the flexor retinaculum and the hamate bone.
   • They are inserted into the little digit as follows:
     – The opponens digiti minimi is inserted into the shaft of the fifth metacarpal bone.

– The flexor digiti minimi is inserted into the medial side of the base of the proximal phalanx of the little finger.
– Abductor digiti minimi is inserted into the medial side of the base of the proximal phalanx of the little finger.
• Hypothenar muscles are supplied by the ulnar nerve.

Note: Regarding the nerve supply of the muscles of the hand, the following five muscles are supplied by the median nerve while all the remaining muscles are supplied by the ulnar nerve.

1. Flexor pollicis brevis (superficial head).
2. Abductor pollicis brevis.
3. Opponens pollicis.
4. First lumbrical.
5. Second lumbrical.

The following muscles of the hand are supplied by the ulnar nerve:

1. Palmaris brevis.
2. Flexor digiti minimi.
3. Abductor digiti minimi.
4. Opponens digiti minimi.
5. Third and fourth lumbricals.
6. Adductor pollicis.
7. Palmar interossei.
8. Dorsal interossei.
9. Flexor pollicis brevis (deep head).

Lumbricals

• There are four lumbricals.
• The lateral two are supplied by the median nerve while the medial two are supplied by the ulnar nerve.
• Lumbricals arise from the tendons of the flexor digitorum profundus.
• Lumbricals are numbered from the lateral to medial side.
• They flex the metacarpophalangeal joint and extend the interphalangeal joints.
• When they are paralyzed, clawing of digits occurs.

Superficial Palmar Arch

- It is formed by the union of superficial branch of ulnar artery with the superficial palmar branch of radial artery (Fig. 2.32).
- Its apex touches the tangent drawn to the convexity of the hyperextended thumb.
- It lies over the long flexor tendons of the palm.
- It gives three common palmar digital arteries.
- Each common digital artery divides into proper digital arteries at the web of the corresponding fingers.

Deep Palmar Arch

- It is formed by the union of the radial artery with the deep branch of the ulnar artery (Fig. 2.32).
- It lies approximately 1 cm proximal to the superficial palmar arch.
- It gives three palmar metacarpal arteries.
- Each palmar metacarpal artery joins the corresponding common palmar digital artery.

APPLIED ANATOMY

There is rich anastomosis between the radial and ulnar arteries in the palm because of the superficial and deep palmar arches. Therefore, whenever a vessel is cut in the palm, the cut ends bleed from both sides. That is the reason why it is impossible sometimes to stop the bleeding by just compressing the radial or ulnar artery. In such cases the compression of brachial artery is preferable.

Interossei Muscles

- There are three palmar (may be four) and four dorsal interossei muscles (Fig. 2.33).
- Palmar interossei are adductors and have one head of origin (PAD).
- Dorsal interossei are abductors and have two heads of origin (DAB).
- PAD and DAB are mnemonics for their actions.
- All interossei are supplied by the ulnar nerve.

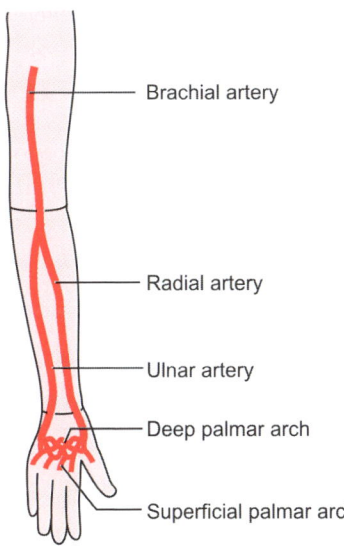

Fig. 2.32: Superficial and deep palmar arch

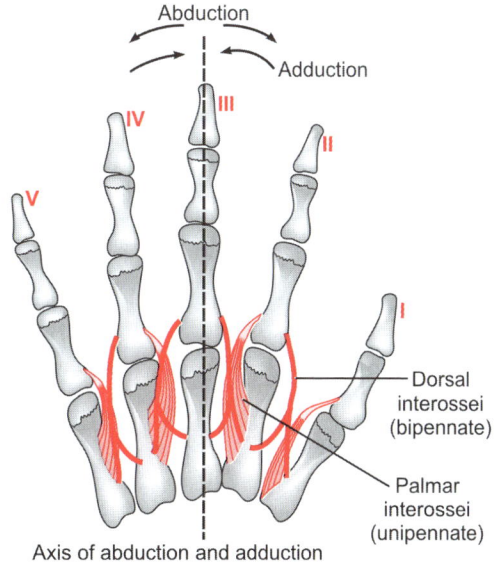

Fig. 2.33: Palmar and dorsal interossei

- The axis of adduction and abduction passes through the middle finger. The middle finger is relatively fixed as two dorsal interossei insert into it.
- They arise from the metacarpal bones and are inserted into the proximal phalanx and into the dorsal digital expansion. Therefore, they flex the metacarpophalangeal joints and extend the interphalangeal joints.

Carpal Bones

- *There are eight carpal bones (Fig. 2.34):*

There are four in the proximal row while the other four are in the distal row.

The four carpals of the proximal row (from lateral to medial) are:
1. Scaphoid.
2. Lunate.
3. Triquetral.
4. Pisiform.

The four carpals of the distal row (from lateral to medial) are:
1. Trapezium.
2. Trapezoid.
3. Capitate.
4. Hamate.

(Mnemonic is "**S**he **L**ooks **T**oo **P**retty **T**ry **T**o **C**atch **H**er").

Extensor Compartment of the Forearm

- It has superficial and deep group of muscles.

Superficial muscles of the back of the forearm: Two muscles of this group arise from the lateral supracondylar ridge.

They are:
1. Brachioradialis.
2. Extensor carpi radialis longus.

The remaining superficial muscles arise from the lateral epicondyle of the humerus by a common extensor tendinous origin.

They are:
1. Extensor carpi radialis brevis.
2. Extensor digitorum.
3. Extensor digiti minimi.
4. Extensor carpi ulnaris.
5. Anconeus.

The following belong to the deep group of muscles of the back of the forearm: The supinator lies deep in the upper part of the back of the forearm.

The other deep muscles (out-crop muscles) that cross the back of the wrist joint are:
1. Abductor pollicis longus.
2. Extensor pollicis brevis.
3. Extensor pollicis longus.
4. Extensor indicis.

Action: Except brachioradialis which is a weak flexor of forearm; all the above mentioned muscles are extensors of forearm.

Anconeus

- Find the anconeus muscle at the lower end of the posterior aspect of the arm.

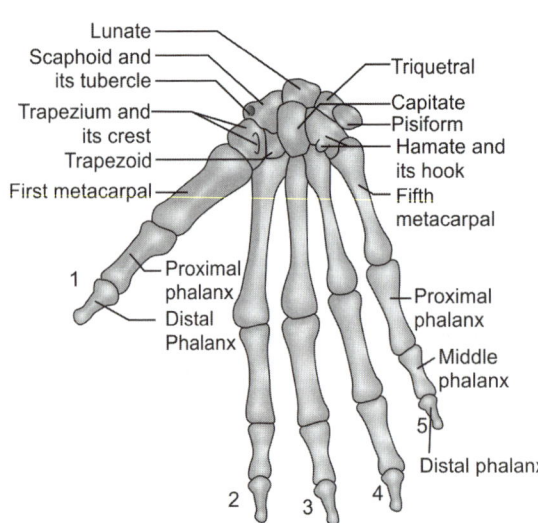

Fig. 2.34: Bones of the hand

Labels: Lunate, Scaphoid and its tubercle, Trapezium and its crest, Trapezoid, First metacarpal, 1, Proximal phalanx, Distal Phalanx, Triquetral, Capitate, Pisiform, Hamate and its hook, Fifth metacarpal, Proximal phalanx, Middle phalanx, 5, Distal phalanx, 2, 3, 4

- It arises from the back of the lateral epicondyle of the humerus and is inserted into the posterior aspect of upper part of ulna. It moors the ulna to the radius during all rotatory movements of the forearm.
- It is supplied by the radial nerve while it is still in the radial groove. This branch traverses the medial head of the triceps before it supplies the anconeus muscle.

Brachioradialis

Origin: From the upper part of the lateral supracondylar ridge.

Insertion: It is inserted into the base of the styloid process of radius.

Nerve supply: It is supplied by the radial nerve. It is the only flexor muscle of the elbow which is grouped under the extensors as it arises from the lateral supracondylar ridge and is supplied by the radial nerve

Action: It efficiently flexes the midprone forearm. Brachioradialis reflex is elicited to test the integrity of C6 spinal segment.

Extensor Carpi Radialis Longus

Origin: It arises from the lower part of the lateral supracondylar ridge.

Insertion: It is inserted into the base of the second metacarpal bone.

Nerve supply: It is supplied by the radial nerve.

Action: It acts as the extensor of the wrist. It also helps in the abduction acting with the flexor carpi radialis and extensor carpi radialis brevis.

Extensor Carpi Radialis Brevis

Origin: It arises from the lateral epicondyle of the humerus by a common extensor tendinous origin.

Insertion: It is inserted into the base of the third metacarpal bone.

Nerve supply: It is supplied by the posterior interosseous nerve (deep branch of the radial nerve).

Action: It acts as extensor of the wrist and also helps in the abduction of the wrist.

Extensor Digitorum

Origin: It arises from a common tendinous origin attached to the lateral epicondyle of the humerus.

Insertion: It divides into four tendons to the lateral four digits and takes part in their extensor expansion. It helps in the extension of metacarpophalangeal and extension of proximal and distal interphalangeal joints through the extensor digital expansion.

Nerve supply: It is supplied by the posterior interosseous nerve (deep branch of radial nerve).

Extensor Digiti Minimi

Origin: It arises from the common extensor tendon attached to the lateral epicondyle of the humerus.

Insertion: It is inserted into the little finger and takes part in its extensor expansion.

Nerve supply: Posterior interosseous nerve (deep branch of radial nerve).

Extensor Carpi Ulnaris

Origin: It arises from the common extensor tendinous origin attached to the lateral epicondyle of the humerus.

Insertion: It is inserted into the base of the fifth metacarpal bone.

Nerve supply: It is supplied by the posterior interosseous nerve (deep branch of radial nerve).

Supinator

Origin: It arises from the lateral epicondyle of humerus and supinator crest of ulna.

Insertion: It is inserted into the lateral side of the upper part of the radius.

Nerve supply: It is supplied by the posterior interosseous nerve. The posterior interosseous nerve (deep branch of radial nerve) pierces the supinator and reaches the back of the forearm. *Note:* This is the position of deep branch of radial nerve entrapment as it passes through the supinator muscle.

Action: It supinates the pronated forearm. It crosses the superior radioulnar joint and acts on that. Supination and pronation take place in the superior and inferior radioulnar joints. These joints are pivot type of synovial joints. Pivot joints are uniaxial but the axis is vertical. The axes of supination and pronation pass through the head of radius and styloid process of ulna.

Abductor Pollicis Longus

Origin: It arises from the posterior surface of the radius, ulna and adjoining interosseous membrane.

Insertion: It is inserted into the base of the first metacarpal bone.

Nerve supply: It is supplied by the deep branch of radial nerve (do not get confused the deep branch of radial nerve and posterior interosseous nerves are interchangeable terms).

Action: It abducts the thumb.

Extensor Pollicis Brevis

Origin: It arises from the posterior surface of the radius and adjoining interosseous membrane.

Insertion: It is inserted into the dorsal part of base of the proximal phalanx of the thumb.

Nerve supply: It is supplied by the posterior interosseous nerve.

Action: It extends the metacarpophalangeal joint of the thumb.

Extensor Pollicis Longus

Origin: It arises from the posterior surface of the ulna and adjoining interosseous membrane.

Insertion: It is inserted into the dorsal part of base of the distal phalanx of the thumb.

Action: It extends the interphalangeal joint of the thumb.

Nerve supply: The posterior interosseous nerve.

Extensor Indicis

Origin: It arises from the posterior surface of the ulna and adjoining interosseous membrane.

Insertion: It takes part in the dorsal extensor expansion of the index finger along with the tendon of extensor digitorum.

Nerve supply: The posterior interosseous nerve.

Action: The extension of the index finger as in pointing something is facilitated by the presence of an extra tendon of extensor indicis apart from the extensor digitorum tendon of this finger.

The following muscles are inserted into the thumb:

- Base of the first metacarpal bone—abductor pollicis longus.
- Lateral part of the base of the proximal phalanx of the thumb—abductor pollicis brevis.
- Lateral part of the base of the proximal phalanx of the thumb—flexor pollicis brevis.
- Medial part of the base of the proximal phalanx of the thumb—adductor pollicis.
- Dorsal part of the base of the proximal phalanx of thumb—extensor pollicis brevis.
- Dorsal part of the base of the distal phalanx of thumb—extensor pollicis longus.
- Anterior part of the base of the distal phalanx of thumb—flexor pollicis longus.
- Shaft of the first metacarpal bone—opponens pollicis.

Extensor Retinaculum of the Wrist

- It is a thickened band of deep fascia on the back of the wrist (Fig. 2.35).
- It is oblique. It is oblique because it is disposed perpendicular to the pull of the tendons of the back of the wrist.

Attachments:

Lateral: Lower end of radius.
Medial: Pisiform and triquetral bones.

- All extensor tendons pass deep to the extensor retinaculum.
- There are six compartments deep to the extensor retinaculum.
- They are usually numbered from the lateral to medial side.

The first compartment contains the following two tendons:

Abductor pollicis longus and extensor pollicis brevis.

The second compartment contains the following two tendons:

- Extensor carpi radialis longus.
- Extensor carpi radialis brevis.

The third compartment contains:

- The tendon of extensor pollicis longus.

The fourth compartment contains the following structures:

- Extensor digitorum.
- Extensor indicis.

- Posterior interosseous nerve.
- Anterior interosseous artery.

The fifth compartment contains:

- The tendon of extensor digiti minimi.

The sixth compartment contains:

- The tendon of extensor carpi ulnaris.

The Anatomical Snuff Box

- This is situated on the lateral side of the wrist (Fig. 2.36).
- Its medial boundary is formed by the extensor pollicis longus.
- The lateral boundary is formed by the tendons of abductor pollicis longus and extensor pollicis brevis.
- The following structures lie in its roof. Skin, fascia, cephalic vein and superficial branch of radial nerve.
- The following structures lie in its floor:
  - Styloid process of radius.
  - Scaphoid bone.
  - Radial artery lies over the floor of the anatomical snuff box.

Dorsum of the Hand

- The skin is loosely attached to the underlying fascia. Swelling on the dorsum of the hand is characteristic because of this.

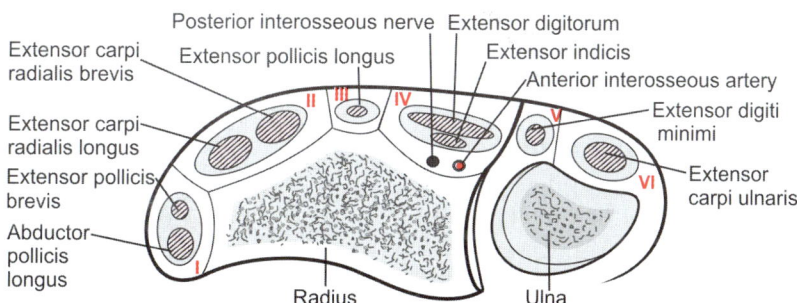

Fig. 2.35: Compartments under the extensor retinaculum

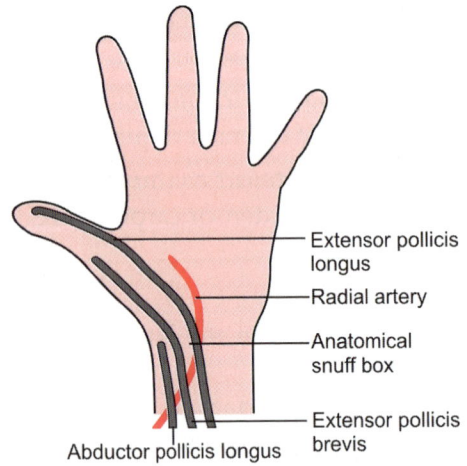

Fig. 2.36: The anatomical snuff box

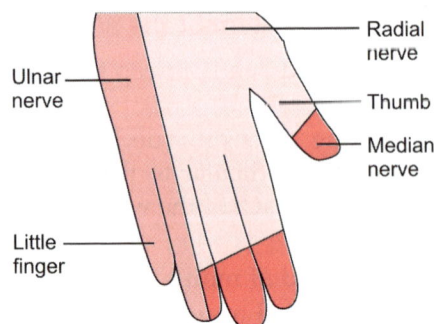

Fig. 2.37: Cutaneous innervation of dorsum of right hand

The structures present in the dorsum of the hand are:

- Dorsal digital veins.
- Dorsal metacarpal veins.
- Dorsal venous arch.
- Cephalic vein begins from the lateral side of the dorsal venous arch while the basilic vein begins from the medial side of the dorsal venous arch.
- Radial artery gives the first dorsal metacarpal artery and then dips into the palm of the hand between the two heads of the first dorsal interosseous muscle.
- Radial artery also gives the dorsal carpal branch which anastomoses with the dorsal carpal branch of the ulnar artery and forms the dorsal carpal arterial arch. This dorsal carpal arterial arch gives three dorsal metacarpal arteries.

The nerve supply of the dorsum of the hand:

- The medial one-third is supplied by the dorsal branches of the ulnar nerve (Fig. 2.37).
- The lateral two-thirds of the dorsum of the hand including the skin over proximal phalanges are supplied by the radial nerve.

- The skin over the middle and distal phalanges of the lateral three and half fingers is supplied by the branches of median nerve.

Extensor Digital Expansion

- Following structures contribute to the extensor expansion (Fig. 2.38):
1. Tendon of extensor digitorum.
2. Lumbrical muscle.
3. Palmar and dorsal interossei.

In the index finger, the tendon of extensor indicis joins the expansion.

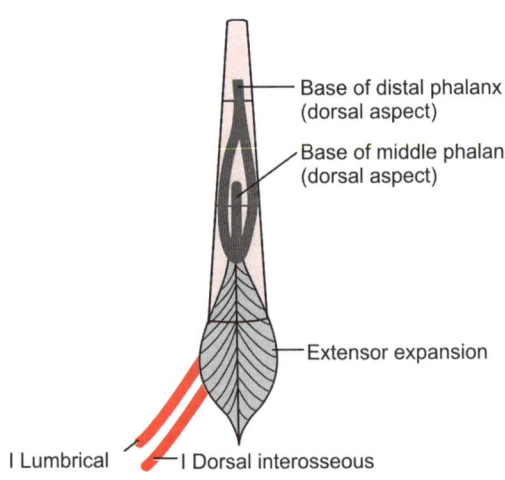

Fig. 2.38: Dorsal digital expansion

In the little finger, the tendon of extensor digiti minimi joins the expansion.

- Hood is an expansion of the tendon of extensor digitorum over the proximal phalanx and metacarpophalangeal joint. It is joined on either side by the lumbrical and interossei.

Then the hood divides into three parts:

- The central part which is attached to the base of the middle phalanx.
- The lateral parts join and form one median part which is inserted into the base of the distal phalanx.

By this arrangement, the lumbricals can flex the metacarpophalangeal joint and extend the interphalangeal joint. This action is assisted by the interossei muscles.

Mallet finger: The extensor tendon insertion to the terminal phalanx might get avulsed resulting in the mallets finger. This happens when direct force hits the terminal phalanx hyperflexing it; when the tendon was extending it.

Fracture of the scaphoid: It is the most commonly fractured carpal bone. Blood supply to its proximal part comes from its distal end. It is usually fractured at the narrow waist in the middle. Following this fracture, the proximal part of the scaphoid may undergo necrosis because of lack of blood supply to it. This is termed "avascular necrosis of scaphoid". When the scaphoid is fractured, there is swelling in the anatomical snuff box.

Axillary Nerve

- It arises from the posterior cord of the brachial plexus (Fig. 2.16).
- Its root value is C5 and C6.
- It lies over the subscapularis muscle.
- It passes through the quadrangular space. As it passes through this space, the shoulder joint lies just superior to it, therefore, it

supplies the shoulder joint. Then it divides into two branches:

- *Anterior branch:* It goes around the surgical neck of the humerus accompanied by the posterior circumflex humeral artery. It supplies the deltoid muscle and a small area of the skin over the lower part of the deltoid muscle.
- *Posterior branch:* It supplies the teres minor muscle, posterior part of the deltoid and becomes continuous as the superior lateral cutaneous nerve of the arm.

CLINICAL ANATOMY

This nerve is injured in the inferior dislocation of the shoulder joint. Deltoid muscle is paralyzed resulting in the flattening of the shoulder. There is also loss of sensation over the distribution of superior lateral cutaneous nerve of arm.

Musculocutaneous Nerve

- This nerve arises from the lateral cord of the brachial plexus (Fig. 2.20).
- It pierces the coracobrachialis muscle.
- *It supplies:* Biceps brachii, coracobrachialis and brachialis (Mnemonic: BBC muscles).
- It continues as the lateral cutaneous nerve of forearm in the roof of the cubital fossa and supplies the skin of the lateral side of the forearm.

Nerve entrapment: Musculocutaneous nerve can be entrapped as it passes through the coracobrachialis muscle.

Signs of musculocutaneous nerve involvement: Weakness of flexion and supination of elbow and loss of sensation over the lateral side of the forearm.

Median Nerve

- Arises from the lateral and medial cords of the brachial plexus (Fig. 2.39).

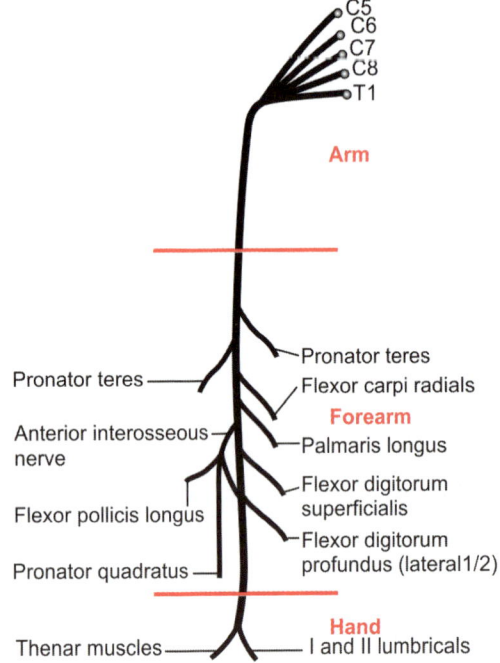

Pronator teres

Anterior interosseous nerve

Flexor pollicis longus

Pronator quadratus

Thenar muscles

C5
C6
C7
C8
T1

Arm

Pronator teres
Flexor carpi radials
Forearm
Palmaris longus
Flexor digitorum superficialis
Flexor digitorum profundus (lateral1/2)
Hand
I and II lumbricals

Fig. 2.39: Muscular branches of median nerve

- It arises from all the roots of the brachial plexus.
- Lateral and medial roots of the median nerve join to form the median nerve.
- It lies lateral to the third part of the axillary artery and brachial artery as far as the insertion of the coracobrachialis.
- It crosses anterior to the brachial artery at this level from the lateral to the medial side.
- It lies medial to the artery below this level.
- It lies in the cubital fossa medial to the tendon of biceps and medial to the brachial artery.
- It does not give any branches in the arm except vascular branches.
- It gives its first motor branch to pronator teres before it passes between the two heads of pronator teres.
- It gives anterior interosseous nerve just distal to the pronator teres and continues

on the deep surface of the flexor digitorum superficialis.
- It supplies the following superficial flexor muscles in the forearm:
  1. Pronator teres.
  2. Flexor carpi radialis.
  3. Palmaris longus.
  4. Flexor digitorum superficialis.
- *Anterior interosseous branch of median nerve supplies the following structures:*
  1. Lateral half of the flexor digitorum profundus.
  2. Flexor pollicis longus.
  3. Pronator quadratus.
  4. Wrist joint.
  5. Intercarpal joint.
- Median nerve runs deep to the flexor retinaculum in the carpal tunnel.
- Before running deep to the flexor retinaculum, it gives palmar cutaneous branch which supplies the lateral part of skin of the palm of the hand.
- At the distal border of the flexor retinaculum, it enters the palm of the hand.
- In the hand it gives sensory fibers to the lateral three and half digits and it also supplies the skin over the dorsum of the middle and distal phalanges of these fingers.

In the hand median nerve supplies the following muscles:
1. Abductor pollicis brevis.
2. Flexor pollicis brevis.
3. Opponens pollicis.
4. First lumbrical muscle.
5. Second lumbrical muscle.

CLINICAL ANATOMY

- Median nerve is frequently slashed in suicidal attempt when the front of the lower end of the forearm is transversely cut.

Note: The thumb looses its important opposition function and it cannot be opposed to other fingers.

- Thumb remains close to the index finger (adducted and laterally rotated) because of the unopposed action of adductor pollicis. This deformity constitutes the so-called "ape-like hand".
- When the patient is asked to make a fist, he ends up making a hand similar to papal benediction, due to paralysis of muscles supplied by median nerve.
- Fine movements of 2nd and 3rd fingers are affected because first and second lumbricals are involved. Higher lesions cause loss of flexion of proximal and distal interphalangeal joints of 2nd and 3rd digits due to involvement of flexor digitorum superficialis and lateral half of flexor digitorum profundus.
- The median nerve can be entrapped as it enters between the two heads of pronator teres resulting in an entrapment syndrome.
- *Carpal tunnel syndrome:*
  - Compression of median nerve in carpal tunnel.
  - May be due to tenosynovitis, fluid retention or inflammation of joints in the viscinity reducing the size of the tunnel.
  - Loss of sensation, abnormal sensation or diminished sensation may be observed in the lateral 3½ digits.

ULNAR NERVE

- It arises from the medial cord of the brachial plexus (Fig. 2.40).
- Its root value is C8 and T1 (sometimes C7).
- It lies between the third part of the axillary artery and axillary vein.
- It runs medial to the brachial artery as far as the insertion of the coracobrachialis.
- At this level it leaves the company of the brachial artery and runs far more medial

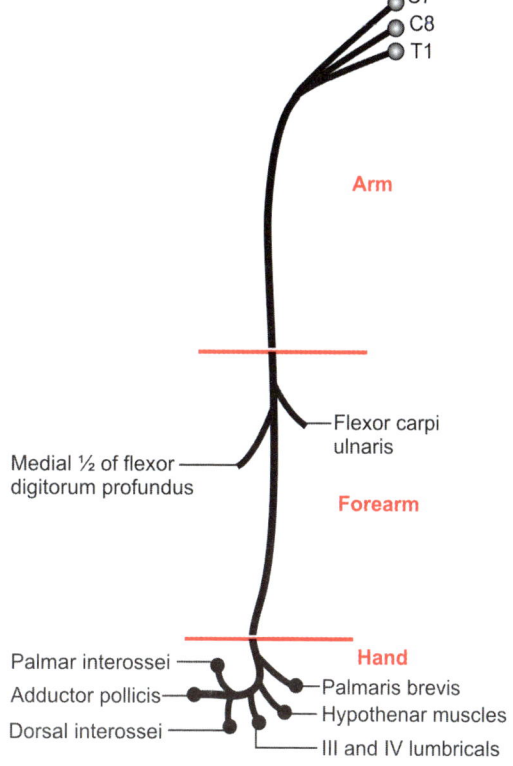

Fig. 2.40: Muscular branches of ulnar nerve

accompanied by the superior ulnar collateral artery.

- It lies behind the medial epicondyle of the humerus (this is the area where it can be injured in the fractures of the medial epicondyle of the humerus).

- It passes between the two heads of the flexor carpi ulnaris.(*Note:* This is the potential area for nerve entrapment).

- It supplies the flexor carpi ulnaris before it passes between its two heads.
- It lies on the medial part of the anterior surface of the flexor digitorum profundus in the forearm covered superficially by the flexor carpi ulnaris.

- It supplies the medial part of the flexor digitorum profundus. These tendons of profundus go to the little and ring fingers.
- It lies medial to the ulnar artery in the lower part.
- It gives a palmar cutaneous branch which crosses superficial to the flexor retinaculum and supplies the medial side of the palm of the hand.
- It gives a dorsal branch which supplies the medial part of the dorsum and one and half fingers on the back of the hand.
- It passes superficial to the flexor retinaculum and is accompanied by the ulnar artery.
- It gives a deep branch which pierces the opponens pollicis and runs under the concavity of the deep palmar arch.

We can simplify the distribution of the ulnar nerve as follows:

- Deep branch supplies all the muscles of the hand except those muscles which are supplied by the median nerve (recollect those five muscles supplied by the median nerve. If you remember those five muscles, the rest is easy. All other muscles of the hand are supplied by the ulnar nerve).
- Superficial branch supplies unimportant palmaris brevis, skin over the medial side of the hand and also supplies the skin of the medial one and half fingers.

CLINICAL ANATOMY

- Ulnar nerve injury is common because it lies relatively superficial.
- When a patient is asked to make a fist, the 2nd and 3rd fingers are flexed by the first and second lumbricals. The 4th and 5th fingers lag behind and they remain extended at the metacarpophalangeal joints because of paralysis of 3rd and 4th

lumbricals and interossei. The thumb is drawn away from the index finger due to the paralysis of the adductor pollicis. This deformity is called "ulnar claw hand". In fact this is a partial claw hand (Fig. 2.41).

- Complete claw hand results when both median and ulnar nerves are involved. In this case, all the four lumbricals are paralyzed.

Ulnar paradox

It is normally logical to think that when a nerve is severed proximally, the symptoms must be severe and a distal injury to a nerve should present less severe symptoms. In the case of ulnar nerve, reverse is true. It means a proximal injury of the ulnar nerve before the branch to flexor digitorum profundus (FDP) is given, presents a less severe symptom. If it is injured distally after the branch to FDP is given, the symptom appears more severe or more disabling. This is because, in both the cases whether the injury is proximal or distal, the claw hand is a must. But the claw appears less disabling if the injury is proximal because in this case FDP to the little and ring fingers is also paralyzed and the finger is relatively extended due to the unopposed action of extensors. If the cut is after the nerve to FDP is given, the intact FDP tendons to ring and little fingers flex it more and the claw appears more disabling. This is called the ulnar paradox.

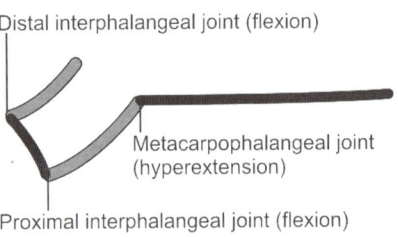

Distal interphalangeal joint (flexion)

Metacarpophalangeal joint (hyperextension)

Proximal interphalangeal joint (flexion)

Fig. 2.41: Claw hand

To test for ulnar nerve integrity

- *Dorsal interossei:* Abduction against resistance.
- *Palmar interossei:* Adduction against resistance.
- *Adductor pollicis:* Piece of paper held between the thumb and index is pulled by the doctor.

Nerve entrapment: Ulnar nerve is entrapped as it passes between the two heads of flexor carpi ulnaris.

RADIAL NERVE

- It arises from the posterior cord of the brachial plexus (Fig. 2.42).
- It has all the roots of the brachial plexus.
- It lies over the subscapularis muscle.
- It passes through the lower triangular space formed by the lower border of teres major, long head of triceps and shaft of the humerus.
- It is accompanied by the profunda brachii (deep artery of the arm) artery.

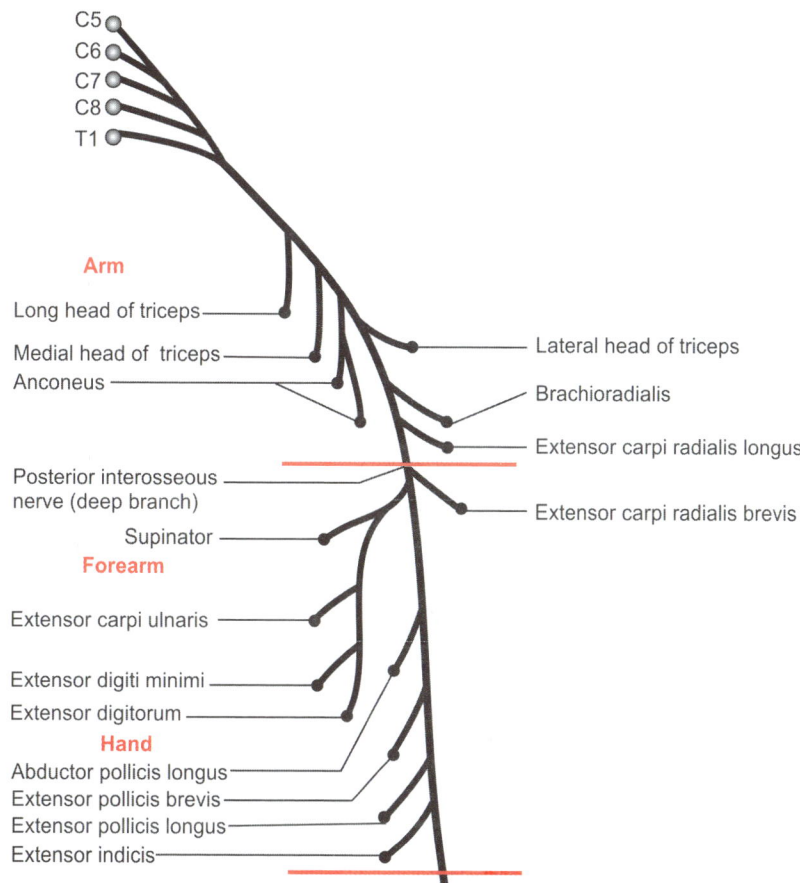

Fig. 2.42: Muscular branches of radial nerve

- It traverses the spiral groove.
- It pierces the lateral intermuscular septum and enters the anterior compartment.
- The part of the nerve which lies superior to the spiral groove gives three branches:
  1. Branch of long head of triceps.
  2. Branch to medial head of triceps.
  3. Posterior cutaneous nerve of arm.
- The part which lies in the spiral groove gives three branches:
  1. Muscular branches to triceps (lateral and medial head) and anconeus.
  2. Lower lateral cutaneous nerve of arm.
  3. Posterior cutaneous nerve of forearm.

The part which lies in the anterior compartment (lower arm) gives three branches:

1. Branch to brachioradialis.
2. Branch to brachialis.
3. Branch to extensor carpi radialis longus.

It lies in the floor of the cubital fossa. It gives a deep branch which is also called the posterior interosseous nerve. It continues as the superficial sensory branch.

Posterior Interosseous Nerve (Deep Branch)

- It is purely a motor nerve.
- It passes through the supinator muscle.
- It supplies the supinator before it passes through that muscle.
- The posterior interosseous nerve supplies all the muscles of the extensor compartment except three which are already supplied by the radial nerve in the arm.

Remember the names of these three muscles of extensor compartment which are supplied by the radial nerve directly:

1. Anconeus.
2. Brachioradialis.
3. Extensor carpi radialis longus.

All the other muscles of the posterior compartment are supplied by the deep branch (posterior interosseous nerve) of the radial nerve.

Superficial Branch of Radial Nerve

- It is purely sensory.
- It runs in the roof of the cubital fossa.
- It supplies the lateral part of the dorsum of the hand except the skin over the middle and distal phalanges which is supplied by the median nerve.

The trunk of the radial nerve can be entrapped in the spiral groove between the lateral and medial heads of triceps or involved in midshaft humeral fractures.

The deep branch of radial nerve can be entrapped as it passes between the two strata of supinator muscle.

CLINICAL ANATOMY

- Radial nerve tends to get compressed in the spiral groove, especially when an inebriated individual falls asleep on the edge of a chair for a long time. Therefore, it is often called "Saturday night palsy".
- Improperly fixed crutch may also compress the radial nerve in axilla (crutch palsy).
- In all such cases there is "wrist drop".
- Wrist drop results even when only the deep branch of radial nerve is injured.
- There is loss of sensation over a small area on the lateral side of the dorsum of the hand when radial nerve trunk or superficial branch of radial nerve is involved.

Nerve Entrapment Syndromes

- Musculocutaneous nerve can be entrapped as it passes through the coracobrachialis muscle.
- *Supinator syndrome:* The deep branch of radial nerve can be entrapped as it passes between the two strata of supinator muscle.
- *Cubital tunnel syndrome:* Ulnar nerve is entrapped as it passes between the two heads of flexor carpi ulnaris.

- *Pronator syndrome:* The median nerve can be entrapped as it enters between the two heads of pronator teres resulting in an entrapment syndrome.

Radial Artery

- It is in line with the brachial artery.
- It arises as one of the small terminal branches of brachial artery at the level of the neck of the radius.
- It gives a radial collateral artery in the cubital fossa.

It lies on the following structures on the lateral side of the front of the forearm.

1. Supinator.
2. Pronator teres.
3. Flexor digitorum superficialis.
4. Flexor pollicis longus.
5. Lower part of the front of the radius (where its pulsations are felt).
   - It is covered superficially by the brachioradialis muscle.
   - It gives superficial palmar branch before it winds round the lower end of the radius.
   - The superficial palmar branch completes the superficial palmar arch on its lateral end.
   - It winds round the lateral side of the wrist, deep to abductor pollicis longus and extensor pollicis brevis tendons.
   - It lies in the floor of the anatomical snuff box.
   - It leaves the back of the hand by passing between the two heads of the first dorsal interosseous muscle.
   - Before dipping to the front, it gives the first dorsal metacarpal artery.
   - In the palm of the hand it gives two branches.
1. Princeps pollicis artery.
2. Radialis indicis artery.
   - Then it passes between the two heads of adductor pollicis and forms the deep palmar arch.

- The deep palmar arch is completed medially by the deep branch of the ulnar artery.
- Deep palmar arch gives three palmar metacarpal arteries.
- Palmar metacarpal arteries join the common palmar digital arteries of the superficial palmar branch.

Ulnar Artery

- It is one of the larger terminal divisions of the brachial artery.
- It is not in line with its parent trunk, the brachial artery.
- It runs downwards and medially.
- It lies deep to the deep head of the pronator teres.
- Deep head of the pronator teres separates this artery from the median nerve.
- It joins the lateral side of the ulnar nerve in the middle of the forearm.

In the proximal part of the forearm, it gives two recurrent branches:

1. Anterior ulnar recurrent.
2. Posterior ulnar recurrent.

It gives a large branch, the common interosseous artery in the upper part of the forearm.

Common interosseous artery divides into two branches:

1. Anterior interosseous artery (anterior to the interosseous membrane).

2. Posterior interosseous artery (posterior to the interosseous membrane).

- Ulnar artery crosses superficial to the flexor retinaculum lateral to the ulnar nerve.
- It divides into superficial and deep branches in the hand.
- The superficial branch continues as the superficial palmar arch after giving a proper digital branch to the medial side of the little finger.
- Superficial palmar arch is completed laterally by the superficial palmar branch of the radial artery.
- Superficial palmar arch gives three common palmar digital arteries which divide into the corresponding proper digital arteries at the web of the fingers.
- Common palmar digital arteries receive the palmar metacarpal arteries of the deep palmar arch.
- The deep branch of the ulnar artery accompanies the deep branch of the ulnar nerve and completes the deep palmar arch on the medial side by joining the radial artery.
- The deep palmar arch gives three palmar metacarpal arteries.

CLINICAL ANATOMY

- Pulsations of ulnar artery can be felt lateral to the pisiform bone.
- Ulnar artery can also be used for arterial punctures.

VEINS OF THE UPPER LIMB

Following are the veins of the upper limb:

Superficial:
1. Cephalic vein.
2. Basilic vein.
3. Median cubital vein.
4. Median vein of forearm.

Deep:
5. Venae comitantes which accompany the large arteries.

Cephalic Vein

- It begins at the lateral end of the dorsal venous arch (Fig. 2.43).
- It lies in the roof of the anatomical snuff box.
- It ascends along the lateral aspect of the forearm and arm.
- It is interconnected with the basilic vein in the roof of the cubital fossa by the median cubital vein.
- It reaches the deltopectoral triangle and pierces the clavipectoral fascia to open into the axillary vein.
- It is accompanied by the lymph vessels which drain the lateral side of the hand (thumb, lateral fingers) and lateral forearm. That is the reason why infection of the thumb can directly spread to the apical group of axillary lymph nodes.
- It is accompanied by the lateral cutaneous nerve of the forearm.
- It bends acutely as it pierces the clavipectoral fascia. This is the reason why it is not a ready choice for cardiac catheterization.

Basilic Vein

- It begins at the medial end of the dorsal venous arch (Fig. 2.43).
- It pierces the deep fascia of the arm at the level of the insertion of the coracobrachialis and ascends deep to the deep fascia superior to that level. At the level of teres major it continues as the axillary vein by receiving the venae comitantes of the brachial artery.
- It is accompanied by the medial cutaneous nerve of the forearm.
- It is one of the choices for cardiac catheterization because of its straight path.

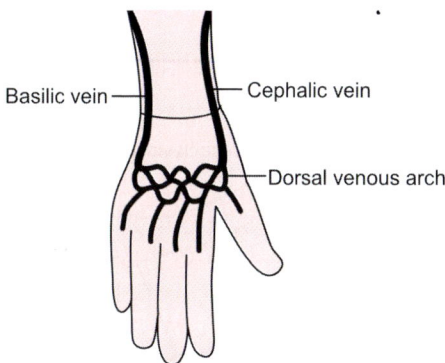

Fig. 2.43: Dorsal venous arch

- The median cubital vein connects the basilic vein with the cephalic vein in front of the elbow.

Median Cubital Vein

- It is the vein of choice for intravenous infusions or venous withdrawal of blood for investigative purposes (Fig. 2.44).

- It is separated from the underlying brachial artery and median nerve by the bicipital aponeurosis.
- Variation of median cubital vein is very common.

Venae Comitantes

- These are the parallel veins which accompany the deep arteries.
- There are interconnections between the two veins which run on either side of the artery.
- The pulsation of the large artery helps in the venous return through these veins.
- The venae comitantes of the brachial artery join the basilic vein to form the axillary vein at the level of the lower border of the teres major muscle.

Lymphatic Drainage of the Upper Limb

It is divided into the superficial and deep lymphatic vessels.

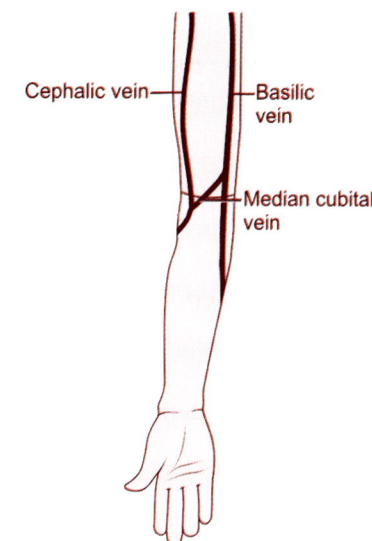

Fig. 2.44: Superficial veins of the upper limb

Superficial Lymph Vessels

- They accompany the cephalic and basilic veins.
- Those lymph vessels which accompany the cephalic vein reach the deltopectoral lymph nodes present in the deltopectoral triangle and later pierce the clavipectoral fascia to reach the apical group of axillary lymph nodes directly.
- Therefore, superficial lymph vessels from thumb and lateral side of the hand reach the apical axillary lymph nodes directly.
- The superficial lymph vessels from the medial side of the upper limb accompany the basilic vein. Majority of these vessels terminate in the cubital lymph node in front of the medial epicondyle and later continue upwards to end in the lateral axillary lymph nodes.

Deep Lymph Vessels

The deep group of lymph vessels accompanies the deep vessels (radial, ulnar and brachial) and reaches the lateral axillary lymph nodes directly.

- Axillary lymph nodes receive all the lymph of the upper limb. That is the reason why you come across edema of the upper limb following resection of axillary lymph nodes in breast cancer.

JOINTS

Sternoclavicular Joint

- *Bones taking part in the joint:* Sternal end of the clavicle articulates with the manubrium of the sternum and first costal cartilage (Fig. 2.45).
- *Type of joint:* Saddle type of synovial joint.
- *Joint cavity:* It is divided into two by the articular disc.
- *Ligaments:*
  - Sternoclavicular ligaments.
  - Interclavicular ligament.
  - Costoclavicular ligament.
- *Nerve supply:* It is supplied by the medial supraclavicular nerve.
- *Movements:* Keep your fingers over the sternal end of the clavicle and take the arm backwards. You find the clavicle moving forwards. Similarly, when you raise your hand, the clavicle is depressed. It allows the elevation, depression, forward, backward movements of the clavicle and also its rotation along its long axis.

- *Clinical:* It is rarely dislocated because it is a very stable joint and protected by strong ligaments.

Acromioclavicular Joint (AC Joint)

- *Bones taking part in the joint:* Acromial end of the clavicle and acromion (Fig. 2.45).
- *Type of joint:* A plane type of synovial joint.
- *Joint cavity:* Contains a small incomplete articular disc.
- *Ligaments:* Acromioclavicular (strengthens the joint superiorly).

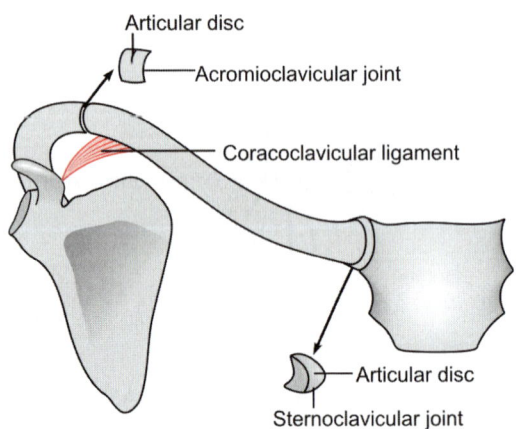

Fig. 2.45: Acromioclavicular and sternoclavicular

- Coracoclavicular (maintains the integrity of the joint).
- *Movements:* Both sternoclavicular and acromioclavicular joints allow movements of scapula (elevation, depression, protraction, retraction, forward rotation and backward rotation) and clavicle (rotation along its long axis, elevation, depression, forward movement or backward movement of its medial and lateral ends). The movements of medial and lateral ends of clavicle are opposite to each other, e.g. when medial end of clavicle moves forwards, lateral end moves backwards and so on.
- *Clinical:* The dislocation of the AC joint is common. This is called shoulder separation. Rupture of the coracoclavicular ligament results in shoulder separation. Lateral end of clavicle runs over acromion.

Shoulder Joint

- *Bones taking part in the joint:* Head of the humerus and glenoid cavity of the scapula (Fig. 2.46).
- *Type of joint:* Ball and socket type of synovial joint.

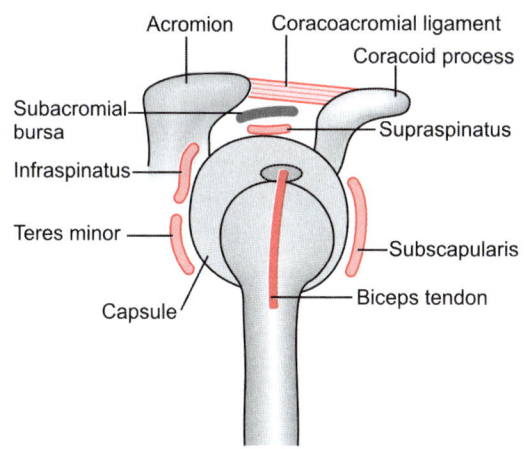

Fig. 2.46: Relations of the shoulder joint

- *Axis:* Multiaxial.
- *Joint cavity:* It contains synovial fluid and does not contain articular disc. Glenoidal labrum lines the margins of the glenoid cavity which increases the depth of glenoid cavity.
- *Fibrous capsule:*
  – It is attached to the margins of the glenoid cavity. It encloses the origin of the long head of the biceps and excludes the origin of long head of triceps.
  – The long head of biceps is intracapsular and extrasynovial.
  – The fibrous capsule is attached to the anatomical neck of the humerus which lies between the head and tubercles of the humerus. The attachment extends 2 cm inferiorly on the medial side which allows the abduction at the shoulder.
- *Ligaments:*
  1. Glenohumeral ligaments.
  2. Coracohumeral ligament.
  Coracoacromial arch (It includes the coracoid process, coracoacromial ligament and acromion. This arch prevents the upward displacement of the head of the humerus).

Movements:

Flexion: Any muscle which crosses anterior to the joint helps in flexion. These muscles are:
1. Pectoralis major.
2. Anterior fibers of deltoid.
3. Coracobrachialis.
4. Biceps brachii.

Extension: Any muscle which crosses posterior to the joint helps in extension. The only massive muscle which comes from behind is latissimus dorsi. Therefore, latissimus dorsi is a powerful extensor of the shoulder joint. Posterior fibers of deltoid also.

Abduction: Any muscle which crosses superior to the joint acts like abductor of the joint. There are two muscles which cross superior to the joint and they are:
- Middle fibers of deltoid and supraspinatus.
- Supraspinatus initiates the abduction and is responsible for the movement between 0 and 15 degrees.
- Deltoid is the main abductor and abducts between 15 and 90 degrees.

Adduction: Muscles which cross the joint from medial to lateral side act as adductors. They are latissimus dorsi, pectoralis major and teres major.

Medial rotators: Subscapularis goes around the front of shoulder joint to the lesser tubercle. Therefore, it acts as a medial rotator. Latissimus dorsi, teres major and pectoralis major.

Lateral rotator: Infraspinatus goes around the back of the shoulder joint to the greater tubercle and, therefore, it acts as the lateral rotator of the shoulder joint.

Muscular Rotator Cuff

- These muscles embrace the shoulder joint more closely and contribute to its stability. They are (Fig. 2.46):
  – Subscapularis.
  – Supraspinatus.

- Teres minor.
- Infraspinatus.
- They envelope the fibrous capsule very closely.

- Tears of the rotator cuff are very common in sports.
- The supraspinatus tendon is more prone to be involved because of its relative avascularity.

Painful arc syndrome: It is the pain during 50–130 degrees of abduction due to subacromial bursitis.

Dislocation of the shoulder joint: The inferior part of the shoulder joint remains unprotected by the rotator cuff muscles and, therefore, it is a weak area. The head of the humerus tends to get dislocated inferiorly. Axillary nerve may be injured during the inferior dislocation of the shoulder joint.

Bursae around the shoulder joint:

1. Subacromial bursa lies under the acromion and does not communicate with the joint cavity.
2. Subscapular bursa lies under the subscapularis and it communicates with the joint cavity.
   Nerve supply of the joint: Axillary, supra-scapular and lateral pectoral nerves supply the shoulder joint.

Elbow Joint

Bones that take part in the joint (Fig. 2.47):
- *Superior:* Trochlea and capitulum of humerus.
- *Inferior:* Trochlear notch of ulna and head of radius.

Type of joint: Hinge type of synovial joint.

Axis: Transverse uniaxial joint.

Joint cavity: Contains only the synovial fluid and there is no articular disc within.

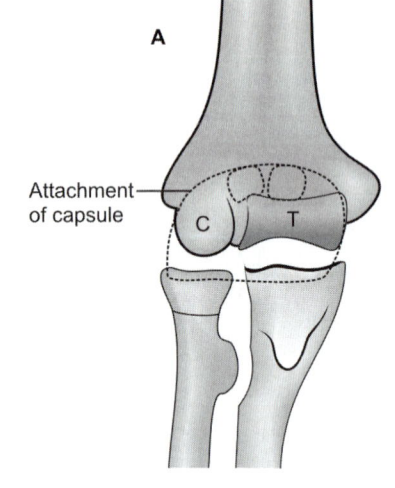

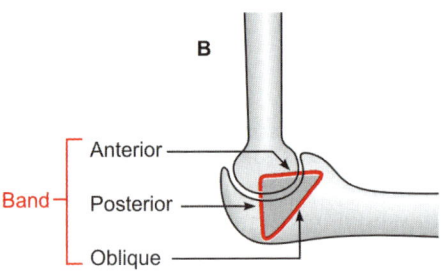

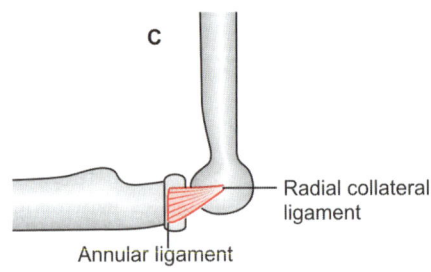

Fig. 2.47: A. Attachment of capsule of right elbow joint (anterior aspect), B. Ulnar collateral ligament (left), C. Radial collateral ligament and annular ligament (left)

Fibrous capsule:
- *Attached superiorly to:* Superior borders of coronoid, radial and olecranon fossae and to the margins of articular surfaces of capitulum and trochlea.

- *Attached inferiorly to:* Anterior surface of the coronoid process of ulna and annular ligament of radius.
- On either side it is continuous with the collateral ligaments (Fig. 2.47).

Ligaments:
- Radial collateral ligament (lateral).
- Ulnar collateral ligament (medial).

The strong medial and lateral collateral ligaments prevent all other rotatory movements and make it a true hinge joint.

Movements:
- Flexion—Muscles which cross in front of it act as flexors and they are brachialis and biceps brachii (brachioradialis acts like an efficient flexor in midprone position of the forearm).
- Extension—Muscle which crosses posteriorly acts like extensor and triceps is the main extensor of the elbow.

Blood supply of the elbow joint: Anastomoses around the elbow.

Nerve supply of the elbow joint: Musculo-cutaneous, ulnar and radial nerves supply the joint.

Superior Radioulnar Joint

Bones taking part in the joint:

Head of the radius, annular ligament of radius and radial notch of ulna (Fig. 2.48).
- *Type of joint:* Pivot type of synovial joint.
- *Axis:* Uniaxial but the axis is vertical.

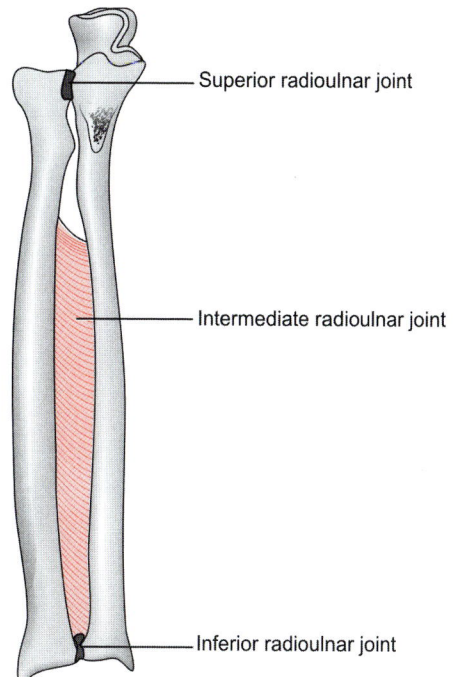

Fig. 2.48: Superior, middle and inferior radioulnar joints

- *Fibrous capsule:* Fibrous capsule of this joint is continuous with the capsule of the elbow joint. The synovial membrane is the lower continuation of the synovial membrane of the elbow joint.
- *Ligaments:* Strong annular ligament forms a collar with the radial notch of ulna.
- *Movements:*
  - Pronation and supination are the two movements which take place at this joint (Fig. 2.49). The axis of pronation and supination passes through the head of the radius and styloid process of ulna. *Note:* It is always the radius which moves during supination and pronation and not ulna. (All the pronators and supinators are inserted into the radius as it is the radius that moves while executing these movements).
  - Supination is produced by the biceps brachii and supinator.

Labels in figure: Superior radioulnar joint; Intermediate radioulnar joint; Inferior radioulnar joint

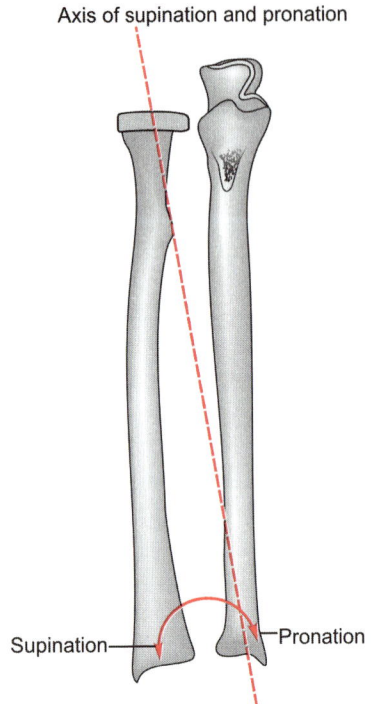

Axis of supination and pronation

Supination — Pronation

Fig. 2.49: Axis of supination and pronation

– Pronation is produced by the pronators teres and pronators quadratus.
- *Nerve supply:* Musculocutaneous, median and radial nerves.

Inferior Radioulnar Joint

- *Bones taking part in the joint:* Head of ulna and ulnar notch of the radius (Fig. 2.48).
- *Type of joint:* Pivot type of synovial joint.
- *Axis:* Vertical axis (uniaxial).

- *Joint cavity:* A fibrocartilaginous articular disc binds the lower ends of radius and ulna. This disc separates the inferior radioulnar joint from the wrist joint. The presence of disc inferiorly in the joint makes the joint cavity L-shaped. The vertical limb of the "L" lies between the lower ends of radius and ulna while the horizontal limb lies between the head of ulna and articular disc.
- *Movements:*
  – The distal end of the radius moves around the stationary head of the ulna during pronation and supination. The two movements permitted by this joint are: supination and pronation.
  – Supinators (biceps and supinator) supinate the forearm and pronators (pronator teres and pronator quadratus) pronate the forearm.
- *Nerve supply:* Anterior and posterior interosseous nerve supplies the inferior radioulnar joint.
- It is also called "distal radioulnar joint".

Wrist Joint

Bones taking part in the joint:
- Proximal—distal end of the radius and articular disc (Fig. 2.50).
- Distal—scaphoid, lunate and triquetrum carpal bones. There are two bones which do not take part in the formation of the wrist joint. They are: head of ulna which is separated by the articular disc and pisiform bone which lies on a more anterior plane. In fact pisiform bone is a sesamoid bone in the tendon of flexor carpi ulnaris.

Type of joint: It is an ellipsoid type of synovial joint. (Place an egg over concave surface and see the different possibilities of movement).
Axis: It is a biaxial joint.
Movements:
- Flexion-extension in one axis.
- Adduction-abduction in another axis.

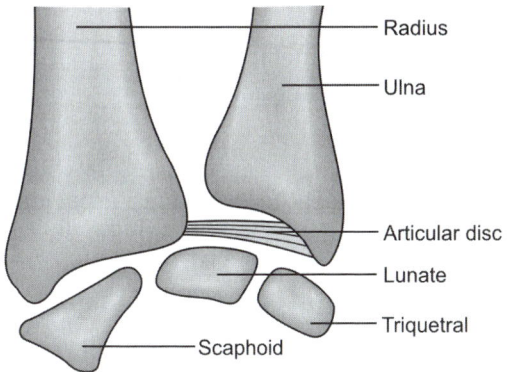

Labels: Radius, Ulna, Articular disc, Lunate, Triquetral, Scaphoid

Fig. 2.50: Wrist joint

- When all the four movements are sequentially performed one after the other, it comes to be called circumduction.
- Muscles responsible for these movements of the wrist joint are:
  - *Flexion:* Flexor carpi ulnaris and flexor carpi radialis acting together. They are assisted by all long flexor tendons which cross anterior to the wrist joint.
  - *Extension:* Extensor carpi radialis longus, extensor carpi radialis brevis and extensor carpi ulnaris. They are assisted by the extensor tendons which cross posterior to the wrist joint.
  - *Adduction:* The two medial muscles are responsible for this movement: Flexor carpi ulnaris and extensor carpi ulnaris.
  - *Abduction:* The tendons which lie lateral to the joint are responsible for this movement. Abductor pollicis longus, extensor carpi radialis longus, extensor carpi radialis brevis and the fourth which joins these tendons during abduction is flexor carpi radialis. Flexor carpi radialis is inserted into the bases of second and third metacarpal bones and thereby counteracts and balances two extensor muscles, the extensor carpi radialis longus and brevis.

How do you mark the wrist joint cavity on the surface?

Join a line connecting the two styloid processes and it represents the level of joint cavity.

Nerve supply of the wrist joint:
1. Anterior interosseous branch of median nerve.
2. Posterior interosseous branch of radial nerve.
3. Branches of ulnar nerve.

CLINICAL ANATOMY

Four very important points to remember:
1. Whenever a person falls on the outstretched hand (forced dorsiflexion of the hand) the lower end of the radius is fractured and the fractured distal segment of radius is displaced dorsally resulting in a clinical condition called the "dinner fork deformity" or "Colle's fracture".
2. Should a person fall on the back of the hand (forced palmar flexion of the hand) the lower end of the radius is fractured but the distal fractured segment is displaced ventrally resulting in a condition called the "Smith's fracture" (opposite of Colle's fracture).
3. Fracture of the scaphoid is common in young adults because of its strategic location of transfer of force to the radius. Whenever the scaphoid is fractured (commonly at the waist) there is a threat of avascular necrosis of the proximal part of the scaphoid because its nourishment comes from the distal part. There is a swelling and pain in the anatomical snuff box as this bone lies in its floor.
4. A fall on the outstretched hand on dorsal aspect may also result in the anterior dislocation of the lunate bone which has potential to compress the median nerve.

Intercarpal Joints

These are group of joints combined together. They are as follows:

1. Joints between the proximal row of carpal bones.
2. Joints between the distal row of carpal bones.
3. Joint between the proximal and distal row of carpal bones (midcarpal joint).

Bones taking part in these joints: Carpal bones.

Type of joints: All these joints belong to plane type of synovial joints.

Axis: All plane joints belong to multiaxial type as they can slide in any direction.

Fibrous capsule: There is a common fibrous capsule and synovial membrane for all these joints.

Ligaments:
- Anterior carpal.
- Posterior carpal.
- Interosseous carpal.

Movements: These joints serve to enhance the movements of wrist joint.

Nerve supply of the intercarpal joints:
Anterior interosseous branch of median nerve, posterior interosseous branch of radial nerve and branches of ulnar nerve.

Carpometacarpal Joints

Bones taking part in these joints:
The four carpal bones of the distal row: From medial to lateral side, they are: Hamate, capitate, trapezoid and trapezium (proximally). Bases of the medial four metacarpal bones (distally).

Types of joints: Plane type of synovial joints.

Axis: Multiaxial (they slide in all directions).

Fibrous capsule: All these joints have a common fibrous capsule and synovial membrane. (Remember that the only joint which is excluded from this complex is: Carpometacarpal joint of the thumb).

Ligaments:
- Palmar carpometacarpal.
- Dorsal carpometacarpal.
- Interosseous.

Movements:
These joints assist the carpometacarpal joint of thumb in grasping objects tightly by the hand.

Nerve supply:
- Anterior interosseous nerve.
- Posterior interosseous nerve.
- Branches of ulnar nerve.

Intermetacarpal Joints

Bones taking part in these joints:
Bases of 2nd–5th metacarpals.

Types of joints: Plane type of synovial joints.

Ligaments:
- Palmar.
- Dorsal.
- Interosseous.

Carpometacarpal Joint of Thumb

- *Bones taking part in this joint:*
  - Base of the first metacarpal bone—distal.
  - Trapezium (carpal bone)—proximal.
- *Type of joint:* Saddle type of synovial joint.
- *Ligaments:* Palmar and dorsal carpometacarpal and lateral ligaments of the thumb.
- *Movements (Fig. 2.51):*
  - Flexion—extension along one axis.
  - Adduction—abduction along another axis.
  - Opposition.
- Whenever a ball is held tightly, there is movement in the carpometacarpal joint of the thumb and this movement is assisted by other carpometacarpal joints as stated above.
- *Nerve supply:*
  - Anterior interosseous nerve.
  - Posterior interosseous nerve.

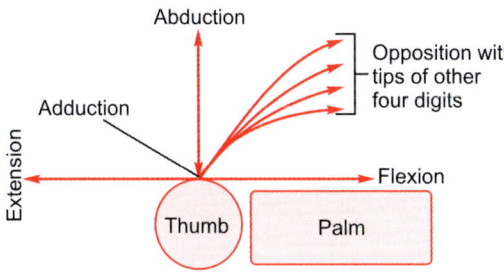

Fig. 2.51: Movements of the left thumb

Metacarpophalangeal Joints

These joints are also called MP joints. These joints are numbered from lateral to medial side

Bones taking part in these joints:
- Proximal—heads of metacarpals.
- Distal—bases of the proximal phalanges of each finger.

There are five metacarpophalangeal joints.

Type of joint: Condyloid type of synovial joint; some authorities feel it is ellipsoid type.

Axis: Biaxial (note all condyloid joints are biaxial).

Ligaments:
- Medial collateral ligament.
- Lateral collateral ligament.
- Palmar ligament.

[Though the collateral ligaments are present, they still permit adduction and abduction when the fingers are in extended position. This is because these collateral ligaments are lax in the extended position of fingers and they permit adduction and abduction. However, abduction and adduction are not permitted when the fingers are flexed because the collateral ligaments are taut in this position. One should know that the first metacarpophalangeal joint (of thumb) behaves like interphalangeal joints. This joint presents only flexion and extension. Do not forget to remember that the adduction and abduction of thumb take place at the carpometacarpal joint of the thumb].

Movements:
- Flexion-extension (along one axis).
- Adduction-abduction (along another axis). (These movements are seen in 2nd to 5th metacarpophalangeal joints only).

Nerve supply: Branches of ulnar and median nerves.

Interphalangeal Joints

These joints are also called IP joints. They are divided into proximal interphalangeal (PIP) and distal interphalangeal (DIP) joints. There are four PIP and four DIP joints in the medial four fingers. However, there is only one interphalangeal joint in the thumb.

- *Bones taking part in these joints:*
  - Heads of phalanges—proximal.
  - Bases of the phalanges—distal.
- *How many interphalangeal joints are there?*
  - Thumb—you have only one interphalangeal joint.
  - The rest of the fingers have two interphalangeal joints for each finger, it means 4 × 2 = 8.
  - Therefore, totally you have nine interphalangeal joints in each hand.
- *Type of joint:* Hinge type of synovial joint.
- *Axis:* Uniaxial and the axis is transverse.
- *Ligaments:*
  - Medial and lateral collateral ligaments; palmar ligaments.
- *Movements:* Only flexion and extension.
- *Nerve supply:* Branches of ulnar and median nerves.

Lower Limb

3

The lower limb has the following parts:
- Gluteal region.
- Thigh.
- Leg.
- Foot.

GLUTEAL REGION

- This is the rounded part on which one sits. It includes hip and buttock. It has a lot of fat and natal cleft is the groove seen between the buttocks.
- There are gluteal muscles in the gluteal region.
- Gluteal muscles are supplied by the gluteal nerves.
- Muscle on the back of the gluteal region extends the thigh at hip joint as it lies posterior to the joint.
- Muscles on the lateral side of the gluteal region are the abductors of the hip joint.

Hip Joint

- The upper joint of the lower limb is hip joint.
- Acetabulum of hip bone and head of femur form the hip joint.
  Thigh is the region between the hip and knee joints.
- The anterior part of the thigh has flexors of the hip joint.
- Flexors of the thigh are supplied by the femoral nerve.

- The medial part of the thigh has adductors of the hip joint.
- Adductors are supplied by the obturator nerve.
- The back of the thigh has extensors of the hip joint.
- Extensors of thigh are supplied by the sciatic nerve.

The part of the lower limb between the knee joint and ankle joint is *the leg*.

Knee Joint

- The knee joint is at the junction of the thigh with the leg.
- It is a synovial joint.
- It is a modified hinge joint.
- Lower end of the femur, patella and the upper end of the tibia take part in its formation.
- It has flexion and extension movements.
- Flexion of the knee is the approximation of the posterior surface of the leg with the posterior surface of the thigh.
- Extension of the knee is the straightening of the leg in line with the thigh.
- The anterior part of the thigh has the extensors of knee and the posterior part of the knee has flexors of the knee.
- The extensors of the knee are supplied by the femoral nerve.
- The flexors of the knee are supplied by the sciatic nerve.

- Tendons which form the flexors of knee, form strings on either side of the knee joint and, therefore, they are called hamstring muscles. Feel for the tendons of the hamstrings in a semiflexed knee on either side of the popliteal fossa on the back of the knee joint.

LEG

- It has two bones—tibia and fibula.
- Tibia is a large bone and it can be felt along the medial side of the front of the leg.
- The lower end of the tibia becomes a medial malleolus.
- Fibula is surrounded by muscles.
- The lower end of the fibula is called the lateral malleolus.

    Identify the great saphenous vein anterior to the medial malleolus and small saphenous vein posterior to the lateral malleolus.

Ankle Joint

- The bones which take part in the formation of the ankle joint are the lower end of the tibia and fibula and the upper part of the talus bone of the foot. It is a synovial joint.
- *There are two movements of the ankle joint:*
    - Dorsiflexion is the approximation of the dorsum of the foot with the front of the leg.
    - Plantar flexion of the ankle is the opposite movement.

The leg has three compartments:

1. The posterior compartment has muscles which plantar flex the ankle joint. Therefore, this compartment is also called the flexor compartment of the leg. This compartment is supplied by the tibial branch of the sciatic nerve.
2. The anterior compartment contains muscles which dorsiflex the foot. These are also called extensors. Therefore, the anterior compartment is also called the extensor compartment. This compartment is supplied by the deep fibular nerve.
3. The lateral compartment contains two muscles which evert the foot. These two muscles are supplied by the superficial fibular nerve.

FOOT

It is made up of the following bones:
- Talus.
- Calcaneum.
- Navicular.
- Cuboid.
- Medial cuneiform.
- Intermediate cuneiform.
- Lateral cuneiform.
- Five metatarsals (metatarsals are numbered from medial to lateral side).
- Great toe has two phalanges (a proximal and a distal).
- Other toes have three phalanges each (a proximal, a middle and a distal).

Talus is the key bone as it forms the link between foot and leg bones. It has a head, neck and body. Calcaneus is the largest tarsal bone. Its medial surface shows a shelf called sustentaculum tali which supports the talus. Undersurface of sustentaculum tali is grooved by flexor hallucis longus tendon. Posterior surface of calcaneus receives tendocalcaneus or Achilles tendon. Cuboid has a groove on its undersurface for peroneus longus tendon. Tuberosity of navicular receives insertion of tibialis posterior tendon. The base of 5th metatarsal has a tuberosity which receives insertion of peroneus brevis and tertius muscles. The 1st metatarsal is thickest.

The following are the joints of the foot:
- Subtalar joint (posterior talocalcaneal joint) is a joint between talus and calcaneus (synovial type of joint).
- Talocalcaneonavicular joint (ball and socket type of synovial joint). It is a compound joint.

- Calcaneocuboid joint (saddle type of synovial joint).
- Cuneonavicular joint (plane type of synovial joint) which connects the cuneiform bones with the navicular bone. It is a compound joint.
- Tarsometatarsal joints (plane type of synovial joints).
- Metatarsophalangeal joints (ellipsoid type of synovial joints).
- Interphalangeal joints (hinge type of synovial joints).

Dorsum of the foot:
- It has dorsal venous arch.
- It has only one muscle over it and that is extensor digitorum brevis and its part going to the great toe is called the extensor hallucis brevis.
- Identify the tendon of extensor digitorum longus which stand in bold relief when you extend the toes.

Sole of the foot:
- Its skin is thick. The deep fascia of the sole of the foot is called the plantar fascia and its central part is thickened to be called plantar aponeurosis.
- The sole of the foot contains the small muscles which move the toes. These muscles are comparable to the muscles of the hand.
- Two nerves which supply all the muscles of the sole of the foot are the medial and lateral plantar nerves.
- The medial and lateral plantar nerves are the terminal branches of the tibial nerve.

The medial plantar nerve is comparable to median nerve (Remember M in medial plantar and M in median nerve). It supplies four muscles of the foot and they are:
1. Abductor hallucis.
2. Flexor digitorum brevis.
3. First lumbrical.
4. Flexor hallucis brevis.

Compare with the muscles supplied by the median nerve in the hand. They are:
1. Abductor pollicis brevis.
2. Flexor pollicis brevis.
3. Opponens pollicis.
4. First lumbrical.
5. Second lumbrical.

All the remaining muscles of the sole of the foot are supplied by the lateral plantar nerve which is similar to ulnar nerve in hand.

The arteries which supply the sole of the foot are the lateral and medial plantar arteries.

Bones of the lower limb:
Identify the following in the lower limb bones:

Hip Bone

- The ilium (Figs 3.1 and 3.2).
- Acetabulum
- Iliac crest
- Anterior superior iliac spine
- Posterior superior iliac spine
- Anterior inferior iliac spine
- Posterior inferior iliac spine
- The ischium
- The body of the ischium
- Ischial tuberosity
- Ischiopubic ramus
- The pubis
- The body of the pubis
- Superior pubic ramus
- Inferior pubic ramus
- Greater sciatic notch
- Lesser sciatic notch
- Hip bone is an irregular bone
- Two hip bones and sacrum form pelvic girdle
- Takes part in 2 joints: sacroiliac and symphysis pubis.

Ilium

- The iliac crest is divided into the ventral segment in anterior 2/3rd and dorsal

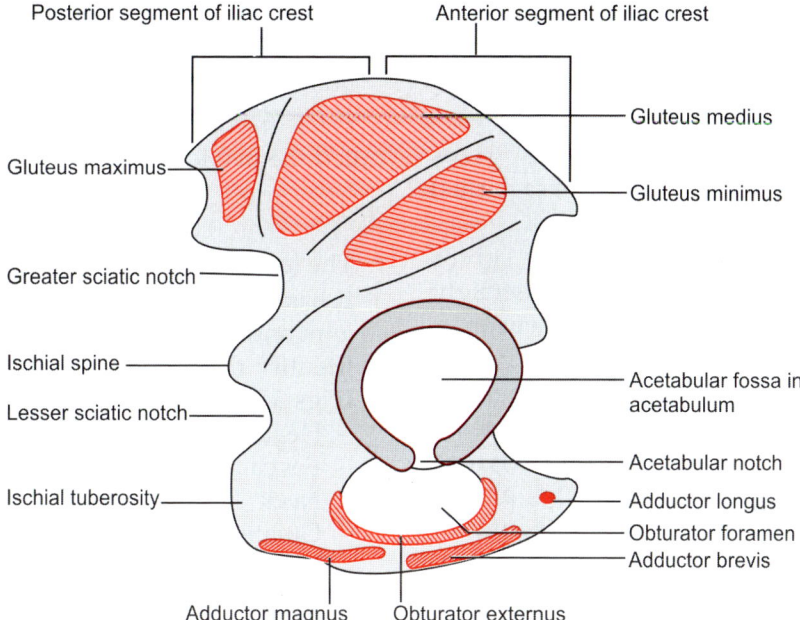

Posterior segment of iliac crest

Anterior segment of iliac crest

Gluteus medius

Gluteus maximus

Gluteus minimus

Greater sciatic notch

Ischial spine

Acetabular fossa in acetabulum

Lesser sciatic notch

Acetabular notch

Ischial tuberosity

Adductor longus

Obturator foramen

Adductor brevis

Adductor magnus   Obturator externus

Fig. 3.1: Lateral aspect of right hip bone

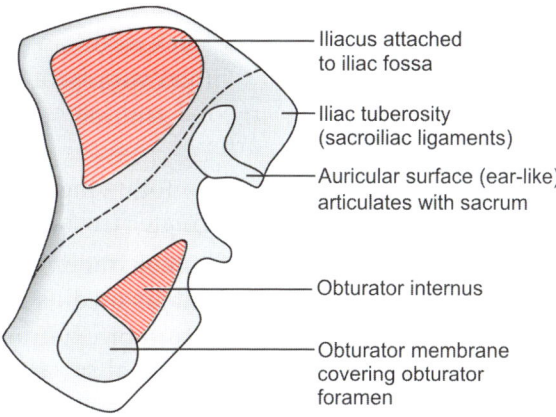

Iliacus attached to iliac fossa

Iliac tuberosity (sacroiliac ligaments)

Auricular surface (ear-like) articulates with sacrum

Obturator internus

Obturator membrane covering obturator foramen

Fig. 3.2: Medial aspect of right hip bone

segment in posterior 1/3rd. The anterior part of the ventral segment provides attachment to tensor fascia lata, external oblique, internal oblique and transversus abdominis. Among these, only external oblique is insertion and the rest are origins. The dorsal part of ventral segment provides origin to latissimus dorsi and quadratus lumborum. The dorsal segment gives origin to gluteus maximus and erector spinae.

- The highest point of iliac crest lies at the level of L4 spine.
- Anterior superior iliac spine gives attachment to 1 muscle (origin of sartorius) and 1 ligament (inguinal).
- Anterior inferior iliac spine gives attachment to 1 muscle (origin of straight head of rectus femoris) and 1 ligament (apex of iliofemoral ligament).
- Gluteal surface of ilium gives origin to 4 muscles: Gluteus maximus behind posterior gluteal line, gluteus medius between posterior and anterior gluteal lines, gluteus minimus between anterior and inferior gluteal lines, reflected head of rectus femoris from a groove just above the acetabulum.
- Medial surface of ilium gives origin to iliacus from iliac fossa and obturator internus from pelvic surface.

Pubis

- Pectineal line (pecten pubis) gives attachment to lacunar and pectineal part of inguinal ligament.
- Pubic tubercle gives attachment to 1 muscle (insertion of cremaster) and 1 ligament (inguinal).
- Pubic crest gives origin to 2 muscles, namely rectus abdominis and pyramidalis of abdomen.
- Front of pubis gives origin to 5 muscles: gracilis, adductor brevis, obturator externus, adductor longus and pubic part of adductor magnus.

Ischium

- Ischial spine gives attachment to 1 muscle (coccygeus) and 1 ligament (sacrospinous).
- The ischial tuberosity gives origin to semimembranosus, semitendinosus, long head of biceps, ischial part of adductor

magnus. Its lateral margin gives origin to quadratus femoris and medial margin gives attachment to sacrotuberous ligament.

Pelvic fracture: Fracture of the hip bone is called the pelvic fracture.

Femur

- The longest bone in the body.
- It has two joints. The upper one is the hip joint and the lower one is the knee joint.
- Identify the following parts of the femur (Figs 3.3 and 3.4):
  - Head.
  - Fovea for the ligament of the head.
  - Neck
  - Greater trochanter
  - Lesser trochanter
  - Linea aspera
  - Gluteal tuberosity
  - Medial femoral condyle
  - Lateral femoral condyle.

Upper End

The neck forms an angle of 125° with shaft.

Blood supply of head is from branches of medial and lateral circumflex and obturator artery.

The following 7 muscles are inserted into the greater trochanter:

- Gluteus minimus into anterior surface.
- Gluteus medius into lateral surface.
- Obturator externus into trochanteric fossa on medial surface.
- Obturator internus, 2 gamelli into medial surface.
- Piriformis into apex.
- The lesser trochanter receives insertion of psoas major and iliacus.
- Intertrochanteric line gives attachment to iliofemoral ligament.
- Quadrate tubercle on intertrochanteric crest receives insertion of quadratus femoris.

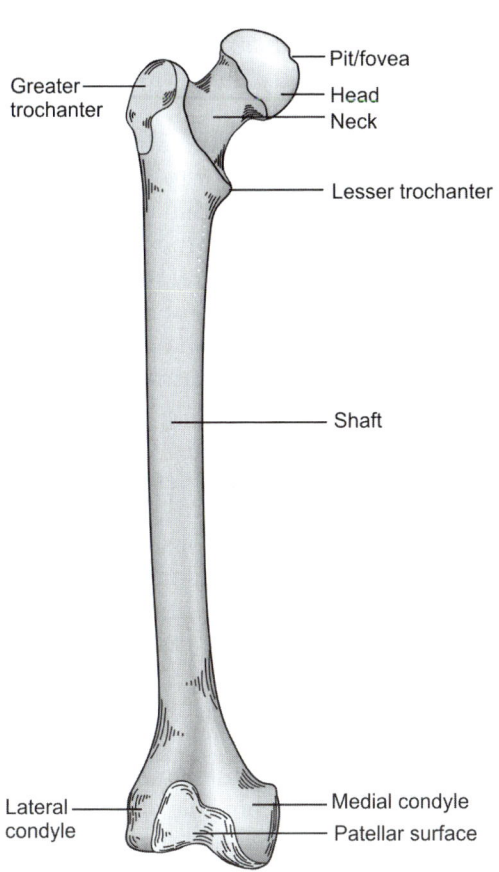

Fig. 3.3: Anterior aspect of right femur

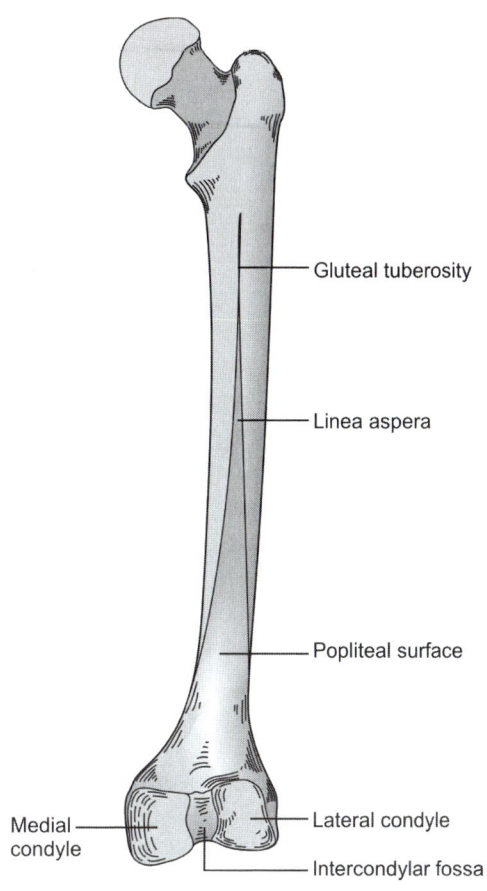

Fig. 3.4: Posterior aspect of right femur

Shaft

Vastus intermedius arises from anterior and lateral surface of shaft. Articularis genu is its detached part.

Along posterior border of shaft is the linea aspera. Structures attached to linea aspera are vastus medialis, medial intermuscular septum, adductor brevis, adductor longus, adductor magnus, posterior intermuscular septum, short head of biceps femoris, lateral intermuscular septum and vastus lateralis.

Gluteal tuberosity receives insertion of gluteus maximus. Spiral line receives insertion of pectineus.

Lower End

Lateral condyle gives attachment to fibular collateral ligament (from lateral epicondyle) and origin to 3 muscles namely popliteus (from anterior end of groove for popliteus), lateral head of gastrocnemius and plantaris.

Medial condyle gives attachment to tibial collateral ligament (from medial epicondyle) and origin to medial head of gastrocnemius and insertion to adductor magnus (into adductor tubercle).

Intercondylar notch or fossa gives attachment to anterior cruciate, posterior cruciate and oblique popliteal ligament.

Patella

- It articulates with the patellar surface of the femur.
- It is a sesamoid bone in the tendon of quadriceps femoris and the tendon is called the ligamentum patella.
- It is triangular with base, apex, 2 borders (medial and lateral) and 2 surfaces (anterior and posterior).
- Base above receives insertion of quadriceps femoris.
- Apex below receives attachment of ligamentum patellae.
- Lateral border receives insertion of vastus lateralis.
- Medial border receives insertion of vastus medialis.
- Anterior surface is subcutaneous.
- Posterior surface articulates with 2 femoral condyles.

Tibia

- This is the weight-bearing medial bone of the leg (Fig. 3.5 A and B).
- Its lower end becomes the medial malleolus.
- It takes part in knee, ankle, superior and inferior tibiofibular joints.

Upper End

- The groove for semimembranosus behind medial condyle receives insertion of semimembranosus.
- Tibial collateral ligament is attached to medial side of medial condyle.

- Lateral condyle articulates with head of fibula to form superior tibiofibular joint.
- Tibial tuberosity gives attachment to ligamentum patellae.
- Intercondylar area gives attachment to 6 structures from anterior to posterior:
  - Anterior horn of medial meniscus.
  - Anterior cruciate ligament.
  - Anterior horn of lateral meniscus.
  - Posterior horn of lateral meniscus.
  - Posterior horn of medial meniscus.
  - Posterior cruciate ligament.

Shaft

- Anterior border is subcutaneous.
- Interosseous or lateral border gives attachment to interosseous membrane.
- Medial surface is subcutaneous and in its upper part receives insertion of sartorius, gracilis and semitendinosus where an anserine bursa is present.
- Lateral surface gives origin to tibialis anterior.
- *Muscles attached to posterior surface include:* Origin of soleus from soleal line, insertion of popliteus above soleal line, origin of tibialis posterior (lateral to vertical ridge) and flexor digitorum longus (medial to vertical ridge) below soleal line.

Lower End

- Is known as medial malleolus.
- Is grooved posteriorly by tibialis posterior tendon.
- Its tip gives attachment to deltoid ligament.
- Its lateral surface articulates with talus.

  Subcutaneous parts of tibia include: anterior border or shin, 2 condyles, tibial tuberosity, medial surface of shaft and medial malleolus.
- *Fracture of the tibia:* Tibia is narrowest at the junction of lower one-third with the middle one-third of its shaft. This is the most frequent site of fracture.

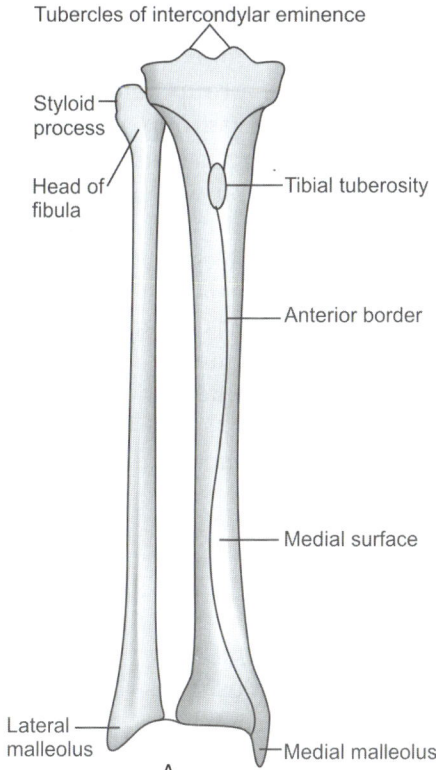 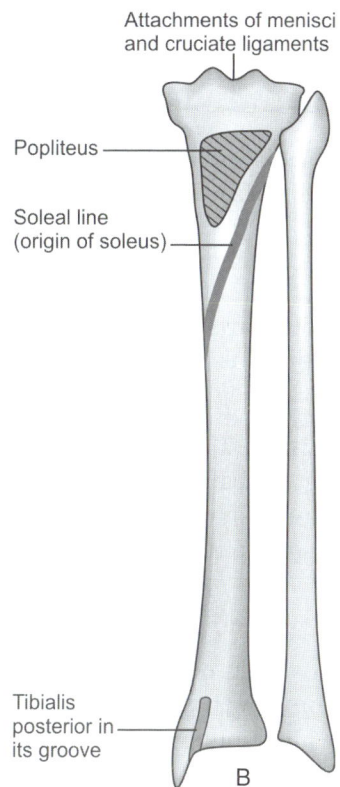

Tubercles of intercondylar eminence

Styloid process

Head of fibula

Tibial tuberosity

Anterior border

Medial surface

Lateral malleolus

Medial malleolus

A

Attachments of menisci and cruciate ligaments

Popliteus

Soleal line (origin of soleus)

Tibialis posterior in its groove

B

Fig. 3.5: A. Anterior aspect of right tibia and fibula, B. Posterior aspect of right tibia and fibula

Fibula

- The lateral bone of the leg (Fig. 3.5A and B).
- It serves mainly for muscle attachment.
- It is not directly involved in weight bearing.
- The shafts of tibia and fibula are inter-connected by an interosseous membrane.
- It forms the following joints: Superior tibiofibular, inferior tibiofibular and ankle joints.
- Its upper end is known as head having a styloid process and a lower end known as lateral malleolus.

Upper End

- It articulates with lateral condyle of tibia to form superior tibiofibular joint.

- Receives insertion of biceps femoris.
- Receives attachment of fibular collateral ligament.
- Common peroneal nerve is related to back of head and neck of fibula.

Shaft

- Anterior surface gives origin to extensor digitorum longus from upper 3/4th, peroneus tertius from lower 1/4th and extensor hallucis longus from middle 1/2.
- Lateral surface gives origin to peroneus longus from upper 2/3rd and peroneus brevis from lower 2/3rd.
- Posterior surface gives origin to soleus from upper 1/3rd, flexor hallucis longus from

lower 2/3rd lateral to medial crest and tibialis posterior medial to medial crest.

Lower End

- Its medial surface articulates with talus.
- Its posterior surface is grooved by tendons of peroneus longus and brevis.
- Its tip gives attachment to lateral ligament of ankle.

Subcutaneous parts of fibula include: head and lateral malleolus.

- *Fractures of fibula:*
  - They occur just proximal to the lateral malleolus and are often associated with the fracture dislocation of the ankle joint.
- Fibula is used for bone grafting.

Lymphatic Drainage of the Lower Limb

- There are two sets of lymph nodes inferior to the inguinal ligament.
- They are called inguinal lymph nodes.
- Inguinal lymph nodes are divided into superficial and deep groups.
- Superficial group of lymph nodes lie in the superficial fascia.
- Deep group of lymph nodes lie deep to the deep fascia.
- Superficial group of lymph nodes are divided into horizontal and vertical groups (see Fig. 3.10).
- Horizontal group is divided into medial and lateral.
- Vertical group accompanies the terminal part of the great saphenous vein.
- Vertical group drains all the superficial structures of the lower limb except the lateral part of the foot and the leg (small saphenous vein territory).
- The medial part of the horizontal superficial group drains the lymph from the anterior abdominal wall below the level of umbilicus.

- The lateral part of the horizontal superficial group drains the gluteal region.
- The superficial groups of lymph nodes drain into the deep group of lymph nodes.
- Deep group of inguinal lymph nodes drains all the deep lymph vessels of lower limb and the superficial lymph from the lateral part of the foot and leg. It also drains lymph from the glans penis and clitoris directly. Deep lymph vessels accompany the deep vessels namely anterior tibial, posterior tibial, fibular, popliteal and femoral.
- From deep inguinal nodes lymph goes to external iliac, common iliac nodes and so on.

Venous Drainage of the Lower Limb

- It has superficial and deep veins (Fig. 3.6).
- Superficial veins are two in number.
  - Great saphenous vein.
  - Small saphenous vein.

Great saphenous vein:
- It begins on the medial side of the dorsal venous arch.
- It ascends anterior to the medial malleolus.
- It passes posterior to the medial condyle of the femur.
- Communicates with the small saphenous vein.

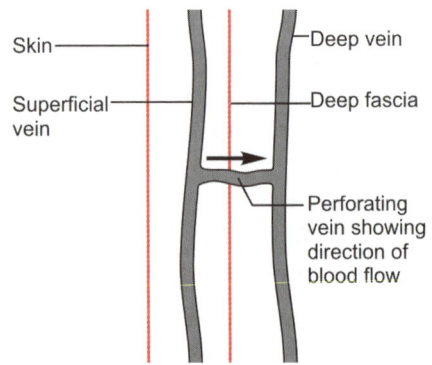

Fig. 3.6: Superficial, perforating and deep veins

- It passes through the saphenous opening of the fascia lata after piercing cribriform fascia.
- It empties into the femoral vein.
- It is accompanied by the saphenous nerve.
- Perforating veins connect the superficial great saphenous vein with the deep veins (Fig. 3.6).
- These perforators contain valves that allow blood to flow only from superficial to deep veins. Perforating veins are compressed whenever pressure increases inside the deep fascia.

- Great saphenous vein is used in coronary bypass. Care is taken to reverse the vein otherwise valves will prevent the blood flow.

- It receives three veins before it pierces the cribriform fascia of saphenous opening. The three veins are:
  - Superficial circumflex iliac.
  - Superficial external pudendal.
  - Superficial epigastric.

Deep veins accompany the major arteries namely anterior tibial, posterior tibial, fibular, popliteal and femoral. The latter two accompanying veins are single but others are in the form of venae comitantes. Finally they continue as femoral vein which continues as external iliac vein.

Deep vein thrombosis (DVT) may occur following long transcontinental flights in aircrafts and more commonly in prolonged immobilization.

Small saphenous vein:
- It arises from the lateral side of the dorsal venous arch.
- It ascends posterior to the lateral malleolus.
- It ascends between the two heads of gastrocnemius.

- It empties into the popliteal vein in the popliteal fossa.
- It drains the lateral side of the foot and leg.
- It is accompanied by the sural nerve.

Varicosities of superficial veins may occur. Femoral vein is used for cannulation and venous catheterization.

Front of the Thigh
Cutaneous Innervation

- The skin of the front of the thigh is supplied by the following dermatomes: L1, L2 and L3.
- The following cutaneous nerves supply the skin of the front of the thigh:
  - Lateral cutaneous nerve of thigh.
  - Femoral branch of genitofemoral nerve.
  - Ilioinguinal nerve.
  - Intermediate cutaneous nerve of thigh.
  - Medial cutaneous nerve of thigh.

Deep fascia of thigh
- It is tough and known as fascia lata. It covers the muscles of thigh and divides the thigh muscles into three compartments.
- The lateral part of the fascia lata is thickened to form iliotibial tract.
- Iliotibial tract extends from the iliac crest to the anterior aspect of the lateral condyle of the tibia.
- Membranous layer of superficial fascia extending inferiorly from the abdomen is fused with the fascia lata along a line near the inguinal ligament. Therefore any extravasated urine will not go below this level of attachment of membranous layer of superficial fascia with the deep fascia.

The muscles of the front of the thigh
Pectineus, iliopsoas (iliacus and psoas major), tensor fascia lata, sartorius, quadriceps femoris.

Pectineus
- *Nerve supply:* Dual nerve supply by femoral and obturator nerve.
- *Special features:* Dealt in adductor region.

Iliopsoas (iliacus and psoas major)
- *Origin:*
  - Psoas major from bodies and transverse processes of all lumbar vertebrae.
  - Iliacus from iliac fossa.
- *Insertion:* Lesser trochanter.
- *Nerve supply:* Femoral.
- *Action:* Flexor of thigh.

Tensor fascia lata
- *Special feature:* Dealt in gluteal region.

Sartorius
- *Origin:*
  - Anterior superior iliac spine.
- *Insertion:* Upper medial surface of shaft of tibia.
- *Nerve supply:* Femoral.
- *Action:* Flexion, abduction and lateral rotation of thigh; flexion of leg.
- *Special feature:* Muscle action responsible for the cross-legged position of the sartors (Latin) for tailors.

Quadriceps femoris
Quadriceps femoris has 4 components—rectus femoris, vastus medialis, vastus lateralis and vastus intermedius.

- *Origin:*
  - Rectus femoris from anterior inferior iliac spine (straight head) and area above acetabulum (reflected head).
  - Vastus medialis from intertrochanteric line and medial lip of linea aspera.
  - Vastus lateralis from greater trochanter and lateral lip of linea aspera.
  - Vastus intermedius from anterior and lateral surfaces of body of femur.
- *Insertion:* Patella and through ligamentum patellae into tibial tuberosity.

- *Nerve supply:* Femoral.
- *Action:* Vastus components act only on knee joint (extension) but rectus femoris also acts on hip joint (flexion). It is the only extensor of knee.

- Patellar tendon reflex (L2–4).
  - Tap the patellar tendon with a tendon hammer.
  - This stretches the patellar tendon.
  - The muscle spindles in the quadriceps are stimulated.
  - Afferent impulses run in the femoral nerve to the spinal cord.
  - Efferent impulses reach the quadriceps in the femoral nerve.
  - Stimulation of the quadriceps causes the leg to kick. Hence, this is also known as knee jerk reflex.
  - This reflex tests the L2–4 segments.

Femoral Triangle
- *Boundaries:* Superiorly the inguinal ligament (Fig. 3.7).

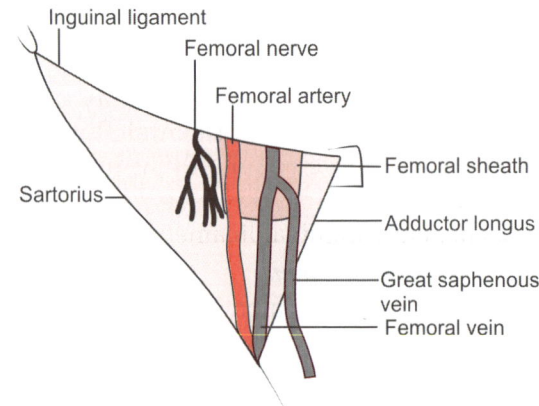

Fig. 3.7: Femoral triangle and its contents (right side)

- Medially the adductor longus.
- Laterally the sartorius.
- Roof—fascia lata.
- Floor (from lateral to medial side).
  - Iliacus.
  - Psoas major.
  - Pectineus.
- *Contents:*
  - Femoral nerve and its branches.
  - Femoral sheath and its contents.
  - Femoral artery and its branches.
  - Femoral vein and its tributaries.
  - Deep inguinal lymph nodes.
- Between the anterior superior iliac spine (ASIS) and pubic tubercle inguinal ligament lies.
  - Femoral nerve is situated midway between these two points.
  - Therefore, it is situated behind mid-point of inguinal ligament.
- Between the ASIS and pubic symphysis inguinal region.
  - Femoral artery is situated midway.
  - Situated behind the midpoint of inguinal region.
  - *Note:* Hence, femoral artery is medial to femoral nerve.

Femoral nerve: Root value L2–4; ventral rami, dorsal division (Fig. 3.9).
- From the trunk it supplies iliacus and pectineus.
  - *Note:* Pectineus is supplied by femoral and obturator nerves.
- Femoral nerve divides into anterior and posterior divisions in the triangle about 2 cm below inguinal ligament.
  - Anterior division:
    - ◆ It gives medial and intermediate cutaneous nerves of thigh.
    - ◆ Supplies the sartorius muscle.
  - Posterior division: supplies muscles mainly.

- ◆ Supplies the quadriceps femoris.
- ◆ The saphenous nerve is cutaneous branch.
- Femoral block is given lateral to the femoral artery just below the inguinal ligament.

Femoral Artery

It is the continuation of external iliac artery behind the midinguinal point.

Branches:
- Superficial circumflex iliac artery.
- Superficial epigastric artery.
- Superficial external pudendal artery.

All these three branches are given by the femoral artery and they lie deep to deep fascia; hence, these 3 arteries pierce the saphenous opening.

Corresponding veins do not pierce the saphenous opening, because they open into the great saphenous vein before it passes through the saphenous opening.

Note: Deep circumflex iliac artery is a branch of the external iliac artery; not a branch of femoral artery.
- Deep external pudendal artery.
  - Does not pierce the saphenous opening (goes more deep and pierces deep fascia).
- Profunda femoris artery (a large branch of femoral artery).
- Descending genicular artery:
  - It descends to supply the knee joint.
  - It also gives a saphenous branch which accompanies the saphenous nerve to medial side of knee.
  - Continues as the popliteal artery in the opening of the adductor magnus.

Relations of the femoral artery:
- Lies in the femoral sheath (Fig. 3.8).
  - Most lateral compartment of femoral sheath contains the femoral artery.
  - Intermediate compartment: femoral vein.

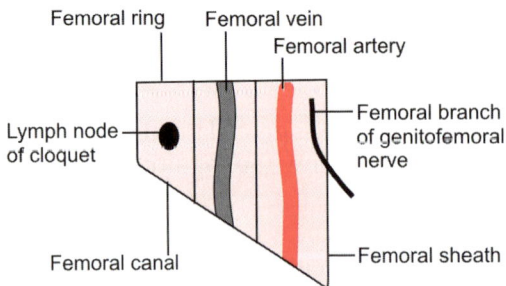

Fig. 3.8: Femoral sheath (left side)

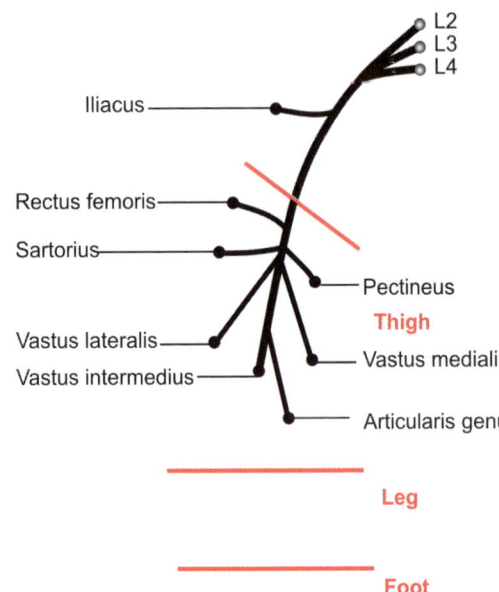

Fig. 3.9: Muscular branches of femoral nerve

– *Medial compartment:* Lymph vessels and lymph node of cloquet.
– *Note:* Femoral branch of genitofemoral nerve accompanies the femoral artery inside the femoral sheath.
  ♦ It supplies the "hands-breadth" area below the inguinal ligament.
– Femoral vein runs medial to femoral artery, then runs behind the femoral artery as it goes down.
– Femoral nerve lies lateral to the femoral artery outside the femoral sheath.

Profunda femoris artery:
• Arises from posterolateral side of femoral artery and then runs posterior to femoral vessels to reach medial side of femur.
• Gives medial circumflex femoral artery and lateral circumflex femoral artery.
• *Note:* Accompanying medial and lateral circumflex femoral veins do not open into profunda femoris vein, but drain into femoral vein.
• Medial circumflex femoral artery has 2 branches:
  – Ascending (trochanteric anastomosis).
  – Transverse (cruciate anastomosis).
• Lateral circumflex femoral artery has 3 branches: Ascending, transverse and descending branches.
  – *Ascending:* Takes part in trochanteric anastomosis in trochanteric fossa of greater trochanter.

– *Transverse:* Takes part in cruciate anastomosis.
– *Descending:* Takes part in anastomosis around knee joint.
• Profunda femoris artery gives 3 perforating arteries. Fourth perforating artery is a continuation of profunda femoris artery. These arteries perforate the adductor magnus muscle and supply the back of the thigh (there are no other arteries at the back of the thigh). They form a chain of anastomoses on the back of the thigh.

CLINICAL ANATOMY
• Femoral pulse can be felt in supine position below the midinguinal point. At this point the artery can also be compressed against the superior pubic ramus or head of femur.
• Femoral artery is used for cannulation and arterial catheterization.

- Femoral artery and vein are close to each other and superficially placed in the femoral triangle. Hence, they are involved in knife and bullet injuries in this region.

Femoral Canal

- Most medial compartment of the femoral sheath (Fig. 3.8).
- Superiorly its continuity with the abdomen at the femoral ring is closed by femoral septum.
- Boundaries of femoral ring:
  - *Anteriorly:* Inguinal ligament.
  - *Posteriorly:* Fascia over pectineus.
  - *Laterally:* Septa which separates it from femoral vein.
  - *Medially:* Base of lacunar ligament (part of inguinal ligament).

  - *Femoral hernia:* Abnormal protrusion of abdominal contents through femoral ring.
    - More common in females, because of wider pelvis.
    - During reduction of hernia, surgeon may come across an abnormal obturator artery (which may be the source of bleeding).
  - *Abnormal obturator artery:* There is an anastomosis of pubic branch of obturator artery and the pubic branch of inferior epigastric artery. When pubic branch of inferior epigastric artery is large it is called abnormal obturator artery.
  - It is in danger of being cut during surgery (femoral hernia reduction) and may cause severe bleeding as it is close to medial border of femoral ring.

Adductor Canal

- Present on the middle of the medial side of the thigh.
- Extends from apex of femoral triangle into the opening of the adductor magnus.
- Formed by adductor longus and magnus posteriorly, vastus medialis anterolaterally and sartorius anteromedially.
- *Another name:* Subsartorial canal; because sartorius lies over the fibrous roof.
- *Contents:* Femoral artery, femoral vein, saphenous nerve and nerve to vastus medialis (Fig. 3.11).
  - No deep vein and artery of the thigh (profunda femoris vessels).
  - No saphenous vein.
  - No femoral nerve.

Medial Compartment of Thigh

- What are the muscles on the medial side of thigh?
  - Adductor longus, brevis, magnus, pectineus and gracilis.
  - All these muscles arise from the pubis and are inserted into the femur.

All adductor muscles are supplied by obturator nerve.

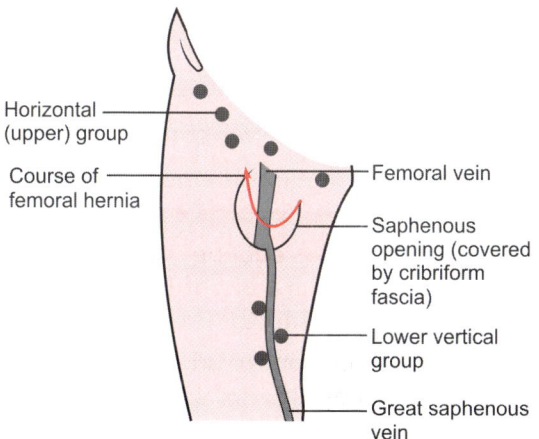

Horizontal (upper) group

Course of femoral hernia

Femoral vein

Saphenous opening (covered by cribriform fascia)

Lower vertical group

Great saphenous vein

Fig. 3.10: Superficial inguinal lymph nodes

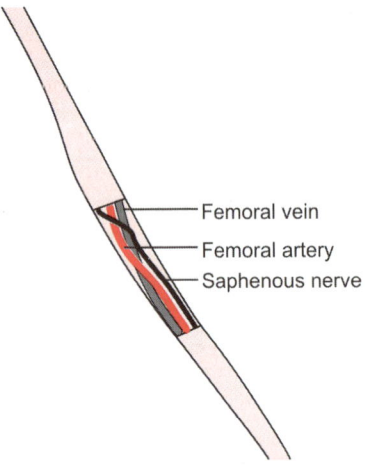

- Femoral vein
- Femoral artery
- Saphenous nerve

Fig. 3.11: Adductor canal

Pectineus
- *Origin:* Superior ramus of pubis.
- *Insertion:* Spiral line of femur.
- *Nerve supply:* Femoral and obturator.
- *Action:* Adducts and flexes the thigh.
- *Special feature:* Dual nerve supply.

Obturator externus
- *Origin:* Obturator membrane and adjacent obturator foramen.
- *Insertion:* Trochanteric fossa.
- *Nerve supply:* Obturator.
- *Action:* Lateral rotation of thigh.

Adductor longus
- *Origin:* Front of body of pubis.
- *Insertion:* Linea aspira.
- *Nerve supply:* Obturator.
- *Action:* Adducts and laterally rotates the thigh.

Adductor brevis
- *Origin:* Front of pubis.
- *Insertion:* Upper part of linea aspira.
- *Nerve supply:* Obturator.
- *Action:* Adducts and laterally rotates the thigh.

Adductor magnus
It has 2 parts: Adductor and hamstring part.

- *Origin:* Adductor part: inferior ramus of pubis and ramus of ischium. Hamstring part from ischial tuberosity.
- *Insertion:* Adductor part into the gluteal tuberosity, linea aspera and medial supra-condylar line while ischial part is into adductor tubercle.
- *Nerve supply:* Dual nerve supply. Adductor part is supplied by obturator and ischial part by tibial part of sciatic nerve.
- *Action:* Adductor part adducts thigh and ischial part extends thigh.

Adductor magnus, as name indicates, is a large muscle.

- Such muscles with dual nerve supply are called hybrid muscles.

- Groin pull in sports involves the origin of adductor muscles.
- Gracilis is used for muscle transplantation.
- Injury to adductor longus may result in rider's strain or sometimes in rider's bone.

Obturator nerve
- L2, 3, 4 (Ventral rami of ventral divisions) (arises from lumbar plexus) (Fig. 3.13).
- Exits the pelvis through obturator foramen.
  - It divides into the anterior and posterior divisions near obturator foramen.
  - Between the anterior and posterior divisions there is obturator externus above and adductor brevis (Fig. 3.12).
  - Muscles in front of adductor brevis are supplied by anterior division.
  - Muscles deep to brevis are supplied by posterior division.

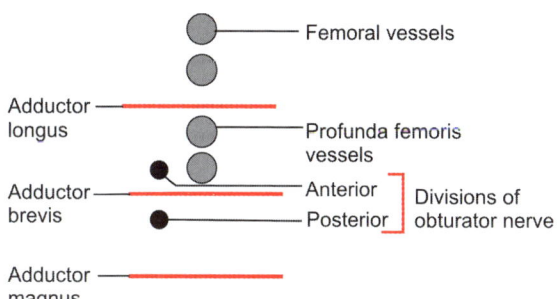

Fig. 3.12: Relation of femoral vessels, profunda femoris vessels and obturator nerve to adductor muscles

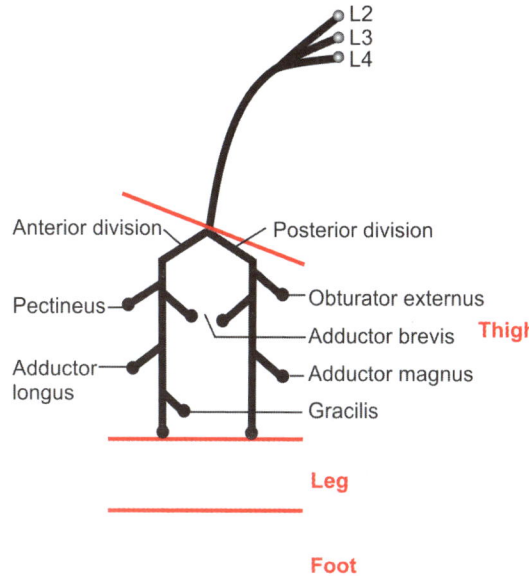

Fig. 3.13: Muscular branches of obturator nerve

Anterior division
- Hip joint.
- Pectineus.
- Adductor longus.
- Gracilis.
- *Note:* Also contributes to a plexus deep to sartorius (known as sub-sartorial plexus) with medial cutaneous and saphenous branches of femoral nerve.

Posterior division
- Obturator externus.
- Adductor brevis (supplied by anterior or posterior division).
- Adductor magnus.
- Supplies knee joint.

When obturator nerve is injured, it results in weakness of the adduction.

Gluteal Region

Cutaneous innervation:
- Cutaneous nerves which supply the skin of gluteal region are called cluneal nerves.
- Superficial gluteal nerves are the cluneal nerves.
- These are the branches of dorsal rami of upper three lumbar (superior cluneal), upper three sacral (middle cluneal) and branches of posterior cutaneous nerve of thigh (inferior cluneal).

Muscles of the gluteal region:
Divided into superficial and deep layers. Superficial layer contains three muscles:

1. Gluteus maximus.
2. Gluteus medius.
3. Gluteus minimus.

Deep layer consists of the following muscles:

1. Piriformis.
2. Obturator internus.
3. Superior gamellus.
4. Inferior gamellus.
5. Quadratus femoris.
Obturator externus and tensor fascia lata are also considered here.

Gluteus maximus:
- It is a large and heavy muscle and it covers all the other muscles of the gluteal region (Fig. 3.14).

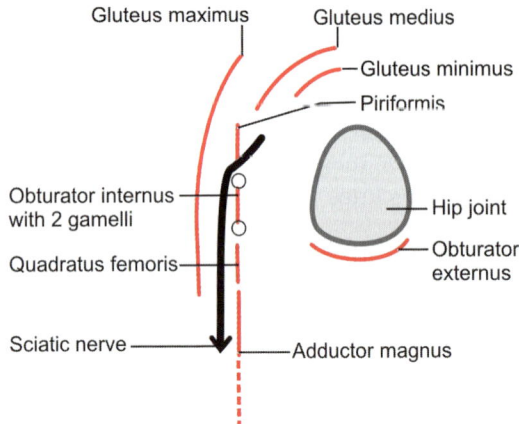

Fig. 3.14: Structures under cover of gluteus maximus

- It arises from the posterior aspect of the ilium, dorsal surface of sacrum and coccyx and sacrotuberous ligament.
- It is inserted into the lateral condyle of tibia through the iliotibial tract and deeper part is inserted into the gluteal tuberosity. It crosses the hip joint. Through iliotibial tract, it makes the extended knee stable.
- *Nerve supply:* Inferior gluteal nerve.
- *Action:* It extends the hip joint. It helps to climb the stairs and while raising from the sitting position.
- While you are sitting, remember that you are sitting on the ischial tuberosity and not on the gluteus maximus.
- *Testing of muscle:* The person lying on prone position is asked to extend the hip joint.
- Two important bursae lie deep to the gluteus maximus.
  1. Trochanteric bursa.
  2. Ischiofemoral bursa.

Gluteus medius: It arises from the ilium between the anterior and posterior gluteal lines. It is inserted into the lateral surface of the greater trochanter.

Gluteus minimus: It arises from the ilium between the anterior and inferior gluteal lines

and it is inserted into the anterior surface of the greater trochanter of the femur.

Action: Both of them abduct and medially rotate the thigh. These two muscles are very important during walking. When one limb is off the ground during walking, the unsupported side is not allowed to sink by the muscles of supported side. During this action, these muscles act at their origin and pull the supported side pelvis down so that the unsupported side does not sink due to weight of the body.

Trendelenburg's sign: If gluteus medius and minimus of one side are paralyzed (due to injury to superior gluteal nerve) and then if the patient is asked to stand on the paralyzed side foot only, the unsupported pelvis sinks to the normal side. This is Trendelenburg's sign positive. If left superior gluteal nerve is cut and if the patient stands on the left leg, the pelvis sinks to the right side when it is off the ground.

Nerve supply: They are supplied by the superior gluteal nerve.

The main action of gluteus medius and minimus is abduction of hip joint.

Tensor fascia lata: This muscle arises from the anterior part of iliac crest and it is inserted into the iliotibial tract. It is supplied by the superior gluteal nerve and it assists the gluteus maximus through the iliotibial tract to keep the knee extended.

Deep short muscles of the gluteal region
These muscles lie deep to gluteus maximus and they lie posterior and across the hip joint. Therefore, they act like lateral rotators of the hip joint. These muscles are:

1. Piriformis.
2. Superior gamellus.
3. Obturator internus.
4. Inferior gamellus.

5. Quadratus femoris.
6. Obturator externus.

- *Piriformis:* It passes through the greater sciatic foramen and is inserted into the apex of the greater trochanter of femur. Direct branches from sacral plexus supply it.
- Superior gamellus lies superior to the obturator internus tendon and is supplied by the nerve to obturator internus.
- Inferior gamellus lies inferior to the obturator internus tendon and is supplied by the nerve to quadratus femoris.
- Quadratus femoris arises from the ischial tuberosity and is inserted into the quadrate tubercle on intertrochanteric crest of femur. It is supplied by the nerve to quadratus femoris.

Piriformis
- *Origin:* Anterior surface of middle 3 pieces of sacrum.
- *Insertion:* Apex of greater trochanter.
- *Nerve supply:* Sacral plexus S1, 2.
- *Action:* Lateral rotation of thigh.

Superior gamellus
- *Origin:* Upper margin of lesser sciatic notch.
- *Insertion:* With obturator internus.
- *Nerve supply:* Nerve to obturator internus.
- *Action:* Lateral rotation of thigh.
- *Special feature:* Gamellus means twins.

Obturator internus
- *Origin:*
  - Inner surface of obturator membrane.
  - Margins of obturator foramen.
  - Pelvic surface of ilium and ischium.
- *Insertion:* Medial surface of greater trochanter.
- *Nerve supply:* Nerve to obturator internus.
- *Action:* Lateral rotation of thigh.

Inferior gamellus
- *Origin:* Lower margin of lesser sciatic notch.
- *Insertion:* With obturator internus.
- *Nerve supply:* Nerve to quadratus femoris.
- *Action:* Lateral rotation of thigh.

Quadratus femoris
- *Origin:* Lateral margin of ischial tuberosity.
- *Insertion:* Quadrate tubercle.
- *Nerve supply:* Nerve to quadratus femoris.
- *Action:* Lateral rotation of thigh.

Obturator externus
- *Special feature:* Dealt earlier.

Structures deep to gluteus maximus.
- *Nerves which lie deep to the gluteus maximus:*
  - Sciatic nerve.
  - Superior gluteal nerve.
  - Inferior gluteal nerve.
  - Posterior cutaneous nerve of thigh.
  - Pudendal nerve.
  - Nerve to obturator internus.
  - Nerve to quadratus femoris.
- *Vessels which lie deep to the gluteus maximus:*
  - Superior gluteal.
  - Inferior gluteal.
  - Internal pudendal.
  - Trochanteric anastomoses.
  - Cruciate anastomoses.
- *Bony prominences which lie deep to the gluteus maximus:*
  - Ischial tuberosity.
  - Greater trochanter.
- *Bursae which lie deep to the gluteus maximus:*
  - Trochanteric bursa.
  - Ischiofemoral bursa.
- *Foramen which lie deep to the gluteus maximus:*
  - Greater sciatic foramen.
  - Lesser sciatic foramen.
- *Joints:*
  - Hip.
  - Sacroiliac.

- *Ligaments:*
  - Sacrotuberous.
  - Sacrospinous.

Structures that pass through the greater sciatic foramen:

Piriformis (key muscle)

- *Above piriformis:*
  - Superior gluteal nerve and vessels.
- *Below piriformis:*
  - Sciatic nerve.
  - Inferior gluteal nerve and vessels.
  - Pudendal nerve.
  - Internal pudendal vessels.
  - Nerve to obturator internus.
  - Nerve to quadratus femoris.
  - Posterior cutaneous nerve of thigh.

Structures that exit through the greater sciatic foramen and enter the lesser sciatic foramen:

(Mnemonic PIN from medial to lateral)

1. Pudendal nerve.
2. Internal pudendal artery.
3. Nerve to obturator internus.

Superior gluteal nerve:

It arises from the sacral plexus. It passes through the greater sciatic foramen superior to the piriformis. It supplies three muscles:

1. Gluteus medius.
2. Gluteus minimus.
3. Tensor fascia lata.

Inferior gluteal nerve:

It arises from the sacral plexus. It passes through the greater sciatic foramen inferior to the piriformis. It supplies gluteus maximus.

Following nerves seen in gluteal region arise directly from the sacral plexus and supply the structures in front of them:

- Nerve to quadratus femoris and inferior gamellus.
- Posterior cutaneous nerve of thigh—supplies more skin than any other

cutaneous nerve. It supplies the skin of perineum, gluteal region, posterior aspect of thigh and upper part of back of leg. Though it is called the cutaneous nerve, most of its course lies deep to deep fascia except its terminal branches.

- Pudendal nerve—exits the greater sciatic foramen and enters the pelvis through the lesser sciatic foramen. It does not supply any structure in the gluteal region. It supplies the perineal structures.
- Nerve to obturator internus—exits the greater sciatic foramen and enters the pelvis through the lesser sciatic foramen. It supplies the obturator internus and superior gamellus.

Following arteries lie in the gluteal region and they arise from the internal iliac artery:

- Superior gluteal.
- Inferior gluteal.
- Internal pudendal.

Internal pudendal artery exits the greater sciatic foramen and enters the pelvis through the lesser sciatic foramen.

CLINICAL ANATOMY

Intramuscular injections in the gluteal region are given in its upper and outer quadrant to avoid injury to sciatic nerve.

Sciatic nerve lesions:

- Though uncommon, a complete section of the sciatic nerve results in paralysis of the muscles of the back of the thigh and all muscles of the leg and foot.

Back of Thigh

What are hamstring muscles?

- Hamstring muscles are those which arise from the ischial tuberosity and cross the knee joint behind.
- Therefore, they mainly act like the flexors of the knee joint. They also assist the extension at the hip joint.

- They are supplied by the tibial component of sciatic nerve.

Following are the hamstring muscles:
1. Semitendinosus.
2. Semimembranosus.
3. Long head of biceps femoris.
4. Ischial head of adductor magnus.

Semitendinosus: Arises from the ischial tuberosity and is inserted into the medial surface of superior part of tibia.

Semimembranosus: Arises from the ischial tuberosity and is inserted into the posterior part of the medial condyle of tibia. It also continues through the oblique popliteal ligament to be attached to the lateral femoral condyle.

Biceps femoris: It has two heads—the long head and the short head.

- Only long head arises from the ischial tuberosity and is supplied by the tibial component of sciatic nerve. Therefore, it is included under the hamstrings.
- The short head arises from the linea aspera and is supplied by the common peroneal component of sciatic nerve. Therefore, it is not included under hamstrings.
- The common tendon of biceps femoris is inserted into the head of the fibula. Fibular collateral ligament splits the biceps tendon.

Action of hamstrings:
- They extend the thigh and flex the leg.
- Biceps femoris laterally rotates the flexed leg.
- Semitendinosus and semimembranosus medially rotate the flexed leg.

Sciatic Nerve

- It arises from all the roots of the sacral plexus (L4–S3) (Fig. 3.15).
- It exits through the greater sciatic foramen.
- At its exits it lies inferior to the piriformis and is the most lateral structure emerging through the greater sciatic foramen.
- It lies midway between the greater trochanter and ischial tuberosity.
- It lies successively on ischium, obturator internus, quadratus femoris and adductor magnus.
- It is supplied by the artery to the sciatic nerve which is a branch of the inferior gluteal artery.

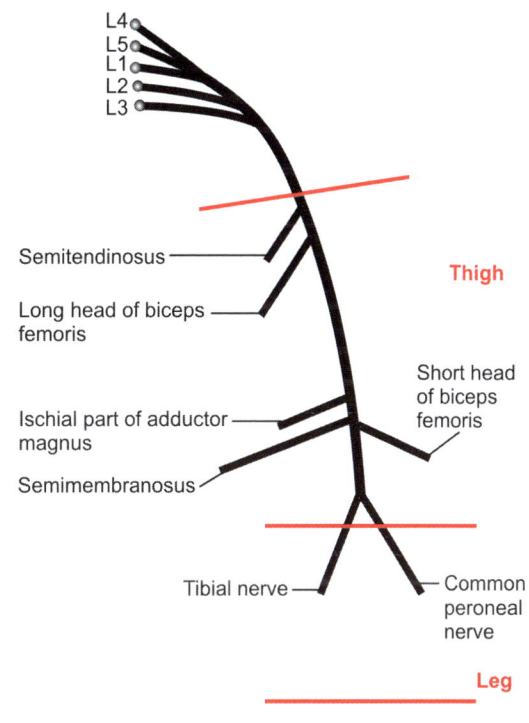

Fig. 3.15: Muscular branches of sciatic nerve

- *It is in fact formed by the union of two nerves:*
  1. Tibial nerve.
  2. Common fibular nerve (common peroneal nerve).

It lies on the back of the thigh and divides into two terminal branches at the level of middle third with the lower one-third of the thigh.

Branches:

- It has no branches in the gluteal region.
- It gives most of its branches on its medial side in the back of the thigh.
- Only one branch is given to short head of biceps on the lateral side and that too at its lower end. Therefore, the medial side of the sciatic nerve is dangerous and the lateral side is safe.

It supplies the following muscles in the back of the thigh:

1. Nerve to semitendinosus.
2. Nerve to semimembranosus.
3. Nerve to long head of biceps femoris.
4. Nerve to hamstring part of adductor magnus.
5. Nerve to short head of biceps femoris. (1–4 from tibial component of sciatic. 5 from common peroneal component of sciatic.)

It divides into two terminal branches:

1. Tibial nerve.
2. Common fibular nerve.

Cruciate anastomosis of the thigh:

It is formed by the following arteries on the back of the thigh:

- Inferior gluteal artery (descending branch).
- Transverse branches of medial and lateral circumflex femoral arteries (Fig. 3.16).
- First perforating artery (ascending branch).

    Gluteal veins: They accompany the corresponding arteries of the gluteal region.

Lymphatic drainage of the gluteal region:

- Superficial lymph is drained into the lateral

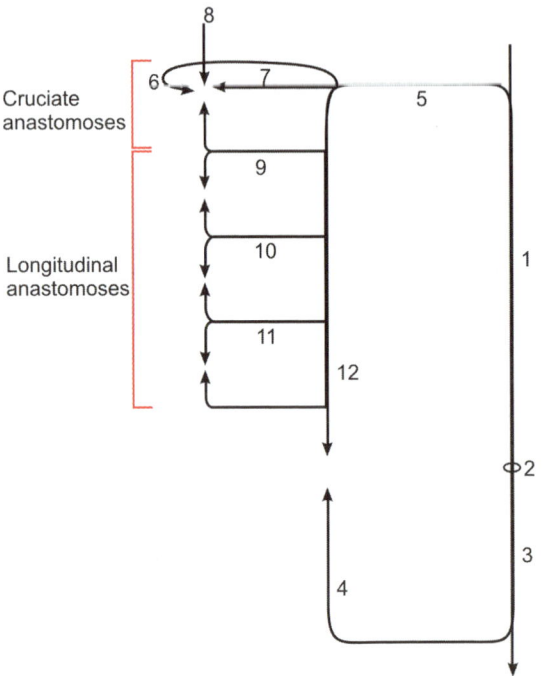

Fig. 3.16: Anastomoses on the back of thigh. 1. Femoral artery, 2. Opening in adductor magnus, 3. Popliteal artery, 4. Superior muscular branch, 5. Profunda femoris artery, 6. and 7. Medial and lateral circumflex femoral, 8. Descending branch of inferior gluteal, 9. I perforating, 10. II Perforating, 11. III perforating, 12. IV Perforating

horizontal group of superficial inguinal lymph nodes.

- Lymph from deep structures is drained into the superior and inferior gluteal lymph nodes and they pass through the greater sciatic foramen to end in internal iliac and common iliac nodes.

Popliteal Fossa

- It is a fossa on the back of the knee.
- It is a diamond-shaped depression (Fig. 3.17).
- The roof of the fossa is formed by the deep fascia called the popliteal fascia and skin.

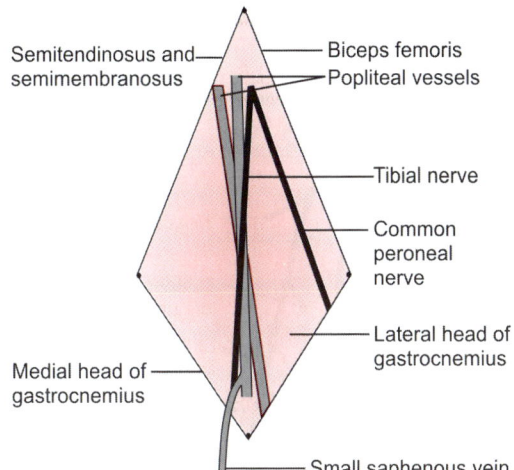

Semitendinosus and semimembranosus

Biceps femoris

Popliteal vessels

Tibial nerve

Common peroneal nerve

Lateral head of gastrocnemius

Medial head of gastrocnemius

Small saphenous vein

Fig. 3.17: Boundaries and contents of popliteal fossa

The roof is pierced by the following structures:
1. Posterior cutaneous nerve of thigh.
2. Short saphenous vein.

Boundaries of the popliteal fossa:
- *Superolateral:* Biceps femoris.
- *Superomedial:* Semitendinosus and semi-membranosus.
- *Inferolateral:* Lateral head of gastrocnemius and plantaris.
- *Inferomedial:* Medial head of gastrocnemius. *Floor of the popliteal fossa is formed by the following:*
1. Popliteal surface of femur.
2. Capsule of knee joint.
3. Fascia over popliteus muscle.

Contents of the popliteal fossa:
1. Popliteal artery and its branches.
2. Popliteal vein and its tributaries.
3. Tibial nerve and its branches.
4. Common fibular nerve and its branches.
5. Popliteal group of lymph nodes.

Popliteal Artery

Branches of popliteal artery:
- It terminates by dividing into anterior and posterior tibial arteries.

The other branches are:
1. Superior medial and lateral genicular arteries.
2. Inferior medial and lateral genicular arteries.
3. Middle genicular artery.
4. Muscular branches.
   - Genicular arteries supply the knee joint. They form the anastomosis around the knee joint.

Popliteal Vein
- It is formed at the distal border of the popliteus muscle by the union of anterior and posterior tibial veins.
- It lies superficial to the popliteal artery.
- It lies between the tibial nerve and popliteal artery. The nerve lies superficial just deep to the roof. Vein lies deep to the nerve. Popliteal artery lies anterior to the vein and is the deepest structure in the popliteal fossa.
- Popliteal vein continues as the femoral vein at the adductor hiatus, an opening in the adductor magnus.
- It receives the short (small) saphenous vein.
- It receives some tributaries from the surrounding muscles and the knee joint (corresponding to arteries).
- Popliteal vein has about 4 valves.

Tibial Nerve
- It is one of the terminal branches of the sciatic nerve at the superior angle of the popliteal fossa (Fig. 3.18).
- It is the medial and larger branch.
- It is the most superficial content of the popliteal fossa. Though it is superficial, it is protected by the gutter-like shape of popliteal fossa.
- It runs vertically in the middle of the fossa.

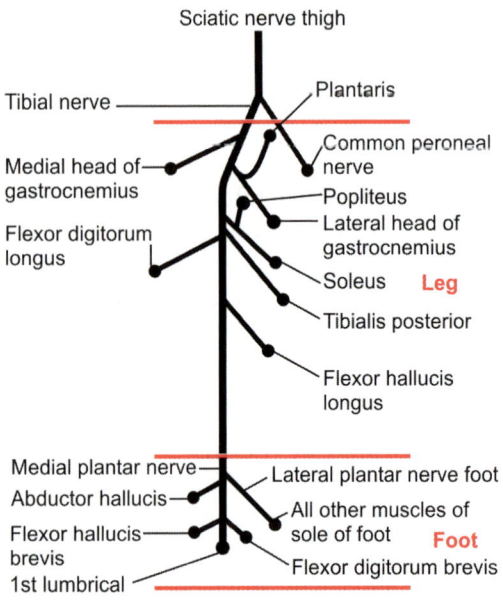

Fig. 3.18: Muscular branches of tibial nerve

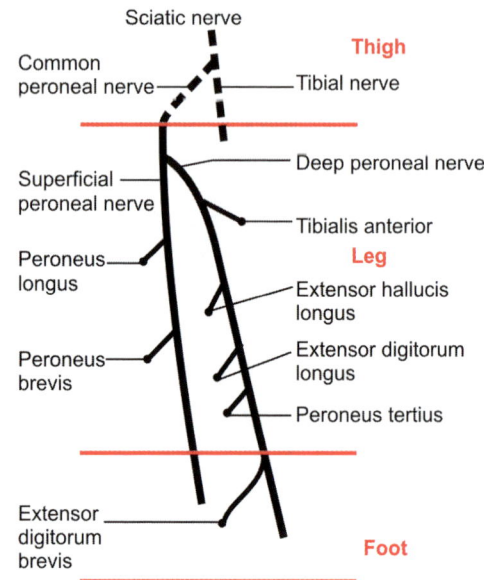

Fig. 3.19: Muscular branches of common peroneal nerve

It gives following branches in the popliteal fossa:
1. To soleus.
2. To gastrocnemius.
3. To plantaris.
4. To popliteus.

It gives a cutaneous branch called sural nerve. Sural nerve is joined by the sural communicating (fibular communicating nerve) of common peroneal (common fibular) nerve.

Common peroneal (common fibular) nerve:
- It is a smaller and lateral terminal branch.
- It begins at the superior angle of the popliteal fossa.
- It follows the superolateral border of the popliteal fossa formed by the biceps femoris.
- It crosses superficial to the lateral head of gastrocnemius and the posterior aspect of head of fibula.
- It winds around the lateral side of the neck of the fibula and divides into two terminal branches (Fig. 3.19):

- Superficial fibular nerve.
- Deep fibular branches.

The posterior cutaneous nerve of thigh:
It has certain peculiarities:
- It supplies more area of skin than any other cutaneous nerve in the body.
- In greater part of its course, it lies deep to deep fascia.
- It is an exclusive cutaneous nerve which exits the greater sciatic foramen.
- It pierces the roof of popliteal fossa and accompanies the termination of small saphenous vein.

Lymph nodes of the popliteal fossa:
- The superficial lymph nodes lie superficially in the fat of the popliteal fossa.
- A lymph node is present at the termination of the small saphenous vein beneath popliteal fascia which receives the superficial lymph vessels from the lateral side of the leg and foot. These lymph vessels accompany the small saphenous vein.

- The deep lymph nodes lie deep in the popliteal fossa and they drain the knee joint and the deep structures of the leg and foot. They accompany the arteries of the leg. They follow the femoral vessels and drain into the deep inguinal lymph nodes.

APPLIED ANATOMY OF THE POPLITEAL FOSSA

- Pus from a popliteal abscess tends to spread superiorly and inferiorly because of tough popliteal fascia.
- Popliteal pulse is difficult to feel because of its deep position. Further, the knee has to be flexed to relax the popliteal fascia and hamstring muscles. The popliteal pulse is best felt in the lower part of the popliteal fossa.
- In popliteal aneurysm (abnormal dilation), the artery can be safely ligated because of the rich genicular anastomosis.
- Tibial nerve may be injured in the deep wounds of the popliteal fossa and in posterior dislocation of knee joint.

Posterior Compartment of the Leg

- The muscles in this compartment are divided into superficial and deep groups by transverse septum.
- The superficial group of muscles in the posterior compartment are:
  1. Gastrocnemius.
  2. Soleus.
  3. Plantaris.

Gastrocnemius: It has two heads:
- Medial head arises from the posterior aspect of medial condyle of femur.
- Lateral head arises from the lateral surface of the lateral condyle of femur.
- It forms the tendocalcaneus along with the soleus.
- Tendocalcaneus is attached to the middle of the posterior surface of the calcaneus.
- *Nerve supply:* It is supplied by the tibial nerve.

- *Action:* It plantar flexes the ankle. Its fibers are mainly vertical, long (strap muscle) and white. Because of white fibers they produce rapid movements as in running or jumping. Therefore, it is called top gear muscle. Because it is strap muscle it increases range of movement but not power. (Long muscles can contract so that their length reduction is more; so more movement). It crosses both the knee and ankle joints. Therefore, it is a weak flexor of the knee joint. However, it cannot exert its full power on both the joints at the same time.

Soleus

- It lies deep to gastrocnemius.
- It joins the gastrocnemius to form tendo-calcaneus.
- It arises from the soleal line of the tibia.
- It arises from the head of the fibula.
- It is a plantar flexor of the ankle joint.
- It is a slow plantar flexor and it overcomes the inertia and therefore, it is called first gear muscle.
- It is an antigravity muscle that contracts alternatively with the anterior muscles of leg to maintain balance.
- It is supplied by the tibial nerve.

Two heads of gastrocnemius and soleus together are sometimes called "triceps surae". Triceps surae helps in the venous return and therefore, it is said to act like a musculovenous pump.

Plantaris

- It is a small muscle with a long thin tendon.
- It lies along the lateral head of gastro-cnemius.
- Arises from popliteal surface of femur just above lateral condyle.
- Its tendon is inserted into back of calcaneus.
- It is often absent.
- This tendon is used for grafting.

- It has high density of proprioceptors and it has been proposed to be an organ of proprioception for the plantar flexors.
- It is supplied by the tibial nerve.
- Helps in plantar flexion of foot.

Popliteus

- It lies in the floor of the popliteal fossa.
- It arises from the popliteal groove on the lateral aspect of the lateral condyle of femur.
- Its origin is intracapsular and extrasynovial.
- The muscle emerges through an opening in the capsule of the knee joint and is inserted into the upper part of the posterior surface of the shaft of the tibia.
- *Nerve supply:* It is supplied by the tibial nerve.
- It is an unlocking muscle of the knee joint.

What is Unlocking of Knee Joint?

At the termination of extension of knee joint, there is slight medial (screw home) rotation, so that all ligaments become taut. This tight packing position of knee joint spares muscular contraction to keep it extended for a long time. However, in the beginning of flexion of knee joint, there is either lateral rotation of femur (foot on ground) or medial rotation of tibia (foot off ground) to unlock the tight packing position. This process is called unlocking of the knee joint. This is done by the popliteus muscle. When a person is standing, the insertion of the popliteus is fixed and it acts at its origin and rotates the femur laterally and this is called

unlocking. However, when person's legs are off the ground, the popliteus acts at its insertion and rotates the tibia medially and this is also unlocking of the knee joint.

Flexor Digitorum Longus

- It arises from the posterior surface of the tibia.
- It lies behind the medial malleolus and divides into four slips in the sole of the foot.
- Each slip is inserted into the distal phalanx.
- Each slip goes to all toes except the great toe as it has its own longus tendon.
- It plantar flexes the foot.
- It plantar flexes the metacarpophalangeal and interphalangeal joints.
- *Nerve supply:* Tibial nerve.

Flexor Hallucis Longus

- It arises from the posterior surface of the fibula.
- It lies below the sustentaculum tali (acts as pulley) and is inserted into the distal phalanx of the great toe.
- Tibial nerve supplies it.
- It plantar flexes great toe.
- It plantar flexes the foot.

Tibialis Posterior

- It lies in the deepest compartment of the back of the leg.
- It arises both from tibia and fibula and intervening interosseous membrane.
- It is mainly inserted into the tuberosity of the navicular bone.
- It gives slips to all tarsal bones except talus.
- It is supplied by the tibial nerve.
- It is an invertor and plantar flexor of the foot.

Posterior Tibial Artery

- It is one of the terminal branches of the popliteal artery.

- It begins at the lower border of the popliteus muscle.
- It terminates behind the flexor retinaculum into medial and lateral plantar arteries.

The following are the branches of the posterior tibial artery:
- Circumflex fibular artery.
- Nutrient artery to tibia.
- Muscular branches.
- Fibular artery.
- Medial plantar.
- Lateral plantar.

The following are the branches of fibular artery:
- Muscular branches.
- Nutrient artery to fibula.
- Perforating branch.

The Tibial Nerve

- It supplies all the muscles of the posterior compartment of the leg.
- It accompanies the posterior tibial artery
- Behind the flexor retinaculum, it divides into lateral and medial plantar nerves.

Anterior Compartment of the Leg

The following four muscles are there in the anterior compartment of the leg:

1. Tibialis anterior.
2. Extensor hallucis longus.
3. Extensor digitorum longus.
4. Fibularis tertius (peroneus tertius).

Note: These muscles cross anterior to the ankle joint and, therefore, they dorsiflex the ankle. The EHL and EDL also extend the toes. They are supplied by the deep fibular nerve.

Tibialis Anterior

- It arises from the lateral surface of the tibia. It is inserted into the medial part of the medial cuneiform and adjacent surface on base of first metatarsal.
- *Action:* It dorsiflexes the foot. It inverts the foot as it crosses the medial border of the foot. It supports the medial arch of the foot.
- *Nerve supply:* Deep fibular nerve.

Extensor Hallucis Longus

- It arises from the medial surface of the fibula and adjacent interosseous membrane. It is inserted into the base of the distal phalanx of the great toe (remember longus, therefore, it goes to the distal phalanx).
- It extends the great toe and dorsiflexes the foot.
- *Nerve supply:* It is supplied by the deep fibular nerve.

Extensor Digitorum Longus

- It arises from the medial surface of fibula and related lateral tibial condyle. It is inserted into the bases of the middle and distal phalanges of the lateral four toes through the dorsal digital expansion.
- It extends the lateral four toes and also dorsiflexes the foot.
- *Nerve supply:* Deep fibular nerve.

Fibularis Tertius

- It arises from the distal part of the medial surface of fibula. It is inserted into the base of the fifth metatarsal. Fifth metatarsal is along the lateral border of the foot and, therefore, it everts the foot but dorsiflexes the foot at ankle.

- *Note:* Out of the four anterior compartment muscles, only fibularis tertius is an evertor.
- Fibularis tertius is often absent.
- It is supplied by the deep fibular nerve.

Anterior Tibial Artery

- It is the artery of the anterior compartment of the leg.
- It is a branch of the popliteal artery and reaches the anterior compartment by passing through the opening in upper part of interosseous membrane.
- It runs in the anterior compartment.
- It crosses anterior to the ankle joint and continues as dorsalis pedis artery on the dorsal aspect of the foot.
- It supplies the muscles of the anterior compartment of the leg.
- At the lower end of the tibia, it gives the medial malleolar and lateral malleolar arteries which form anastomosis around the ankle, along with the perforating branch of fibular artery, branches of posterior tibial and medial and lateral tarsal branches of dorsalis pedis artery.

Deep Fibular Nerve

- It is the nerve of the anterior compartment of the leg.
- It is one of the terminal branches of the common fibular nerve (Fig. 3.19).
- It supplies all the four muscles of the anterior compartment of the leg.
- It continues into the dorsum of the foot and supplies one muscle on the dorsum of the foot and that is extensor digitorum brevis. Later it supplies the skin between the great and second toes.
- It is called nervi hesitans because though it accompanies the anterior tibial vessels it hesitates to cross them.

CLINICAL ANATOMY

Injury to common peroneal nerve results in:
- i. Foot drop.
- ii. Paralysis of muscles of anterior and lateral compartments of leg.
- iii. High stepping gait.

Lateral Compartment of the Leg

There are two muscles in this compartment:
- Fibularis longus.
- Fibularis brevis.

Fibularis Longus

- It arises from the upper 2/3rd of lateral surface of fibula. It is inserted into the lateral sides of medial cuneiform and base of first metatarsal.
- It is supplied by the superficial fibular nerve.
- It plantar flexes and everts the foot.
- It supports the arches of the foot.
- Note two important points about its course: It passes posterior to the lateral malleolus and occupies the groove of the cuboid bone.

Fibularis Brevis

- It arises from the lower two-thirds of the lateral surface of the shaft of the fibula.
- It passes behind the lateral malleolus.
- It is attached to the tubercle at the base of the fifth metatarsal bone.
- It everts the foot.
- It is supplied by the superficial fibular nerve.

Note: No major artery lies in this compartment. It is mainly supplied by the fibular artery of the posterior compartment of the leg.

Superficial Fibular Nerve

- This nerve is associated with the lateral compartment of the leg.

- It is one of the terminal branches of the common fibular nerve (Fig. 3.19).
- It supplies the two muscles of the lateral compartment of the leg.
- It becomes cutaneous in the lower part of leg and supplies the skin of the greater part of the dorsum of the foot except the following:
  - The web space between the great and second toes (supplied by the deep fibular nerve).
  - The lateral side of the little toe and foot (supplied by the sural branch of tibial nerve).
  - Medial border of the foot (supplied by the saphenous nerve).

Retinacula around the Ankle

- These are thickening of the deep fascia designed to hold the structures in place.
- Following retinacula are seen around the ankle:
  - Flexor retinaculum—1.
  - Extensor retinaculum—2 (superior and inferior).
  - Fibular retinaculum—2 (superior and inferior).

Flexor Retinaculum

- It bridges the gap between the medial malleolus and medial surface of calcaneus (Fig. 3.20).
- It is continuous superiorly and inferiorly with the rest of the deep fascia.
- Posterior tibial artery and tibial nerve divide into medial and lateral plantar arteries and nerves behind the flexor retinaculum and enter the sole of the foot.
  Note: Pulsations of posterior tibial artery can be felt deep to the flexor retinaculum.
- *Structures present deep to the flexor retinaculum:* (from medial to lateral side) Remember mnemonic **T**om **D**ick **AN**d **H**arry.

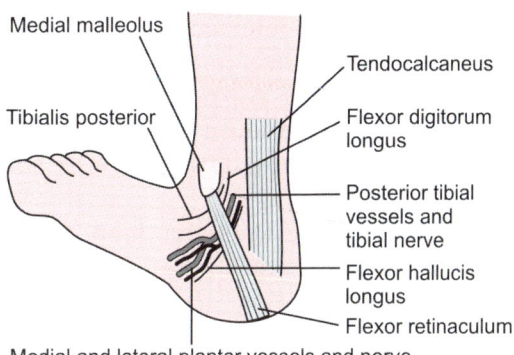

Fig. 3.20: Flexor retinaculum

T—Tibialis posterior tendon
D—Flexor digitorum longus tendon
A—Artery posterior tibial
N—Nerve tibial
H—Flexor hallucis longus tendon

Extensor Retinaculum

It straps the tendons of extensor muscles to the front of the ankle region (Fig. 3.21). They are two:

1. Superior extensor retinaculum.
   - Extends between lower ends of tibia and fibula.

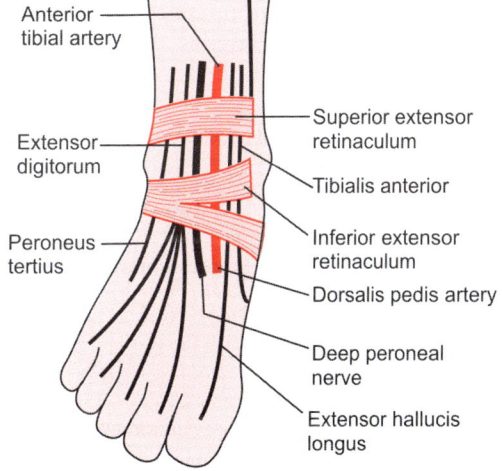

Fig. 3.21: Extensor retinaculum

2. Inferior extensor retinaculum
  • Y shaped. Stem laterally attached to anterosuperior surface of calcaneus. Upper limb and lower limb attached to medial malleolus and fascia of sole respectively.

Following structures lie deep to the extensor retinaculum in that order from medial to the lateral side:
• Tibialis anterior tendon.
• Extensor hallucis longus tendon.
• Anterior tibial artery and accompanying vena comitantes.
• Deep fibular nerve.
• Extensor digitorum longus.
• Fibularis tertius.

Fibular Retinaculum (Superior and Inferior)

They are two (Fig. 3.22):
1. Superior fibular retinaculum
  • Extends between lateral malleolus and lateral surface of calcaneus.
2. Inferior fibular retinaculum
  • Extends between anterosuperior surface of calcaneus and lateral surface of calcaneus.
  • It binds two tendons behind and below the lateral malleolus.

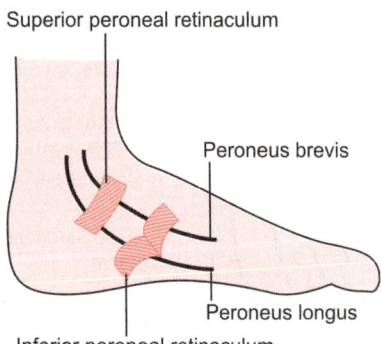

Superior peroneal retinaculum

Peroneus brevis

Peroneus longus

Inferior peroneal retinaculum

Fig. 3.22: Peroneal retinaculum

• The two tendons are:
  – Fibularis longus.
  – Fibularis brevis.
• There are no vessels and nerves behind this retinaculum.

Dorsum of the Foot

The sensory nerve supply of the dorsum of the foot is as follows:
• *Medial border of the foot:* Saphenous nerve.
• *Adjacent sides of the great and second toes:* Deep fibular nerve.
• *Lateral border of the foot and the lateral side of the little toe:* Sural nerve.
• *Medial three and half nail beds:* Medial plantar nerve.
• *Lateral one and half nail beds:* Lateral plantar nerve.
• *Rest of the skin of the dorsum of the foot:* Superficial fibular nerve.

Muscles: Only one muscle is present in the dorsum of the foot and that is extensor digitorum brevis. Medially it gives rise to extensor hallucis brevis to great toe.

Veins: Dorsal venous arch which receives dorsal metacarpal veins from the toes and is drained into the great saphenous vein on the medial side and into short saphenous vein on the lateral side.

Tendons present:
• Tibialis anterior.
• Extensor hallucis longus.
• Extensor digitorum longus.
• Fibularis tertius.

Arteries:
• All arteries are the branches of the dorsalis pedis artery which is the continuation of the anterior tibial artery.
• Pulsation of the dorsalis pedis artery can be felt against the tarsal bone between the extensor hallucis longus and tendon of extensor digitorum longus to the second toe.

- It gives the following branches:
  - Medial tarsal artery.
  - Lateral tarsal artery.
  - Arcuate artery.
  - First dorsal metatarsal artery.

Dorsal digital expansion:
- Like in hand; has 1 central and 2 lateral slips.
- Central slip attaches to dorsal aspect of base of middle phalanx.
- The 2 lateral slips unite and attach to base of distal phalanx of the toe.

Sole of the Foot

The skin of the sole of the foot is supplied by the medial and lateral plantar nerves.

- Medial plantar nerve supplies the medial part of the sole of the foot and medial three and half toes including nail beds.
- Lateral plantar nerve supplies the lateral part of the sole of the foot and the lateral one-third of the toes including nail beds.

CLINICAL ANATOMY

- Plantar reflex
  - Tests L4–S2 segments.
  - The skin of the sole is stroked, starting from the heel, across the lateral border of the sole, to the base of the great toe.
  - Normal response to this is flexion of toes.
  - Abnormal response (Babinski sign positive) is dorsiflexion of great toe and spreading apart of the other toes.
  - Abnormal response indicates neuro-logical damage.

Deep fascia is thickened to form the plantar fascia.

It is thickened in the middle part to form the plantar aponeurosis.

Plantar Aponeurosis

- It is attached to the calcaneus posteriorly and divides into five slips one each for one toe. These slips are interconnected by the transverse metatarsal ligaments.
- Plantar aponeurosis maintains the arches of the foot.
- This aponeurosis might get inflamed by running resulting in plantar fascitis. This is a painful condition.

Muscles of the Sole of the Foot

They are divided into four layers (Fig. 3.23). First layer of the sole of the foot: It contains the following muscles (3 muscles):
1. Abductor hallucis.
2. Flexor digitorum brevis.
3. Abductor digit minimi.

Abductor Hallucis

- Arises from the medial tubercle of the calcaneus and is inserted into the medial side of the base of the proximal phalanx of the great toe.
- *Action:* Abduction of the great toe.
- *Nerve supply:* Medial plantar nerve.

Flexor Digitorum Brevis

- Arises from the medial tubercle of the calcaneus and is inserted into both sides of the middle phalanges of lateral four toes.
- *Action:* Flexes lateral four digits at MP and PIP joints.
- *Nerve supply:* Medial plantar nerve.

Abductor Digiti Minimi

- Arises from both medial and lateral tubercles of the calcaneum and is inserted into the lateral side of the base of the proximal phalanx of the little toe.
- *Nerve supply:* Lateral plantar nerve.
- *Action:* Abduction of the little toe.

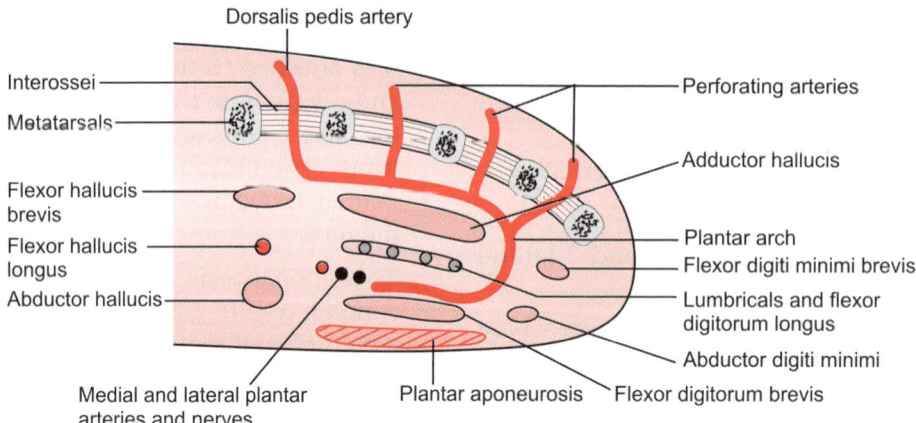

Fig. 3.23: Layers of the sole of the foot

Lateral and medial plantar nerves and accompanying arteries lie between the first and second layers of the sole of the foot.

Second layer of the sole of the foot:
It contains the following: (2 muscles; 2 tendons)
- Quadratus plantae.
- Lumbricals.
- Tendon of flexor hallucis longus.
- Tendon of flexor digitorum longus.

Quadratus Plantae

- It arises from the medial and lateral sides of plantar aspect of calcaneus and is inserted into the lateral side of the tendon of flexor digitorum longus.
- *Action:* It pulls the flexor digitorum longus tendon in line with the toes and makes it an efficient flexor.
- *Nerve supply:* Lateral plantar nerve.

Lumbricals

- They are four in number.
- They are numbered from medial to lateral side.
- They arise from the tendon of flexor digitorum longus and are inserted into the digital expansion of lateral four toes.

- *Action:* They flex the metatarsophalangeal joints and extend the proximal and distal interphalangeal joints of lateral 4 toes.
- *Nerve supply:* The first lumbrical is supplied by the medial plantar nerve and the remaining lateral three lumbricals are supplied by the lateral plantar nerve.

Third layer of the sole of the foot:
It contains the following muscles: (3 muscles)
1. Flexor hallucis brevis.
2. Adductor hallucis.
3. Flexor digiti minimi brevis.

Flexor Hallucis Brevis

- It arises from the plantar surface of cuboid and lateral cuneiform bones and is inserted into both sides of the base of the proximal phalanx of the great toe (2 sesamoid bones present here).
- *Action:* It flexes the proximal phalanx of the great toe.
- *Nerve supply:* It is supplied by the medial plantar nerve.

Adductor Hallucis

- It has two heads of origin—oblique head and transverse head.

- The oblique head arises from the bases of metatarsal bones (2–4).
- The transverse head arises from the plantar ligaments of the metatarsophalangeal joints (2–4).
- Both the heads join together and are inserted into the lateral side of the base of the proximal phalanx of the great toe.
- *Action:* Adduction of the great toe.
- *Nerve supply:* It is supplied by the lateral plantar nerve.

Flexor Digiti Minimi Brevis

- It arises from the base of the fifth metatarsal. It is inserted into the base of the proximal phalanx of little toe.
- *Action:* It flexes the proximal phalanx of the little toe.
- *Nerve supply:* It is supplied by the lateral plantar nerve.

Plantar arterial arch and deep branch of lateral plantar nerve lie between the third and fourth layers of the sole of the foot.

Fourth layer of the sole of the foot: (2 muscles; 2 tendons)

It contains the plantar and dorsal interossei; tendons of tibialis posterior and peroneus longus.

Plantar Interossei

- They are three in number.
- They arise from the medial sides of third, fourth and fifth metatarsals.
- They are inserted into medial sides of the bases of proximal phalanges of lateral three toes.
- There are no plantar interossei for first and second toes.
- Second toe is the axis of the adduction and abduction.
- Plantar interossei are adductors (PAD) and they have one head of origin.

- They are supplied by the lateral plantar nerve.

Dorsal Interossei

- They are four in number.
- They have two heads of origin. Arise from adjacent sides of 2 metatarsals and insert into base of proximal phalanx of toes 2–4.
- Dorsal interossei abduct the toes (DAB)
- There is no dorsal interosseous for the great toe and second toe has two dorsal interossei.
- The third and fourth dorsal interossei are on the medial sides of the fourth and fifth metatarsals.
- *Nerve supply:* They are supplied by the lateral plantar nerve.

Compared with hand little/no attachment of interossei into extensor expansion, so they flex the MP joints but usually do not extend the IP joints.

Medial plantar nerve: (similar to median nerve in hand)

- It is similar to the median nerve of the upper limb.
- Medial plantar nerve supplies the following muscles:
  – Abductor hallucis.
  – Flexor digitorum brevis.
  – Flexor hallucis brevis.
  – First lumbrical.

It also supplies the medial three and half toes and the nail bed and skin of the medial side of the sole of the foot.

Lateral plantar nerve: (similar to ulnar nerve in hand)

- It supplies all the muscles of the foot except the four muscles shown above.
- Therefore, it supplies the following muscles:
  – Abductor digit minimi.
  – Adductor hallucis.
  – Flexor digiti minimi brevis.

– Quadratus plantae.
– Lateral three lumbricals.
– Three plantar interossei.
– Four dorsal interossei.

Medial plantar artery:
- It is smaller terminal branch of the posterior tibial artery.
- It supplies the medial side of the skin of sole of the foot and gives muscular branches to adjoining muscles.
- Its digital branches accompany the digital branches of the medial plantar nerve (Fig. 3.23).

Lateral plantar artery:
- It is larger terminal branch of the posterior tibial artery.
- It accompanies the lateral plantar nerve (Fig. 3.23).
- It forms the plantar arch. The plantar arch is completed by the union of lateral plantar artery with the continuation of the dorsalis pedis artery.
- Plantar arterial arch gives four plantar metatarsal arteries each of which divides into 2 plantar digital arteries.

Note: There are 2 neurovascular planes; between 1st and 2nd layers and between 3rd and 4th layers of the sole of foot respectively.

Wounds of plantar arterial arch:

They bleed profusely, typically from both ends cut. Ligature of the artery is difficult as it is very deeply placed.

Note: There is a slight difference in arterial arches of sole of foot (1 arch) and palm of hand (2 arches) and also in the terminologies awarded to their branches and in the connections between them.

Veins of the Sole of the Foot

Superficial and deep.

Superficial: In the form of superficial plantar venous cutaneous arch along the roots of toes

and plantar venous network (plexus) along the entire area of sole proximal to the plantar venous cutaneous arch. They drain along medial and lateral border of sole of foot into the dorsal venous arch.

Deep: Medial and lateral plantar veins (vena comitantes along respective arteries) join to form posterior tibial veins.

Joints of the Lower Limb

Hip Joint

Articular surfaces: Head of femur (ball) and acetabulum (socket) of hip bone.

Type: This is a ball and socket synovial joint.

Capsule: Encloses joint. Medially attached to acetabular labrum (deepens socket) and laterally in front to intertrochanteric line and behind halfway along the neck of femur.

Ligaments:
1. Iliofemoral ligament—very strong, Y- shaped, prevents hyperextension of hip joint.
2. Pubofemoral ligament—prevents hyper-abduction of hip joint.
3. Ischiofemoral ligament—prevents hyper-extension of hip joint.

Synovial membrane: Lines the capsule.

Nerve supply: Femoral, obturator, sciatic and nerve to quadratus femoris.

Blood supply: Medial and lateral circumflex femoral, obturator, superior and inferior gluteal.

Important relations (Fig. 3.14):
- Anteriorly—iliopsoas and pectineus separate femoral nerve and vessels from hip joint.
- Posteriorly—short lateral rotators of hip and sciatic nerve.
- Inferiorly—obturator externus.
- Superiorly—gluteus minimus, medius and piriformis.

Movements:
- Flexion—iliopsoas, rectus femoris.

- Extension—hamstrings and gluteus maximus.
- Abduction—gluteus medius and minimus.
- Adduction—adductor brevis, longus and magnus.
- Medial rotation—gluteus minimus, anterior fibers of gluteus medius, tensor fascia lata.
- Lateral rotation—short lateral rotators of hip (obturator externus, internus with 2 gamelli, piriformis, quadratus femoris, gluteus maximus).

1. Hip replacement by using prosthesis.
2. Fractures of femoral neck can damage the blood vessels supplying femoral head causing avascular necrosis. The neck of the femur is commonly fractured in the elderly, especially in individuals suffering from osteoporosis. (Ligament of the head of femur connects the pit over the head of femur with the acetabular margin. It carries an artery which is a branch of the obturator artery. This artery supplies the head of femur. But the area of head of femur supplied by this artery is very little and is not sufficient to keep the head of femur alive in case of fracture of neck of femur).
3. *Referred pain:* Obturator nerve supplies both hip and knee joints. So pain in one joint may be referred to other.
4. *Congenital dislocation:* Acetabulum not well developed so head of femur dislocates.
5. *Posterior dislocation of the hip joint:* It is very common during automobile accidents and it is also called the dashboard dislocation. The thigh is shortened and medially rotated by the gluteus medius and minimus. The sciatic nerve may be involved. It results in the weakness of hamstring muscles, leg muscles and foot. There is also loss of sensation over the parts of leg and foot.

Knee Joint

Articular surfaces: Femoral and tibial condyles, patella.

Type: This is a modified hinge synovial joint (because some rotation takes place).

Capsule: Encloses joint.

Ligaments:

- Extracapsular—ligamentum patellae, tibial and fibular collateral ligament, oblique popliteal ligament.
- Intracapsular—anterior and posterior cruciate ligaments (named based on their attachments to tibia) and menisci (medial and lateral) meaning crescent-shaped or C-shaped (Figs 3.24 to 3.26).

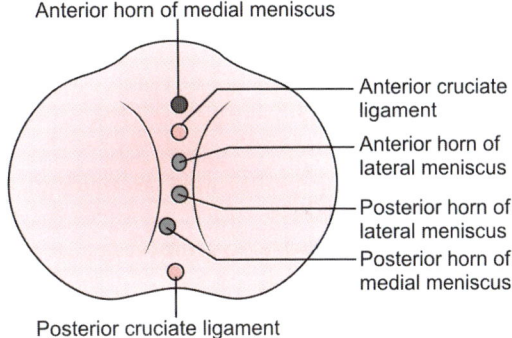

Anterior horn of medial meniscus

Anterior cruciate ligament

Anterior horn of lateral meniscus

Posterior horn of lateral meniscus

Posterior horn of medial meniscus

Posterior cruciate ligament

Fig. 3.24: Attachments to intercondylar area of tibia

Synovial membrane: Lines the capsule.

Important bursae: Suprapatellar and popliteal which communicate with knee joint cavity.

Nerve supply: Femoral, obturator, tibial and common peroneal nerve.

Blood supply: Anastomoses around knee (branches of femoral, popliteal and anterior tibial).

Important relations:

- Anteriorly—prepatellar bursa.
- Posteriorly—popliteal vessels, tibial and common peroneal nerves.

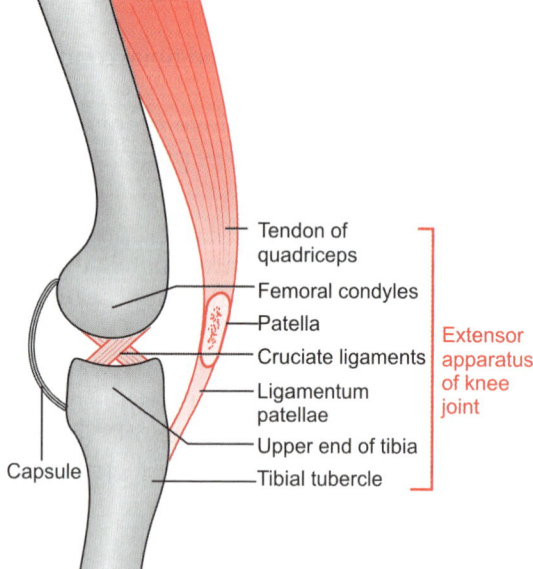

Fig. 3.25: Extensor apparatus and cruciate ligaments of knee joint

Movements:

* Flexion—semimembranosus, semitendino-sus, biceps femoris.
* Extension— quadriceps femoris.

* Medial rotation—sartorius, gracilis, semitendinosus.
* Lateral rotation—biceps femoris.

CLINICAL ANATOMY

1. Knee replacement by using prosthesis in osteoarthritis.
2. Cruciate ligament tears (anterior common, posterior rare).
3. *Referred pain:* Obturator nerve supplies both hip and knee joints. So pain in one joint may be referred to other.
4. Injury to medial and lateral menisci.
5. Injury to medial (more common) and lateral collateral ligaments (less common).
6. Arthroscopy is viewing interior of a joint. Common in knee joint.
7. Knee aspiration—excess fluid in joint cavity seen in infections and inflammation is aspirated.

Note:

1. Superior tibiofibular joint—plane synovial joint.

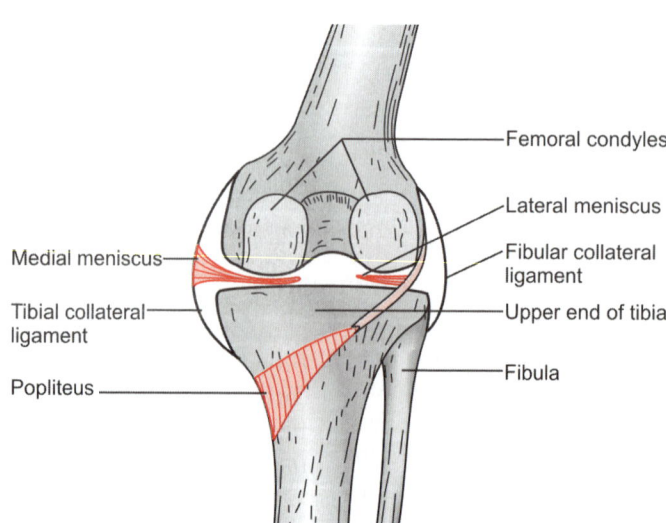

Fig. 3.26: Menisci

2. Middle tibiofibular joint (interosseous membrane)—fibrous joint of syndesmosis variety.
3. Inferior tibiofibular joint—fibrous joint of syndesmosis variety.

Ankle Joint

Articular surfaces: Distal ends of tibia and fibula and talus forming tibiofibular mortise.

Type: This is a hinge synovial joint.

Capsule: Encloses joint.

Ligaments:
- Lateral—parts are anterior and posterior talofibular and calcaneofibular.
- Medial—(deltoid) parts are tibionavicular, tibiocalcaneal, anterior and posterior tibiotalar (Fig. 3.27).

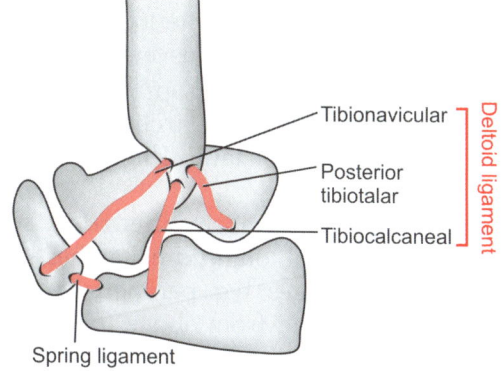

Fig. 3.27: Deltoid and spring ligament

Tibionavicular
Posterior tibiotalar
Tibiocalcaneal
Deltoid ligament
Spring ligament

Synovial membrane: Lines the capsule.
Nerve supply: Tibial and deep peroneal nerve.
Blood supply: Anastomoses around ankle (branches of fibular, posterior and anterior tibial).

Important relations:
- Anteriorly—structures deep to extensor retinaculum.
- Posteriorly—achilles tendon and plantaris.

- Posteromedially—structures deep to flexor retinaculum.
- Posterolaterally—structures deep to peroneal retinaculum.

Movements:
- Plantar flexion—gastrocnemius, soleus, tibialis posterior, FDL, FHL, peroneus longus and brevis.
- Dorsiflexion—tibialis anterior, EDL, EHL, peroneus tertius.

Subtalar Joint

Articular surfaces: Inferior surface of talus and superior surface of calcaneus.

Type: This is a plane synovial joint.

Capsule: Encloses joint.

Synovial membrane: Lines the capsule.
Movements:
- Inversion—by tibialis anterior and posterior.
- Eversion—peroneus longus, brevis and tertius.

Talocalcaneonavicular Joint

Articular surfaces: Head of talus (ball) and socket by navicular bone, spring ligament (plantar calcaneonavicular ligament) and sustentaculum tali.

Type: This is a ball and socket synovial joint.
Capsule: Encloses joint.
Synovial membrane: Lines the capsule.
Movements: Allow gliding and rotation to enable inversion and eversion.

Arch	Medial	Lateral	Transverse
Components	Medial 3 metatarsals, 3 cuneiforms, navicular, talus, calcaneus	Lateral 2 metatarsals, cuboid, calcaneus	Bases of metatarsals, 3 cuneiforms, cuboid
Summit Pillars	Superior surface of talus Anterior formed by heads of medial 3 metatarsals. Posterior formed by medial tubercle of calcaneus	At level of subtalar joint Anterior formed by heads of lateral 2 metatarsals. Posterior formed by medial tubercle of calcaneus	Formed by medial and lateral aspects of respective longitudinal arches
Plane	Sagittal	Sagittal	Coronal

Table 3.1: Classification of arches of foot

Arches of Foot

Foot is not flat, more so the bones of foot do not form a flat surface. Bones of the foot are engineered as arches (Fig. 3.28).

Functions:
1. Distribute body weight.
2. Concavity thus created protects underlying vessels and nerves.

3. Being segmented improves maneuverability.
4. Helps walking on uneven surfaces.

Classification: Longitudinal (medial and lateral) and transverse (Table 3.1).

Supports of the Arches

1. Shape of bones—wedged interlocking bones, e.g. cuneiform bones of transverse arch.
2. Intersegmental staples, e.g spring ligament of medial longitudinal arch and short plantar ligament of lateral longitudinal arch.
3. Bowstrings—plantar aponeurosis for medial and lateral longitudinal arches.
4. Suspension bridges, e.g. peroneus longus and brevis pulling from above for lateral longitudinal arch.

The relative importance of different factors maintaining arches varies in different arches.

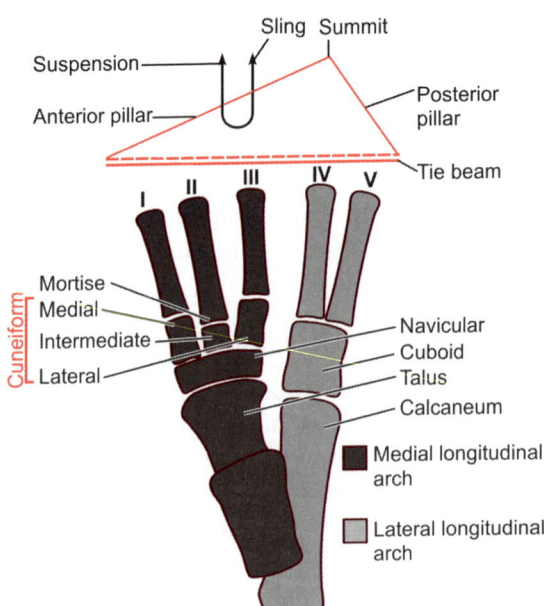

Fig. 3.28: Arches of foot

Thorax

- It is the bony cage which encloses heart and lungs.
- Thoracic bony cage is made up of 37 bones.

Sternum	1
Ribs 12 pairs	24
Thoracic vertebrae	12
Total	37

BOUNDARIES OF THORAX

- *Anterior:* Sternum and costal cartilages.
- *Posterior:* Thoracic vertebrae and intervening intervertebral discs.
- *On either side:* Ribs and intercostal spaces.
- *Superior:* Inlet of thorax formed by the first rib, upper border of sternum and first thoracic vertebra.
- *Inferior:* Diaphragm.

General Features of Vertebrae

Identify the following parts of the vertebra:
- Body.
- Spine.
- Pedicle.
- Lamina.
- Transverse process.
- Superior articular process.
- Inferior articular process.
- Inferior and superior vertebral notches.

Vertebrae are of three types:
- Cervical vertebrae.
- Thoracic vertebrae.
- Lumbar vertebrae.
- Cervical vertebrae have foramen transversarium in the transverse process.
- Thoracic vertebrae have no foramen transversarium but have articular facets on the side of the body near the pedicle for the heads of ribs.
- Lumbar vertebrae have no foramen transversarium and no articular facets on the sides of the body.

Ribs

- There are twelve pairs of ribs.
- Each typical rib has the following parts:
  - Head, neck, tubercle, angle, shaft and costal groove.
  - Head of the rib has two articular facets separated by a crest. It articulates with two vertebrae, the corresponding vertebra and vertebra immediately above that. The crest between the two articular facets is attached to the intervertebral disc.
  - Tubercle has an articular facet which articulates with the transverse process of the corresponding vertebra.
- Joint between the head of the rib and the body is the "costovertebral joint".
- Joint between the tubercle of the rib and the corresponding transverse process is the "costotransverse joint".

Thoracic Vertebrae

- They are twelve in number.
- Each vertebra has superior and inferior articular processes at the junction of the pedicle with the lamina on each side.
- They are divided into typical and atypical thoracic vertebrae.

Typical Thoracic Vertebrae

These have the following characteristics:
- Two demifacets, one at the upper end of the posterior part of the body and the other at the lower end of the posterior part of the body.
- There is an articular facet on the transverse process.
- Superior vertebral notch is not deep.
- Inferior vertebral notch is deep.

Following are the typical thoracic vertebrae:
T2, T3, T4, T5, T6, T7, T8 (2–8)

Atypical thoracic vertebrae (1, 9–12)
These do not have all the characteristics of a typical vertebra.

First thoracic vertebra
- A complete facet at its upper end (since first rib articulates only with the first thoracic vertebra).
- Demifacet at the lower end of the body for the upper demifacet of the head of the second rib and a facet over the transverse process for the tubercle of the first rib.
- Spine is horizontal similar to cervical vertebra.

T9 vertebra
- It has only a demifacet at the upper end of the body for the lower demifacet of the head of the 9th rib.
- There is no facet at the lower end.
- There is a facet on the transverse process for the tubercle of the 9th rib.

T10 vertebra
- There is a complete articular facet on the side of the upper end of the body extending on to the root of the pedicle.
- Body has no articular facet at its lower end.
- There is a facet over the transverse process of the vertebra for the tubercle of the corresponding rib.

T11 vertebra
- There is a complete articular facet for the head of the corresponding rib extending over the pedicle.
- Transverse process of this vertebra does not have an articular facet.

T12 vertebra
- The shape of the body, pedicles, transverse process and spine are similar to the lumbar vertebra.
- It has a complete articular facet for the head of the corresponding rib which lies more on the pedicle than on body.
- Transverse process has no facet.

Vertebral foramen
Boundaries:
- *Anterior:* Body of the vertebra.
- *Lateral:* Pedicle of the vertebra.
- *Posterior:* Lamina of the vertebra.

Contents: Spinal cord and spinal meninges.

Intervertebral foramen
It lies between the superior and inferior vertebral notches of two adjacent vertebrae.

Boundaries
- *Anterior:* Intervertebral disc and parts of the bodies of vertebra.
- *Posterior:* Zygapophyseal (facet) joint.
- *Superior:* Inferior vertebral notch.
- *Inferior:* Superior vertebral notch.

What are the structures which pass through the intervertebral foramen?
- Spinal nerve (segmental).

- Spinal branches of intersegmental arteries and corresponding veins.
- Connections between internal and external vertebral venous plexus.

Ribs

There are twelve pairs of ribs. They are divided into three groups:

1. Vertebrosternal ribs (1st to 7th ribs which articulate with the sternum through the costal cartilages) or true ribs.
2. Vertebrochondral ribs (8th, 9th and 10th ribs) the costal cartilages of these ribs articulate with the costal cartilages of the ribs superior to them at interchondral joints (false ribs).
3. Vertebral ribs (11th and 12th which are free anteriorly) (false ribs).

They are also divided into typical and atypical ribs.

Typical Ribs

A typical rib has the following characteristics:
- Head has two articular demifacets, one demifacet for the corresponding thoracic vertebra and the other for the vertebra immediately above it (Fig. 4.1).
- Tubercle is divided into articular and nonarticular parts. Articular part has a facet which articulates with the transverse process of corresponding thoracic vertebra.

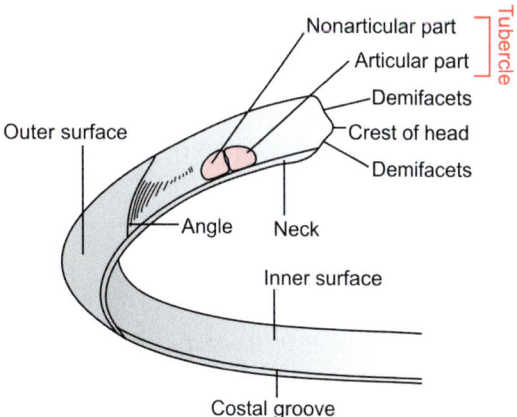

Fig. 4.1: Typical rib

- It presents an angle about 5 cm lateral to the tubercle where it is twisted.
- It has a well defined costal groove.
- It has outer and inner surfaces.

The typical ribs are: 3rd, 4th, 5th, 6th, 7th, 8th and 9th (3–9).

Atypical Ribs

These ribs do not have the characteristics of typical ribs. Atypical ribs are: 1st, 2nd, 10th, 11th and 12th.

First rib: It is atypical because:
- Its angle corresponds to the tubercle.
- There is only one facet over its head which articulates with the first thoracic vertebra.
- It has superior and inferior surfaces instead of outer and inner surfaces.
- No costal groove.
- No twist.

Side identification: When the rib is placed on a horizontal surface with head posteriorly and superior surface with shallow grooves facing upwards, both the anterior and posterior ends touch the surface. The convex border tells you the side of the rib. If it is placed wrongly, head of the rib remains raised above the horizontal surface.

It has superior (upper), inferior (lower) surfaces and inner and outer borders.

Structures related to the First Rib

Neck of the first rib is related to the following:
1. Sympathetic trunk.
2. First posterior intercostal vein.
3. Superior intercostal artery.
4. Ventral ramus of first thoracic nerve.

Upper surface is related to the following structures from before backwards:
1. Subclavius muscle (origin).
2. Costoclavicular ligament.
3. Subclavian vein.
4. Scalenus anterior muscle is inserted into the tubercle on its inner border.
5. Subclavian artery.
6. Lower trunk of brachial plexus.
7. Scalenus medius muscle (insertion).

Inner border is concave and gives attachment to the suprapleural membrane.

Lower surface is related to costal pleura. Outer border gives origin to the first digitation of the serratus anterior.

Second Rib

- Its curvature is like the first rib but it is twice the length of the first rib.
- It has no twist, therefore, its side can be identified by placing it on a horizontal surface with head posteriorly. If both ends touch the surface, the convex border determines the side of the bone.
- Shaft has external and internal surfaces.
- It has a very shallow costal groove.
- External surface has a prominent tubercle near its middle. This tubercle gives origin to the serratus anterior.

Tenth Rib

- It has a single facet on its head which articulates with the side of the body of 10th thoracic vertebra. Other features are similar to a typical rib.

Eleventh Rib

- It has a single facet on its head, which articulates with the body of 11th thoracic vertebra. It has no tubercle and no neck. It has a shallow costal groove and slight angle.

Twelfth Rib

- It has a single facet on its head, which articulates with twelfth thoracic vertebra. It has no neck, no tubercle, no angle and no costal groove.
- It is shorter than the eleventh rib.

Sternum

- It has three parts: Manubrium, body and xiphoid process. It looks like a sword, the manubrium being its handle (Fig. 4.2).
- Manubrium has a free concave upper margin called "suprasternal notch".

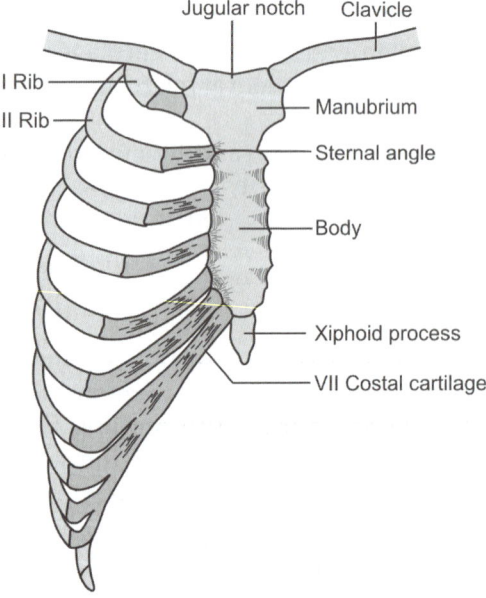

Fig. 4.2: Sternum showing its articulations

- Inferiorly, manubrium articulates with the body at the manubriosternal joint.
- Superolaterally, it articulates with the clavicle to form sternoclavicular joint.
- Second chondrosternal joint lies at the junction of the manubrium with the body. This joint has two joint cavities—one with the manubrium and the other with the body of the sternum.

Anterior surface of the manubrium gives origin to two muscles:

- Sternocleidomastoid and pectoralis major.

Posterior surface gives origin to two muscles:

- Sternothyroid and sternohyoid.

Posterior surface of the manubrium forms the anterior wall of the superior mediastinum and is related to the arch of aorta and its branches and remains of thymus.

- Manubrium lies at the level of third and fourth thoracic vertebrae.
- Manubriosternal joint lies at the level of lower border of fourth thoracic vertebra and it is called "sternal angle" (angle of Louis).

Body of Sternum

- It is made up of four sternebrae. At its upper end it articulates with the manu-brium at the manubriosternal joint and at its lower end it joins the xiphoid process at the xiphisternal joint.
- Part of the second costal cartilage articulates with it at its junction with the manubrium and part of the seventh costal cartilage articulates with it at its junction with the xiphoid process.
- The third, fourth, fifth and sixth costal cartilages articulate on its side at the corresponding chondrosternal joints.
- Anteriorly, it is directly related to the fascia and skin. On either side of the midline, it gives origin to the pectoralis major (1 muscle).

- Posterior surface of the body gives origin to sternocostalis muscle (1 muscle). It is related to pleura, lungs and pericardium.
- Body of the sternum lies at the level of 5th, 6th, 7th and 8th thoracic vertebrae.

Xiphoid Process

- This is the pointed lower end of the sternum. It lies at the level of 9th thoracic vertebra. It joins superiorly with the body of the sternum at the xiphisternal joint.
- Superolaterally, it carries a demifacet for the 7th costal cartilage.
- *Anterior surface gives attachment to two muscles*—external oblique muscle and rectus abdominis muscles of abdomen.
- *Posterior surface gives attachment to 2 muscles:* Lower fibres of sternocostalis and diaphragm.
- Linea alba is attached to its lower end.

CLINICAL ANATOMY

Since it is easy to access, the sternum is a common site for bone marrow biopsy.

The sternum may also be split, to gain access to the heart and great vessels by the cardiothoracic surgeons. After the surgery the split sternum is stapled together.

Joints of Thorax

- Costovertebral joint.
  - Between the head of the rib and the side of the body of thoracic vertebra.
  - These are synovial joints.
  - Each joint cavity has two plane synovial joints with the sides of two adjacent vertebrae. They have a common fibrous capsule. The two joints are separated by an intra-articular ligament. This ligament is attached to the crest of the head of rib between the two articular surfaces laterally and to the intervertebral disc

medially. Second to ninth costovertebral joints follow this pattern. First, tenth, eleventh and twelfth costovertebral joints have one articular facet and have no intra-articular ligament.

- Costotransverse joint.
  - Between the tubercle of the rib and the transverse process of the corresponding vertebra.
  - Plane synovial joint.
  - They are 10 on each side.
- Costochondral joint.
  - Between the rib and its costal cartilage.
  - Primary cartilaginous joint.
- Chondrosternal joints.
  - Chondrosternal joint of the first rib: Primary cartilaginous joint.
  - Other chondrosternal joints from 2nd to 7th costal cartilages: Synovial joints.
- Interchondral joints between 5th and 9th costal cartilages are synovial joints except the interchondral joint between the 9th and 10th costal cartilages which is fibrous (syndesmosis).
- *Manubriosternal joint:* Secondary cartilaginous joint.
- *Xiphisternal joint:* Primary cartilaginous joint.

Intervertebral Joints

- Intervertebral joint of body.
  - This is a median unpaired joint between the bodies of vertebrae.
  - It is a secondary cartilaginous joint which is permanent.
- Joints of the vertebral arches or neural arches.
  - Lamina and pedicle of a vertebra constitute "vertebral or neural arches".
  - Joints of vertebral arches are the "intervertebral joints of facets" (zygapophyseal joints).

- Zygapophyseal joints: These joints connect the articular facets of adjacent vertebrae. These are paired synovial joints (plane type).

Intervertebral Disc

- Present between 2 adjacent vertebrae (Fig. 4.3)
- *Consists of following parts:*
  - Nucleus pulposus in the centre. Its mucoid content is gradually replaced by fibrocartilage with age.
  - An outer ring of annulus fibrosus made of collagen fibers.
- *Functions:*
  - Give flexibility to the vertebral column.
  - Act as shock absorber.

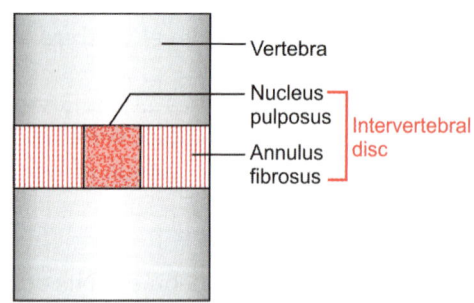

Fig. 4.3: Intervertebral disc

Ligaments of Thoracic Vertebrae

- Anterior longitudinal ligament (lies along the anterior surface of the body of the vertebra).
- Posterior longitudinal ligament (lies along the posterior surface of the body of the vertebra).
- Supraspinous ligament (connects the tips of adjacent spines of vertebrae).
- Interspinous ligament (connects the adjacent spines in front of their tips).
- Ligamenta flava (singular ligamentum flavum) (connect the adjacent lamina).

- Intertransverse ligament (connects the transverse processes of adjacent vertebrae).

Ligaments between the Ribs and Thoracic Vertebrae

- Radiate ligament (connects the anterior part of head of the rib with the bodies of 2 thoracic vertebrae and the intervening intervertebral disc).
- Superior costotransverse ligament (connects the superior border of the neck of the rib with the transverse process of the vertebra above).
- Inferior costotransverse/costotransverse ligament (connects the back of the neck of the rib with the transverse process of the corresponding vertebra).
- Lateral costotransverse ligament (connects the nonarticular part of the tubercle of the rib with the lateral part of the transverse process of the corresponding vertebra).

Respiratory Movements

- Lungs expand during inspiration and retract during expiration. This rhythmic movement is possible because of thoracic cavity and its bony construction.
- During inspiration the capacity of thorax increases, brought about by the movements of thoracic wall and contraction of diaphragm. The movements of thoracic wall result in the increase in its anteroposterior, transverse and vertical diameters. The increase in these diameters of thorax increases the volume of thorax. Increase in the volume of thoracic cavity creates a negative thoracic pressure which helps the air to be sucked into the lungs.
- During expiration the diaphragm relaxes and there is elastic recoil of lungs and thoracic wall. It is mainly a passive process.

Anteroposterior Diameter

- The mechanism of increase of this diameter is called "pump handle movement" (Fig. 4.5).
- In this movement 2nd to 6th ribs take part.
- Articular surfaces of the heads of the ribs forming these joints are convex.
- Anteriorly, these ribs articulate with the sternum through their costal cartilages.
- Movements at the costovertebral joints move anterior ends of the ribs and the body of sternum up and down. When the anterior ends of the ribs move up and anteriorly, thereby carrying the body of the sternum forwards, it increases the antero-posterior distance between the sternum and the vertebral column. This movement is called "pump handle movement". Axis of movement passes through centres of costovertebral and costotransverse joints along neck of rib through opposite costo-chondral junction.

Transverse Diameter

- The mechanism of increase of this diameter is called "bucket handle movement". Vertebrochondral ribs are mainly responsible for this movement (Fig. 4.4).
- Seventh to 10th ribs mainly take part.
- Articular surfaces of the heads of the ribs forming these joints are plane.

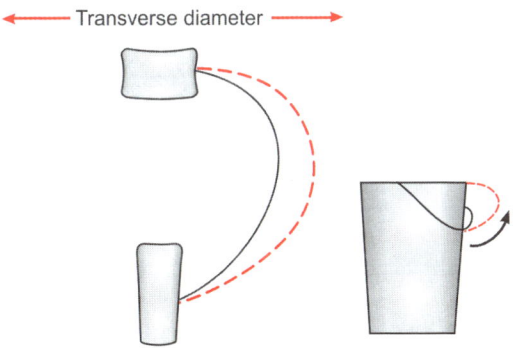

←———— Transverse diameter ————→

Fig. 4.4: Bucket handle movement

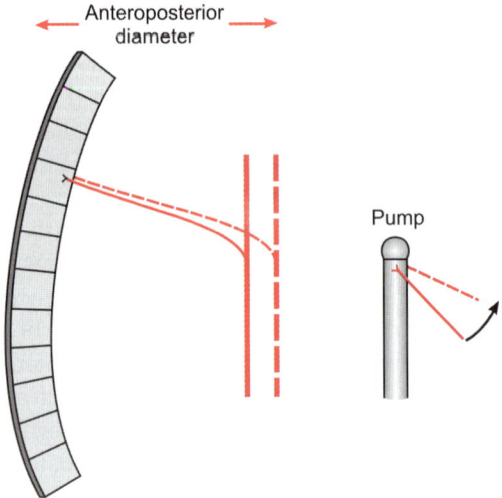

Fig. 4.5: Pump handle movement

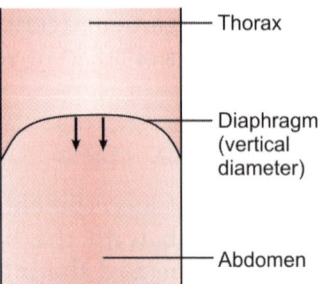

Fig. 4.6: Piston movement

- First rib and manubrium do not move during quiet respiration.
- Seventh to 10th ribs are responsible for the increase in the transverse diameter.
- Contraction of diaphragm increases the vertical diameter.

Deep and Forced Inspiration

- All the above movements take place with increased efficiency.
- First rib and manubrium are also elevated by the scalene and sternocleidomastoid muscles.

Expiration

- *Quiet expiration:* The elastic recoil of the chest wall and pulmonary alveoli expels air.
- *Deep and forced expiration:* Brought about by the contraction of abdominal muscles.

  Note: During quiet breathing range of diaphragmatic movements is about 1.5 cm and in forced ventilation it ranges from 6–10 cm.

- Therefore, they just glide. Anteroposterior axis of movement of these joints passes through the costovertebral and costosternal joints of same side. The middle of the shaft of the rib lies at a lower level than this anteroposterior axis passing through the joints of two ends of the rib. Therefore, during elevation of these ribs, the shaft moves outwards. This helps to increase the transverse diameter of thorax. This movement is called "bucket handle movement".

Vertical Diameter

- The movement which increases this diameter is called the "piston movement" (Fig. 4.6).
- It is brought about by the contraction of diaphragm and its descent. In this movement the lower ribs are fixed.

Inspiration

Quiet Inspiration

- Body of the sternum and 2nd to 6th ribs are responsible for the increase in the anteroposterior diameter.

CLINICAL ANATOMY

Rib fractures may injure the underlying lungs. Also rib fractures below the level of nipple may injure the abdominal viscera like liver, lung and spleen.

Flail chest: In multiple rib fractures, the ribs may be fractured at 2 or more sites. The thoracic wall involving the fractures rib segments (flail segment) then shows paradoxical movement, that is to say the flail segment moves in with inspiration and moves out with expiration. This is reverse of what happens normally.

Cervical rib:

- Seen in 0.5% of population.
- Arises from 7th cervical vertebra.
- It may exert pressure effects on overlying subclavian artery and lower trunk of brachial plexus (which run above the cervical rib) resulting in nervous and vascular symptoms in upper limb.

Intercostal Spaces

- There are eleven intercostal spaces.
- Thorax resembles a truncated cone and the diameter is increased as you proceed downwards. Therefore, spaces become longer as they are traced down.
- Tenth space between the 10th and 11th ribs and the 11th space between the 11th and 12th ribs are open anteriorly and are continuous with the anterior wall of the abdomen.
- Each intercostal space has three layers of muscles (Fig. 4.7):
  1. The outer layer of muscle is called "external intercostal".

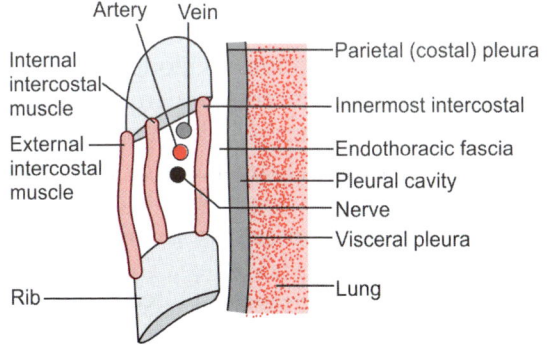

Fig. 4.7: Intercostal space

2. The intermediate layer of muscle is called "internal intercostal".
3. The innermost layer is discontinuous and is called "transversus thoracis".

Transversus thoracic has three parts:

Most anteriorly   Sternocostalis
Middle 1/2 of the space Intercostalis intimi
Posteriorly   Subcostalis

External Intercostal

- This muscle extends from the costochondral junction anteriorly to the tubercle of the rib posteriorly.
- External intercostal membrane (anterior intercostal membrane) replaces it between the costochondral junction and the side of the sternum.
- Posteriorly, the muscle is continuous with the posterior layer of superior costotransverse ligament. The fibres are directed anteroinferiorly.
- *Origin:* Lower border of the upper rib.
- *Insertion:* Outer lip of the upper border of the rib below.
- *Nerve supply:* Corresponding intercostal nerve.
- *Action*
  1. Helps in inspiration.
  2. Prevents bulging out of intercostal spaces in inspiration or caving in during expiration.

Internal Intercostal Muscle

- It extends from the sternum to the angle of the rib. Internal intercostal membrane replaces it posteriorly between the angle of the rib and the superior costotransverse ligament. It is continuous with the anterior layer of superior costotransverse ligament.
- Fibres are directed posteroinferiorly (opposite of externus).
- *Origin:* Floor of the costal groove of the upper rib.

- *Insertion:* Inner lip of the upper border of the rib below.
- *Nerve supply:* Corresponding intercostal nerve.
- *Action*
  1. Prevents bulging out or caving in of the intercostal space.
  2. Interchondral part of the muscle helps in inspiration.

Intercostalis Intimi

- This is the innermost layer occupying the middle 1/2 of the space. The direction of the fibres is same as internal intercostal.
- *Origin:* Inner surface of the rib above.
- *Insertion:* Inner surface of the rib below.
- *Nerve supply:* Corresponding intercostal nerve.
- *Action:* Similar to internal intercostal.

Neurovascular plane: The space between the internal intercostal and intercostalis intimi is called "neurovascular plane". It contains the intercostal vessels and nerve.

Sternocostalis is present in the anterior parts of upper intercostal spaces only. It crosses more than one space.

Subcostalis is present in the posterior parts of the lower spaces only. It crosses more than one space.

Typical Intercostal Nerve

- A typical intercostal nerve is the ventral ramus of a thoracic spinal nerve.
- It should supply only the thorax.
- It should have all the following branches:
  1. Lateral cutaneous branch given near the angle.
  2. Collateral branch given near the angle.
  3. Anterior cutaneous branch given in the anterior part of the space.
  4. Muscular branches to the muscles of the space.

- First intercostal nerve is not a typical nerve because greater part of it contributes to brachial plexus.
- Second intercostal nerve is also not typical because its lateral cutaneous branch supplies the upper arm (intercostobrachial nerve).
- Seventh to 11th intercostal nerve is not typical because they spill over the anterior abdominal wall.
- Only 3rd to 6th intercostal nerves are typical intercostal nerves.
- A typical intercostal nerve exits through the respective intervertebral foramen, then passes in the endothoracic fascia between the internal intercostal membrane and the pleura; enters the neurovascular plane that lies between the internal intercostal and the intercostalis intimi.
- It passes along the costal groove lying inferior to the corresponding artery and vein. The relationship of VAN is maintained. Vein superior, nerve inferior and artery lies in between (Fig. 4.7). It gives two branches near the angle of the rib.
  1. Lateral cutaneous branch.
  2. Collateral nerve.
- Collateral nerve passes along the upper border of the lower rib and lies in the same neurovascular plane as the main trunk and continues into the anterior part of the space. It joins the main trunk. Sometimes it may emerge as an additional anterior cutaneous branch.
- The main trunk continues along the lower border of the corresponding rib and terminates as "anterior cutaneous nerve".
- Dorsal ramus, lateral and anterior cutaneous branches of ventral ramus join with each other to supply a strip of skin along the intercostal space. This strip of skin is called "dermatome". Note: Dorsal ramus is not a part of intercostal nerve; only ventral ramus is.

- Lateral cutaneous branch pierces the intercostal muscles and other muscles of the body wall along the midaxillary line and divides into anterior and posterior branches before supplying the skin.
- Anterior cutaneous branch emerges on the side of the sternum after piercing internal intercostal, anterior intercostal membrane, pectoralis major and divides into lateral and medial branches.

- *Intercostal nerve block*
  - The intercostal nerve should be attacked before the origin of the lateral cutaneous branch at the midaxillary line.
  - The needle is inserted near the lower border of the rib and anesthetic is injected.

Intercostal Vessels

In each intercostal space, arteries are arranged in two groups:
1. Anterior intercostal arteries.
2. Posterior intercostal arteries.

Anterior Intercostal Arteries

- There are two anterior intercostal arteries in each space. The last two spaces (10th and 11th) have no anterior intercostal arteries as they open into the anterior abdominal wall.
- Anterior intercostal arteries of upper six spaces arise from the internal thoracic artery.
- Anterior intercostal arteries of 7th, 8th and 9th spaces arise from the musculophrenic artery.
- The upper anterior intercostal artery courses along the lower border of the corresponding rib and anastomoses with the main trunk of the posterior intercostal artery.

- The lower anterior intercostal artery of each space courses along the upper border of the rib below to anastomoses with the collateral branch of the posterior intercostal artery.

Posterior Intercostal Arteries

- There are 11 posterior intercostal arteries, one for each space. The first and second posterior intercostal arteries are the branches of superior intercostal artery.
- The remaining 9 posterior intercostal arteries for 3rd to 11th spaces arise from the descending thoracic aorta.
- Right posterior intercostal arteries are longer than the left posterior intercostal arteries. This is because the thoracic aorta lies slightly to the left of the median plane.
- Right posterior intercostal arteries arise from the posterior aspect of the aorta and course to the right side behind:
  1. Oesophagus.
  2. Thoracic duct.
  3. Azygos vein.
  4. Sympathetic trunk.
- The left posterior intercostal arteries arise from the back of the thoracic aorta and course to the left side behind:
  1. Hemiazygos veins.
  2. Sympathetic trunk.
- In the posterior part of the intercostal space, the artery lies between the vein and the nerve and the relation from above downwards is VAN.
- To start with, posterior intercostal artery lies between the internal intercostal membrane and costal pleura.
- Later, near the angle of the rib, it lies in the costal groove between the internal intercostal and intercostalis intimi (neurovascular plane).
- Anteriorly, it anastomoses with the upper anterior intercostal artery.

- Near the angle, it gives a collateral branch which runs along the upper border of the rib below and anastomoses with the lower anterior intercostal artery.
- Near the angle, it also gives a lateral cutaneous branch which accompanies the nerve of the same name.

Branches of the posterior intercostal artery

1. Dorsal branch which supplies the muscles and the skin of the back.
2. Collateral branch.
3. Muscular branches to the intercostal muscles and superficial muscles of thorax (serratus anterior and pectoral muscles).
4. Lateral cutaneous branch.

Intercostal Veins

- They correspond to their arteries .There are two anterior intercostal veins in each space and one posterior intercostal vein.
- Anterior intercostal veins of upper six spaces open into the "internal thoracic vein".
- Anterior intercostal veins of 7th, 8th and 9th spaces open into the "musculophrenic veins".

Posterior Intercostal Veins

They are different on right and left sides.

Right Posterior Intercostal Veins

- The first right posterior intercostal vein: It ascends in front of neck of the first rib.
- It arches forwards superior to the apex of the lung and suprapleural membrane and opens into the right brachiocephalic vein.
- The second and third and sometimes the fourth right intercostal veins join together to form a right superior intercostal vein. It opens into the arch of vena azygos.
- Fifth to 11th right posterior intercostal veins open into the vertical part of the azygos vein.

Left Posterior Intercostal Veins

- The first left posterior intercostal vein: The same course as the right one and opens into the left brachiocephalic vein.
- The 2nd, 3rd and 4th veins join to form the left superior intercostal vein. It crosses superficial to arch of aorta and opens into left brachiocephalic vein.
- The 5th, 6th, and 7th independently open into the superior hemiazygos vein.
- Eighth to 11th posterior intercostal veins open independently into the inferior hemiazygos vein.

Lymphatic Drainage of Intercostal Spaces

1. Lymphatics from the anterior part of the spaces are drained into the anterior intercostal nodes that lie along the internal thoracic vessels. Finally, they drain into bronchomediastinal trunk. This trunk joins the right lymphatic duct on the right side and thoracic duct on the left side. Variations are seen in its termination.
2. Lymphatics from the posterior part of the spaces are drained into the "posterior intercostal nodes" that lie on the heads and the necks of ribs.
   - Efferents from lower four to seven spaces drain into cisterna chyli.
   - Efferents from upper spaces on the right side drain into right lymphatic duct.
   - Efferents from upper spaces on the left side drain into thoracic duct.

Internal Thoracic Artery

- It is a branch of the first part of the subclavian artery in the neck.
- It arises 2 cm above the sternal end of the clavicle.
- It runs downwards and medially behind:
  1. Sternal end of the clavicle.
  2. Brachiocephalic vein.

3. First costal cartilage.

4. Phrenic nerve.

- It runs vertically behind the upper six costal cartilages about 1 cm from the margin of the sternum.
- It divides into its two terminal branches:
  1. Superior epigastric.
  2. Musculophrenic at the sixth intercostal space after giving two anterior intercostal arteries to the 6th space.
- The artery is accompanied by two venae comitantes up to the level of 3rd costal cartilage where they unite to form one internal thoracic vein.
- The artery is also accompanied by the internal thoracic chain of lymph nodes.
- It lies between the sternocostalis and internal intercostal muscles.

Branches

1. Pericardiacophrenic accompanies phrenic nerve.

2. Mediastinal.

3. Anterior intercostal arteries for the upper six spaces.

4. Perforating arteries accompany the anterior cutaneous branches of corresponding intercostal nerves. In female, 2nd, 3rd and 4th perforating arteries are large and supply the breast.

5. Musculophrenic artery.

6. Superior epigastric artery.

Azygos Vein (Means Unpaired)

- It is a venous channel of the right side of posterior wall of thorax (Fig. 4.8).
- It is an important channel connecting the superior and inferior vena cava.
- Usually, it is formed in the abdomen by the lumbar azygos (which is connected to the back of the inferior vena cava).
- If lumbar azygos vein is not present, the right subcostal vein and right ascending lumbar vein unite to form the azygos vein.

- It passes through the aortic opening at the level of T12.
- It ascends in the posterior mediastinum till T4 vertebra where it arches forwards over the root of the right lung to open into the superior vena cava .

Tributaries

1. Right superior intercostal vein.

2. Fourth to 11th right posterior intercostal veins.

3. Superior hemiazygos vein.

4. Inferior hemiazygos vein.

5. Oesophageal, mediastinal and some peri-cardial veins.

6. Trunk formed by the right subcostal and right ascending lumbar veins may be the first tributary when azygos vein arises as lumbar azygos.

7. Right bronchial vein (usually, the last tributary).

Superior Hemiazygos Vein (Accessory Azygos Vein)

- It is a venous channel of the upper part of the left side of posterior wall of thorax (Fig. 4.8).
- It is also called "accessory hemiazygos vein".
- It drains the left 5th, 6th, 7th and 8th posterior intercostal veins.
- Crosses from left to right side at the level of T8 vertebra (sometimes T7) behind the following structures:
  – Thoracic aorta.
  – Thoracic duct and opens into the azygos vein.

Left bronchial veins open into it.

- It descends on the left side of the vertebral column from 4th or 5th space till it crosses to the right side at the level of T8 vertebra.

Inferior Hemiazygos Vein (Hemiazygos Vein)

- It is also called hemiazygos vein (Fig. 4.8).

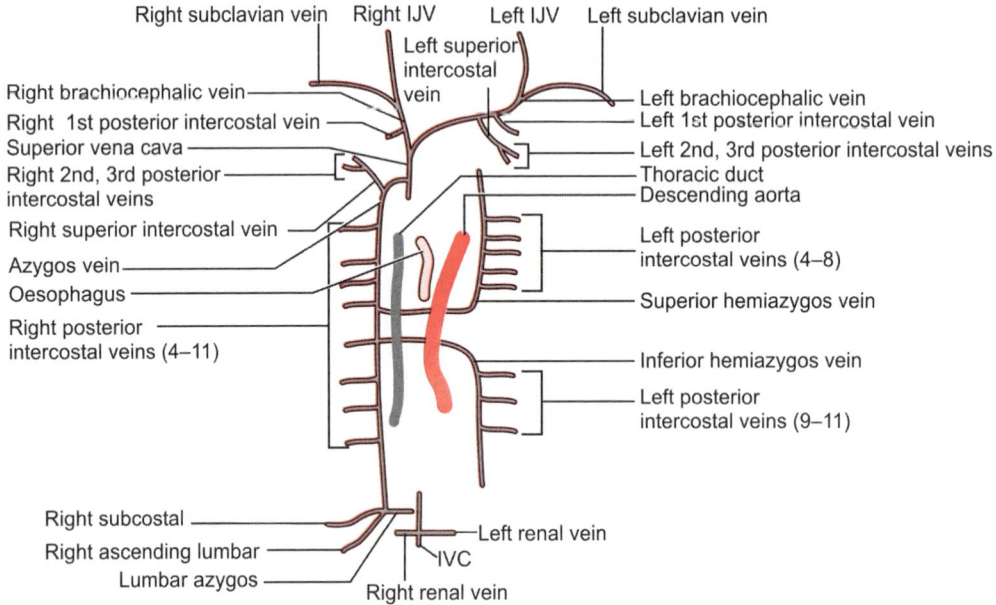

Fig. 4.8: Azygos system of veins

- It usually begins by the union of left ascending lumbar vein with the left subcostal vein.
- It pierces the left crus of the diaphragm.
- It ascends on the left side of the vertebral column behind the aorta.
- At the level of T9 vertebra, (sometimes T8) it crosses from left to right side behind:
  1. Thoracic aorta.
  2. Oesophagus.
  3. Thoracic duct and opens into the azygos vein.

Tributaries: Left 9th, 10th and 11th posterior intercostal veins.

Pleura

Pleura is a serous sac which covers the lung (Fig. 4.9).
- It has two layers—the outer and the inner layer (continuous with each other).
- The outer layer lines the body wall and, therefore it is called parietal layer.

- The inner layer covers the outer surface of the lung and, therefore, it is called the visceral layer.
- The space between the parietal and visceral layers is called the pleural cavity which contains a thin film of fluid called "pleural fluid".
- This helps to prevent the friction generated by the continuous expansion and contraction of the lungs.

Visceral Pleura

- It covers the lung very closely and fuses with the connective tissue of the lung (Fig. 4.9).
- It is not present at the hilum and pulmonary ligament of lung.
- It is developed from the splanchnic mesoderm.
- It is insensitive to pain.
- Autonomic nerves supply it.
- It is also called pulmonary pleura.
- It enters the fissures of the lungs and lines them.

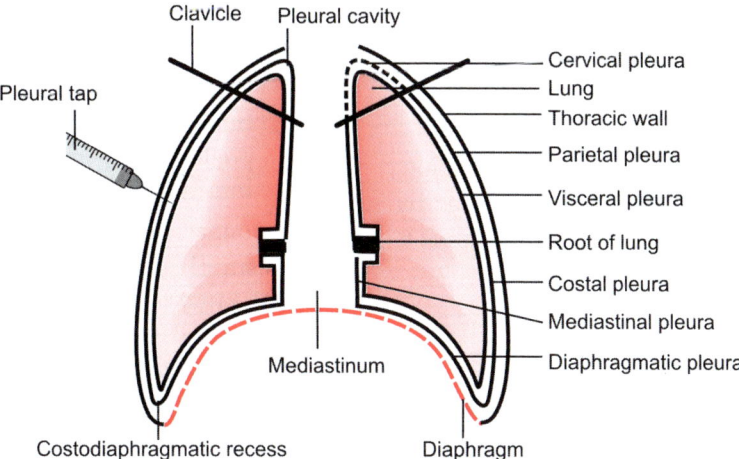

Fig. 4.9: Reflections of pleura

Parietal Pleura

- It is the outer layer and is thicker than the pulmonary pleura (Fig. 4.9).
- It is developed from the somatic mesoderm.
- It is supplied by the somatic nerves (intercostal and phrenic).
- It is supplied by the somatic vessels.
- It is divided into four parts: (Fig. 4.9)
  1. Costal.
  2. Diaphragmatic.
  3. Mediastinal.
  4. Cervical.

Costal Pleura

- Line the inner side of the ribs and intercostal spaces of the thoracic wall.
- "Endothoracic fascia" (loose areolar tissue) lies between the thoracic wall and the costal pleura.
- The line along which the costal pleura becomes continuous with the mediastinal pleura anteriorly is called "costomediastinal line of reflection" (sternal line of pleural reflection). Similarly, the costodiaphragmatic and costovertebral lines (vertebral line of pleural reflection) of reflection are there inferiorly and posteriorly respectively.
- *Nerve supply:* Intercostal nerves.

Mediastinal Pleura

- This extends from the costomediastinal reflection to the costovertebral reflection.
- It forms the lateral wall of the mediastinum (a space between the right and left mediastinal pleurae).
- For the purpose of description, it is divided into three parts:
  1. Above the level of the root of the lung.
  2. At the level of the root of the lung.
  3. Below the level of the root of the lung.
- Above the level of the root of the lung: It is a continuous sheet from the costomediastinal to costovertebral reflections.
- At the level of the root of the lung: It is interrupted and it encloses the structures of the root of the lung like a sleeve.
- Below the level of the root of the lung: Interrupted and it forms a double layer of pleura called "pulmonary ligament".
- *Nerve supply*: Phrenic nerve.

Diaphragmatic Pleura

- It covers the corresponding dome of diaphragm.
- It is continuous with the costal pleura at the costodiaphragmatic line of pleural reflection.

  Nerve supply: Peripheral part is supplied by the intercostal nerves while the central part is supplied by the phrenic nerve.

Cervical Pleura

- It extends into the neck.
- It extends about 1 inch above the level of the medial 1/3rd of the clavicle.
- It is covered by the suprapleural membrane.
- Posteriorly, it does not rise above the level of the upper border of the neck of the first rib.

Suprapleural Membrane

- It extends from the transverse process of the 7th cervical vertebra to the inner border of the first rib. It protects the apex of the lung. All the structures related to the apex of the lung must lie superior to the supra-pleural membrane (Sibson's fascia).

Important Structures related to the Cervical Pleura

- *Anteriorly:* Subclavian artery.
- *Posteriorly:* Neck of the first rib and structures related to it.

Blood Supply and Lymphatic Drainage of Pleura

- Parietal pleura
  - Is supplied by the intercostal, internal thoracic, musculophrenic, bronchial, mediastinal, subclavian arteries and microcirculation of diaphragmatic muscle.
  - Veins drain into internal thoracic veins anteriorly; into azygos, superior hemiazygos and inferior hemiazygos veins posteriorly.
  - Lymphatics
    - Drain into internal thoracic nodes anteriorly.
    - Into posterior intercostal lymph nodes posteriorly.
    - Into diaphragmatic nodes inferiorly.
- Pulmonary pleura
  - Is supplied by the bronchial vessels like the lung.
  - Lymph vessels of this pleura drain into bronchopulmonary lymph nodes.

Pulmonary Ligament

- Parietal pleura covers the root of the lung like a loose sleeve and not like a circular tube. Therefore, it extends inferiorly beyond the root as a double layer. This fold of pleura is called the "pulmonary ligament" (Fig. 4.10).
- This contains loose areolar tissue with a few lymphatics.
- It provides "dead space" for the pulmonary veins, which can occupy this space when they happen to bring more blood as in strenuous exercise.
- It lies between the side of the oesophagus and the medial side of the corresponding lung inferior to the hilum.

Recesses of Pleura

At some places, parietal pleura extends beyond the margin of the lung. This creates an extra reserve space between the lung and pleura. The lung can expand into it during deep inspiration.

There are two recesses in the parietal pleura:

1. Costomediastinal recess.
2. Costodiaphragmatic recess.

- Costomediastinal recess lies between the costal and mediastinal pleurae. It lies behind the sternum and costal cartilages along the costomediastinal reflection.

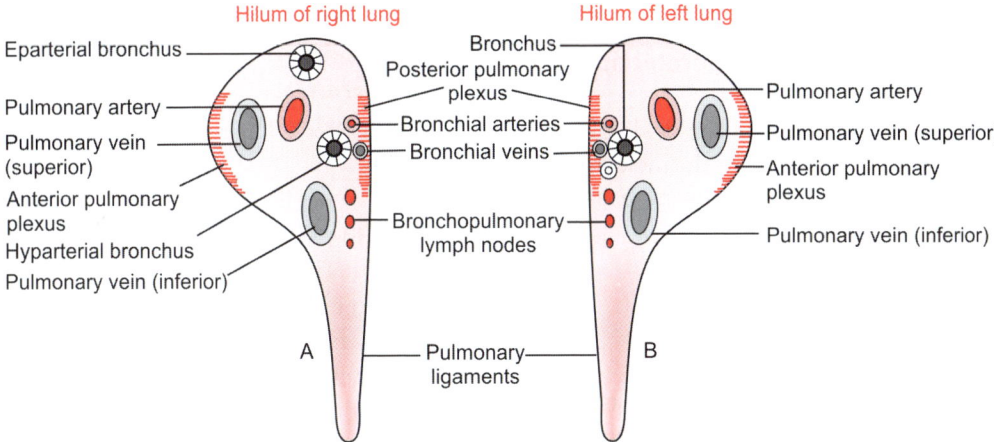

Eparterial bronchus
Pulmonary artery
Pulmonary vein (superior)
Anterior pulmonary plexus
Hyparterial bronchus
Pulmonary vein (inferior)

Hilum of right lung

Bronchus
Posterior pulmonary plexus
Bronchial arteries
Bronchial veins

Hilum of left lung

Pulmonary artery
Pulmonary vein (superior)
Anterior pulmonary plexus
Pulmonary vein (inferior)

Bronchopulmonary lymph nodes

Pulmonary ligaments

A   B

Fig. 4.10: Lung root constituents

This recess is particularly well defined in relation to the cardiac notch of the left lung.

- Costodiaphragmatic recess lies between the costal and diaphragmatic pleura along the costodiaphragmatic line of reflexion (Fig. 4.9). The lung is at the level of 8th rib in the midaxillary line whereas pleurae extend to the level of 10th ribs. The space between the 8th and 10th ribs in the midaxillary line is the extra space called costodiaphragmatic recess.

Pleural effusion fills up this space first.

Surface Marking of the Pleura

Cervical pleurae are marked by a curved line from the junction of medial third with the lateral two-thirds of the clavicle to the sternal end of the clavicle. The top of the convexity should be one inch above the clavicle.

Costomediastinal line of pleural reflection: (common to right and left sides)

- From the sternoclavicular joint to the midpoint of the sternal angle.
- A vertical line from the midpoint of the sternal angle to the level of fourth costal cartilage.

From here it is different on two sides.

Right side: It continues vertically to the midpoint of xiphisternal joint.

Left side: It arches laterally and descends along the sternal margin up to the 6th costal cartilage.

Costodiaphragmatic line of pleural reflection:

- This reflection is same on both sides except that the right pleura crosses the right costoxiphoid angle while left pleura does not cross.
- The reflection is marked by selecting the following points and joining them together:
  - Eighth rib in the midclavicular line.
  - Tenth rib in the midaxillary line.
  - Two cm lateral to the spine of 12th thoracic vertebra.
  - Posteriorly, it crosses the 12th rib and descends inferior to it medially.
- Therefore, it crosses the costovertebral angles inferior to the medial end of 12th rib (behind the upper poles of the kidneys).
- It is important to note that pleura descend below the costal margin at three places:

1. Right costoxiphoid angle.
2. Right costovertebral angle.
3. Left costovertebral angle.

Costovertebral Reflection of Pleura

A vertical line is drawn connecting the following two points:

1. Two cm lateral to the 7th cervical spine.
2. Two cm lateral to the 12th thoracic spine.

The costal pleura becomes mediastinal pleura along this line.

APPLIED ANATOMY

- *Pleural effusion:* Collection of fluid in the pleural cavity.
- *Paracentesis thoracis (pleural tap):* Aspiration of fluid from pleural cavity. The needle is inserted at the upper border of the rib to avoid the main intercostal vessels and nerves. The small collateral vessels and nerves at the upper border of the rib are not of much significance.
- *Pleurisy:* The inflammation of pleura.
- *Empyema:* Presence of pus in the pleural cavity.
- *Pneumothorax:* Presence of air in pleural cavity.
- *Hemothorax:* Presence of blood in pleural cavity.

THE LUNGS

- The lungs are a pair of respiratory organs that exchange oxygen with the carbon dioxide of the blood.
- They are present in the thoracic cavity surrounded by the pleura.
- Mediastinum is the space between the right and left pleurae.
- The lungs are spongy in structure.
- Right lung is heavier than the left lung.

External features of lungs

Each lung has an:

1. Apex.
2. A base.
3. Medial surface.
4. Costal surface and

Three borders:

1. Anterior.
2. Posterior.
3. Inferior.

Apex of the Lung

- It extends into the neck above the level of sternal end of the clavicle.
- The cervical pleura and suprapleural membrane cover it.
- The subclavian artery grooves it.

The other relations are same as the cervical pleura.

APPLIED ANATOMY

A tumor of the apex of the lung may compress the structures around the apex. Following are its symptoms:

1. Enlargement of veins of upper limb and neck (because of the compression of brachiocephalic veins).
2. Diminished pulse at the wrist (because of the compression of the subclavian artery).
3. Paralysis of the corresponding side of the diaphragm (due to the involvement of phrenic nerve).
4. Hoarseness of voice (due to compression of left recurrent laryngeal nerve).

This syndrome is also called "thoracic inlet syndrome".

Base of the lung

- It is concave and is related to the diaphragm.
- Right diaphragm separates the base of right lung from the right lobe of liver.
- Left diaphragm separates the base of the left lung from the left lobe of liver, fundus of stomach and spleen.

Mediastinal surface differs in two lungs:

Mediastinal surface of right lung

It is related to the following:

- Right atrium and its auricle.
- Lower part of the right brachiocephalic vein.
- Superior vena cava.
- Azygos vein.
- Oesophagus.
- Inferior vena cava.
- Trachea.
- Right vagus nerve.
- Right phrenic nerve.

Hilum is present on the mediastinal surface and it contains the following structures: (Fig. 4.10)
- Eparterial bronchus (upper lobar bronchus).
- Pulmonary artery.
- Right principal bronchus (hyparterial bronchus).
- Inferior pulmonary vein.
- Superior pulmonary vein.
- Bronchial vessels.

Pulmonary ligament: It lies inferior to the hilum of the right lung.

Mediastinal surface of the left lung: It is related to the following structures:
- Left ventricle, left auricle.
- Arch of aorta.
- Descending thoracic aorta.
- Left subclavian artery.
- Thoracic duct.
- Oesophagus.
- Left brachiocephalic vein.
- Left vagus nerve.
- Left phrenic nerve.
- Left recurrent laryngeal nerve.

Hilum of the left lung lies on the mediastinal surface and contains the following structures: (Fig. 4.10)
- Pulmonary artery.
- Left principal bronchus.
- Inferior pulmonary vein.
- Superior pulmonary vein.
- Bronchial vessels.

Pulmonary ligament: It lies inferior to the hilum of left lung.

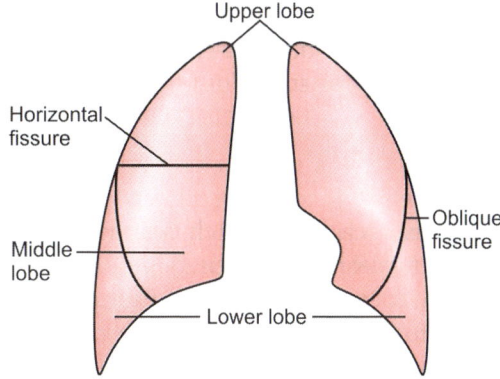

Fig. 4.11: Lobes and fissures of the lungs

Lobes and fissures of the lungs
- Right lung has three lobes and two fissures (oblique and horizontal fissures) (Fig. 4.11).
- Left lung has two lobes and one fissure (oblique fissure) (Fig. 4.11).

Oblique Fissure

- It is deep and, therefore, it cuts the whole lung except at the hilum.
- It acts as a plane of separation so that the upper part of the lung can expand forward and laterally when the ribs are elevated.

It is marked on the surface as follows: Three points are taken.
1. The first point: 2 to 2.5 cm lateral to the 3rd thoracic spine.
2. The second point: 5th rib in the midaxillary line.
3. The third point: 6th costal cartilage about 3 inches from the midline.

A line joining these three points represents the oblique fissure on both sides. When the arm is raised above the head, the medial border of the scapula roughly corresponds to the oblique fissure.

Horizontal Fissure

- It is present only in the right lung.
- A line drawn horizontally at the level of the 4th costal cartilage from the anterior border

of right lung to the oblique fissure in the midaxillary line (5th rib) represents the horizontal fissure.

Surface Marking of Lungs

Apex of the lung

A convex arch of one inch height, over the medial third of the clavicle.

Anterior border of the right lung: (corresponds to costomediastinal line of pleural reflection).

Following points are joined serially from above downwards:

1. Sternoclavicular joint.
2. Median plane at the sternal angle.
3. Median plane at the xiphisternal joint.

Anterior border of the left lung: (Corresponds to the costomediastinal pleural reflection only up to 4th costal cartilage).

Below this level it presents a cardiac notch.

Anterior border of the lung can be marked by selecting the following points:

1. Left sternoclavicular joint.
2. Median plane at the sternal angle.
3. Median plane at the level of left 4th costal cartilage.
4. A point over left 5th costal cartilage about 3.5 cm from the margin of the sternum.
5. A point over the left 6th costal cartilage about 4 cm from the median plane.

The 3rd, 4th and 5th points are joined by a curved line that represents the cardiac notch.

Note: In the region of cardiac notch, the pericardium is covered only by a double layer of pleura. This area is called the "area of superficial cardiac dullness", as it is dull on percussion. (Resonance offered by lung is absent)

Inferior Border of Both the Lungs

It lies two ribs higher than the pleural reflection. The following points are selected to mark it on the surface:

1. Sixth rib in the midclavicular line.
2. Eighth rib in the midaxillary line.
3. Two cm lateral to the 10th thoracic spine.

A line connecting the above points represents the inferior border of the lung.

Posterior Border of Both the Lungs

This border corresponds to the costovertebral pleural reflection from above till the level of the spine of 10th thoracic vertebra. Two points are selected:

1. A point 2 cm lateral to 7th cervical spine.
2. A point 2 cm lateral to the spine of 10th thoracic vertebra.

These two lines are joined by a vertical line which represents the posterior border of the corresponding lung.

Root of the Lung

It connects the medial surface of the lung to the mediastinum. It contains:
- A tube carrying air (bronchus).
- An artery carrying deoxygenated blood (pulmonary artery).
- Two veins carrying oxygenated blood from the lung (two pulmonary veins).
- Lymph vessels from the lung and lymph nodes (bronchopulmonary).
- Plexus of autonomic nerves which are going to supply the lung (anterior and posterior pulmonary plexuses).
- Blood vessels of parenchyma of the lung (bronchial artery and bronchial vein).
  Note:
  One bronchial artery on the right side.
  Two bronchial arteries on the left side.
  Usually two bronchial veins on each side.
- Connective tissue.
- All these structures are covered by a tubular sheath of mediastinal pleura to form root of lung.
- Root of the lung lies at the level of the bodies of the 5th, 6th and 7th thoracic vertebrae.

Arrangement of Structures in the Root

Right lung:

From above downwards:
- Eparterial bronchus (upper lobe bronchus).
- Pulmonary artery.
- Right principal bronchus (hyparterial).
- Inferior pulmonary vein.

From front to back: (VAB)
- Superior pulmonary vein.
- Pulmonary artery.
- Principal bronchus with bronchial vessels posterior to the bronchus.

Left lung: (No upper lobar bronchus in the left lung)

From above downwards:
- Pulmonary artery.
- Principal bronchus.
- Inferior pulmonary vein.

From front to back: (VAB)
- Superior pulmonary vein.
- Pulmonary artery.
- Principal bronchus with bronchial vessels.

Relations of the Root

Root of the right lung:

Anterior:
- Superior vena cava and part of the right atrium.
- Right phrenic nerve.
- Right pericardiacophrenic vessels.
- Anterior pulmonary plexus.

Posterior:
- Right vagus nerve.
- Posterior pulmonary plexus.

Superior: Arch of vena azygos.

Inferior: Pulmonary ligament.

Root of the left lung:

Anterior:
- Left phrenic nerve.
- Left pericardiacophrenic vessels.
- Anterior pulmonary plexus.

Posterior:
- Left vagus nerve.
- Posterior pulmonary plexus.
- Descending thoracic aorta.

Inferior: Pulmonary ligament.

Arterial supply of the lungs:
- Bronchial arteries supply the bronchial tree and pulmonary tissue.
- There is one bronchial artery on the right side and this artery arises from the right 3rd posterior intercostal artery.
- There are two bronchial arteries on the left side. They arise from the descending thoracic aorta.
- Respiratory part of the lung is also supplied by the pulmonary arteries through the pulmonary capillary plexus.
- There is anastomosis between the bronchial and pulmonary arteries. This anastomosis becomes enlarged when one of the vessels is obstructed.

Venous drainage of the lungs:
- Veins of the lung are divided into pulmonary and bronchial veins.
- Bronchial veins are 2 on each side. They drain only a part of the area supplied by bronchial arteries near the root of the lung and open into arch of vena azygos on the right side and left superior intercostal vein or superior hemiazygos vein on the left side.
- Rest is drained by pulmonary veins.

Lymphatic drainage of the lungs:
There are superficial and deep sets of lymph vessels in each lung.
- *Superficial lymph vessels:* Superficial lymph vessels drain the pulmonary pleura and peripheral lung tissue and reach the hilum. They open into the bronchopulmonary nodes which are present in the hilum.
- *Deep lymph vessels:* They drain the bronchial tree, pulmonary vessels and surrounding connective tissue and open into the broncho-pulmonary lymph nodes which are present in the hilum of the lung.

Table 4.1: Differences between lungs		
	Right lung	*Left lung*
	Shorter, wider and heavier (about 700 gm)	Longer, narrower, less heavy (about 600 gm)
Lobes and fissures	Three lobes and two fissures	Two lobes and one fissure
Base	Base more concave (because of liver)	Base shallow
Cardiac notch	No cardiac notch (no lingula)	Cardiac notch is present with lingula
Eparterial bronchus	Eparterial bronchus present	No eparterial bronchus in the hilum
Cardiac impression	Cardiac impression shallow	Cardiac impression deep
Bronchial artery	Supplied by one bronchial artery	Supplied by two bronchial arteries

Note: This means the bronchopulmonary lymph nodes receive both superficial and deep lymph vessels of the lungs but their origin and path to bronchopulmonary lymph nodes differ.

Nerve supply of the lungs:

Supplied by the autonomic nerves which include sympathetic and parasympathetic nerves.

- *Sympathetic nerves:*
  - They are derived from the spinal segments of T2 to T5.
  - They are inhibitory to the smooth muscle of the bronchial tree. Therefore, they bring about bronchodilatation. They are inhibitory to the glands of the bronchial tree. Hence sympathomimetic drugs which mimic sympathetic are used in asthma associated with spasm of bronchi and bronchioles.
- *Parasympathetic nerves:*
  - They are derived from the vagus nerve.
  - They are motor to the smooth muscle of the bronchus.
  - They are secretomotor to the glands of the bronchial tree.
  - They also carry sensory fibres from the lung which help in cough reflex.

Differences between right and left bronchi	
Right bronchus	*Left bronchus*
Short (one inch)	Long (two inches)
Straight	Oblique
Wider	Narrower

Swallowed foreign objects tend to enter the right bronchus because it is more in line with trachea.

Bronchopulmonary Segments

- These are the areas of the lung supplied by one segmental (tertiary) bronchus.
- The lung tissue of one bronchopulmonary segment is pyramidal in shape.
- The base is towards the periphery and the apex is directed towards the hilum.
- It has its own branch of pulmonary artery.
- It is limited by the surrounding connective tissue which is continuous with the pulmonary pleura.
- They are independent respiratory units.
- The connective tissue septae between the bronchopulmonary segments contain the pulmonary veins. The pulmonary veins do not correspond to the bronchopulmonary segments. Therefore, pulmonary veins are intersegmental in their position.

- Bronchopulmonary units are not broncho-vascular units as pulmonary veins do not correspond to the segments.
- Usually, there are 10 bronchopulmonary segments in each lung. Sometimes the left lung may have only 8 or 9 segments (Fig. 4.12).

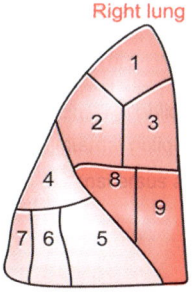 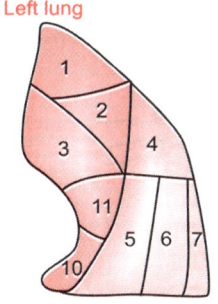

1. Apical, 2.Posterior, 3. Anterior, 4.Apical, 5. Anterior basal, 6.Lateral basal, 7.Posterior basal, 8.Lateral, 9. Medial, 10.Inferior lingular, 11,Superior lingular

Fig. 4.12: Bronchopulmonary segments of right and left lung (Medial basal not shown)

Bronchopulmonary segments of right lung:
1. Upper lobe has three segments:
   a. Apical
   b. Anterior
   c. Posterior
2. Middle lobe has two segments:
   a. Medial
   b. Lateral
3. Lower lobe has five segments:
   a. Apical
   b. Anterior basal
   c. Posterior basal
   d. Medial basal
   e. Lateral basal

Bronchopulmonary segments of left lung:
1. Upper lobar bronchus has two divisions: Upper division and lower division.
   - *Upper division usually has three segments:*
   a. Apical.

   b. Posterior.
   c. Anterior.
   - *Lower division has two segments:*
   a. Superior lingular.
   b. Inferior lingular.
2. Lower lobar bronchus usually has five segments:
   - Apical.
   - Anterior basal.
   - Posterior basal.
   - Lateral basal.
   - Medial basal.
     – Medial basal may not be represented in the left lung because of the projection of the heart to the left side.

APPLIED ANATOMY

- Infection is usually limited to the broncho-pulmonary segment although some like tuberculosis may spread from one bronchopulmonary segment to the other.
- Cancer spreads across the segments.
- Knowledge of the segments is important in surgical resection (removal of segments) and in drainage of infections by putting the patient in a particular posture which aids drainage.

Mediastinum (Middle Septum)

- It is the space between the right and left pleurae (Fig. 4.13).
- It lies between the anterior and posterior bony walls of thorax.
- It extends from the thoracic inlet superiorly to the diaphragm inferiorly.
- It is bounded by the sternum anteriorly and the thoracic vertebral column posteriorly
- On either side it is bounded by the mediastinal pleura which cover the medial surface of the lung.

Divisions:

- It is divided into superior and inferior mediastinum.

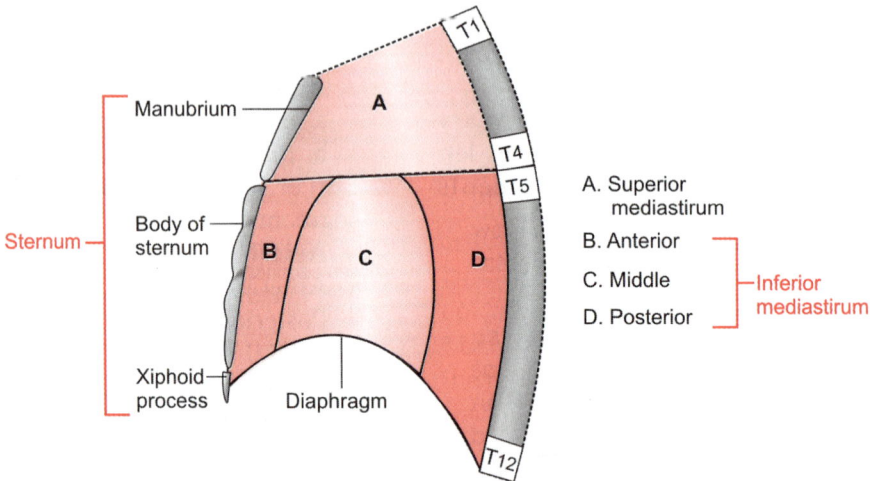

Fig. 4.13: Mediastinum and its subdivisions

- Inferior mediastinum is further subdivided into:
  1. Anterior mediastinum.
  2. Middle mediastinum.
  3. Posterior mediastinum.

Inlet of thorax which is bounded anteriorly by the upper border of manubrium sternum, on either side by the inner border of the first rib, posteriorly by the upper border of the body of the first thoracic vertebra.

Superior Mediastinum

- It lies superior to the transverse thoracic plane (obtained by joining the sternal angle with the lower border of the body of the 4th thoracic vertebra).

Boundaries

- *Anterior:* Posterior surface of the manubrium sterni.
- *Posterior:* Upper four thoracic vertebrae and intervening intervertebral disc.
- *Inferiorly:* It is separated from the inferior mediastinum by the transverse thoracic plane.

- *Lateral:* Bounded by the right and left mediastinal pleurae.
- *Superior:* Inlet of thorax.

Contents

Two muscles anteriorly:
1. Sternohyoid.
2. Sternothyroid

Two tubes:
1. Trachea.
2. Oesophagus.

Four arteries:
1. Arch of aorta.
2. Brachiocephalic artery.
3. Left common carotid artery.
4. Left subclavian artery.

Four veins:
1. Right brachiocephalic vein.
2. Left brachiocephalic vein.
3. Upper half of superior vena cava.
4. Left superior intercostal vein.

Four nerves:
1. Vagus (bilateral).
2. Phrenic (bilateral).

3. Cardiac nerves (bilateral).
4. Left recurrent laryngeal nerve (unilateral).

Four other structures:

1. Thoracic duct.
2. Remains of thymus.
3. Lymph nodes.
4. Connective tissue.

Anterior Mediastinum

It is a narrow space between the heart and sternum.

Boundaries

- *Anterior:* Body of the sternum.
- *Posterior:* Pericardium.
- *Superior:* Imaginary plane connecting the manubriosternal angle with the lower border of the body of fourth thoracic vertebra.
- *Inferior:* Superior surface of the diaphragm.
- *Lateral:* Mediastinal pleura.

Contents

1. Superior and inferior sternopericardial ligaments.
2. Lymph nodes and lymphatics.
3. Connective tissue.

Middle Mediastinum

Heart and its covering pericardium occupy the middle mediastinum.

Boundaries

- *Anterior:* Anterior mediastinum.
- *Posterior:* Posterior mediastinum.
- *Lateral:* Mediastinal pleura. Between the mediastinal pleura and fibrous pericardium, phrenic nerve and the pericardiacophrenic vessels of the corresponding side are present.

Contents

- *Heart with its pericardium.*

- *Two nerves:*
  1. Phrenic nerve.
  2. Deep cardiac plexus placed at the bifurcation of trachea.
- *Two other structures:*
  1. Tracheobronchial lymph nodes.
  2. Connective tissue.
- *Three tubes:*
  1. Bifurcation of trachea.
  2. Right main bronchus.
  3. Left main bronchus.
- *Four arteries:*
  1. Ascending aorta.
  2. Pulmonary trunk.
  3. Right pulmonary artery.
  4. Left pulmonary artery.
- *Four veins:*
  1. Lower half of superior vena cava.
  2. Terminal part of azygos vein.
  3. Right pulmonary veins.
  4. Left pulmonary veins.

Posterior Mediastinum

It lies posterior to the middle mediastinum. Its boundaries are:

- *Anterior:* Pericardium, bifurcation of trachea, pulmonary vessels of the middle mediastinum.
- *Posterior:* Lower eight thoracic vertebrae and intervening intervertebral discs.
- *Lateral:* Mediastinal pleura of right and left sides.

Contents

- *One tube:* Oesophagus.
- *One artery:* Descending thoracic aorta and its branches.
- *One duct:* Thoracic duct.
- *One group of lymph nodes:* Posterior mediastinal lymph nodes. Along the thoracic aorta.
- *Two nerves:*
  1. Vagus.
  2. Splanchnic nerves.

- *Three veins:*
  1. Azygos vein.
  2. Superior hemiazygos vein.
  3. Inferior hemiazygos vein.

Infection of the neck can spread to the superior and inferior mediastina. Compression of mediastinal structures by tumors can give rise to specific symptoms known as "mediastinal syndrome". In Hodgkin's disease mediastinal lymph nodes are enlarged. The following are the symptoms of the mediastinal syndrome:

- Dilatation of the veins of upper half of the body because of the compression of superior vena cava.
- Dyspnoea (difficulty in breathing) caused by the compression of trachea.
- Dysphagia (difficulty in swallowing) caused by the pressure over oesophagus.
- Hoarseness of voice because of involvement of left recurrent laryngeal nerve.
- Paralysis of the corresponding half of the diaphragm because of involvement of phrenic nerve.
- Pain over the thoracic dermatomes because of involvement of intercostal nerves.

The Pericardium

- It is a fibroserous sac containing heart and the roots of the great vessels (Fig. 4.14).
- It is situated in the middle mediastinum behind the body of sternum and 2nd to 6th costal cartilages.
- It consists of outer fibrous pericardium and inner serous pericardium.
- It is as though heart is placed inside the fibrous pericardium and pushed from above and behind towards the serous pericardium. Thereby, serous pericardium is folded inwards to form two layers. The outer layer lines the inner surface of the fibrous

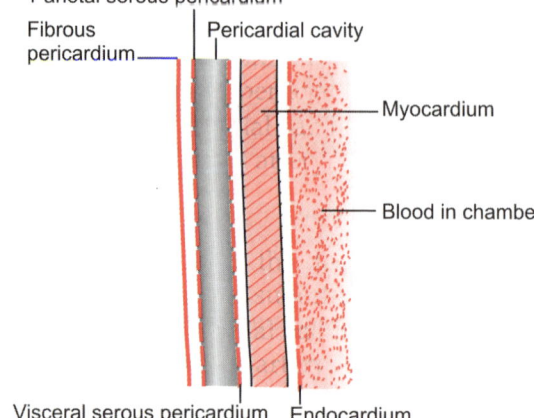

Fig. 4.14: Layers of pericardium and heart

pericardium. It is called "parietal layer of the serous pericardium". The inner layer covers the heart and is called "visceral layer of serous pericardium". The space between the parietal and visceral layers of serous pericardium is called the "pericardial cavity".

Fibrous Pericardium

- It is cone-shaped.
- Its apex is directed superiorly and fuses with the external coats of the roots of ascending aorta and pulmonary trunk.
- Its base fuses with the upper surface of diaphragm. This fusion takes place because both the fibrous pericardium and the diaphragm are developed from the same source, the "septum transversum".

Anteriorly, it is connected to the upper and lower ends of the body of sternum by superior and inferior sternopericardial ligaments.

Posteriorly, it forms the anterior boundary of the posterior mediastinum and is related to the following structures:

- Right and left bronchi.
- Oesophagus with oesophageal plexus of nerves.

- Descending thoracic aorta.
- Thoracic duct.
- Azygos and hemiazygos veins.

Laterally, it is separated from the mediastinal pleura by the phrenic nerve and pericardiacophrenic vessels.

Structures which pierce the fibrous pericardium:
- Superior vena cava.
- Inferior vena cava.
- Right and left pulmonary arteries.
- Four pulmonary veins.

Serous Pericardium

- It is a closed serous sac.
- It lies inside the fibrous pericardium.
- It is divided into two layers. The outer parietal and the inner visceral layers.
- Pericardial cavity is a potential space between the parietal and visceral layers. It contains a thin layer of fluid which helps to reduce the friction.
- The visceral layer lines the outer surface of the heart and forms the epicardium of the heart. Along the cardiac grooves the visceral layer is separated from the heart by the blood vessels.

Parietal layer lines the inner surface of the fibrous pericardium. The visceral and parietal layers are continuous with each other at the entry and exit of the vessels of the heart. Along this continuity, pericardial cavity presents two sinuses (Fig. 4.15).
1. Transverse sinus.
2. Oblique sinus.

Transverse Sinus

- It is a transverse gap between the arterial and venous ends of the heart tube.
- It is lined by visceral layer only.
- Ascending aorta and pulmonary trunk form its anterior boundary (both derived from the common source, truncus arteriosus).

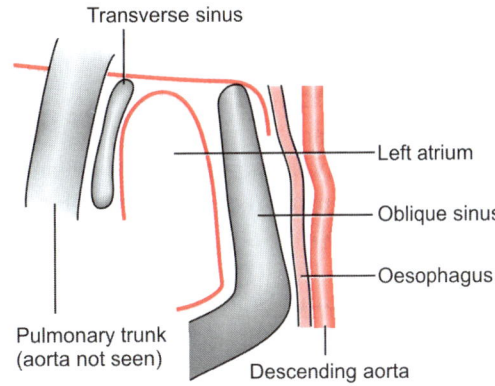

Fig. 4.15: Oblique and transverse sinuses

- Posteriorly, it is bounded by the superior vena cava and below by left atrium (venous end of the heart tube).
- *Applied anatomy:* Transverse sinus may be used to pass a ligature aorta and pulmonary trunk during cardiac surgery.

Oblique Sinus

- It is a blind sac which opens at one end. It lies behind the left atrium.
- It lies between the parietal and visceral layers of pericardium.
- It lies within the J-shaped attachment of serous pericardium to the pulmonary veins and inferior vena cava. It lies between parietal and visceral layers.

Boundaries

- *Anterior:* Left atrium.
- *Posterior:* Posterior part of fibrous pericardium.
- *Right side:* Right superior and inferior pulmonary veins and inferior vena cava.
- *Left side:* Left superior and inferior pulmonary veins.
- *Superior:* Upper margin of left atrium.
- It opens below and left into the rest of the pericardial cavity.

Note: Upper margin of left atrium lies between the roof of oblique sinus and the floor of transverse sinus.

- *Arterial supply:*
  - Fibrous and parietal layers of serous pericardium are supplied by the branches of:
    1. Internal thoracic.
    2. Descending thoracic aorta.
  - Visceral layer is supplied by coronary arteries.
- *Venous drainage:*
  - Fibrous and parietal layers are drained into internal thoracic veins and azygos veins.
  - Visceral layer drains into coronary sinus.
- *Nerve supply:*
  - Fibrous and parietal layers are supplied by the phrenic nerves.
  - Visceral layer is supplied by the autonomic nerves through coronary plexus.
- *Development:*
  - Fibrous pericardium is developed from the septum transversum.
  - Parietal layer of serous pericardium is developed from the somatopleuric mesoderm.
  - Visceral layer is developed from the splanchnopleuric layer of mesoderm.

APPLIED ANATOMY

- Parietal layer is sensitive to pain.
- Pain of pericarditis originates in the parietal layer.
- Pain of the heart as in angina or myocardial infarction (heart attack) originates in cardiac muscle or vessels of the heart.
- Pericardial effusion: Collection of abnormal amount of fluid in the pericardial cavity. It can be drained by two routes:
  1. Puncturing left 5th or 6th intercostal space near the sternum.
  2. Subcostal route: A needle may be inserted through left costoxiphoid angle posterosuperiorly and fluid can be drained.
- When a large pericardial effusion impinges on the heart and interferes with its filling in diastole, it is called cardiac tamponade.

THE HEART

- It is a hollow muscular organ situated in the middle mediastinum.
- It is enclosed within the pericardium.
- It pumps deoxygenated blood to the lungs and oxygenated blood to all parts of the body.
- Two-thirds of the heart is to the left of the median plane and one-third of the heart is to the right of the median plane.
- It weighs about 300 gm in males and about 250 gm in females.

  Usually, it is said to be of the size of the fist of one's hand.

Basic Plan of the Heart

- Heart has four chambers—two atria and two ventricles.
- Right atrium and right ventricle are on the right side while left atrium and left ventricle are on the left side.
- Right atrium lies anterior and to the right of left atrium.
- Right ventricle lies anterior and to the right of the left ventricle.
- Interatrial septum separates the right and left atria.
- Interventricular septum separates the right and left ventricles.
- Venous blood of the upper half of the body reaches the right atrium through the superior vena cava.
- Venous blood from the lower half of the body reaches the right atrium through the inferior vena cava.

- Therefore, right atrium is the receiving station of the deoxygenated blood.
- This blood is pumped into the right ventricle through the right atrioventricular orifice during atrial systole.
- The right ventricle pumps blood to the lungs through pulmonary trunk and pulmonary arteries during ventricular systole.
- Lung oxygenates the blood and drains it into left atrium through four pulmonary veins.
- Left atrium pumps this oxygenated blood to the left ventricle through left atrioventricular orifice during atrial systole.
- Left ventricle pumps the blood through aorta to be distributed all over the body during ventricular systole.
- Systolic blood pressure is generated by the contraction of the left ventricle.
- During ventricular diastole, elastic recoil of large arteries generates diastolic blood pressure.

External Features of the Heart

The heart has an apex, base, anterior surface, inferior surface and left surface. It has lower, right and left borders.

Apex

- It is directed downwards, forwards and to the left.
- It is formed by the left ventricle.
- It is covered by the left lung and left pleura.
- It lies 9 cm away from the median plane in the left 5th intercostal space.

Base of the Heart

- It is directed to the right and posteriorly.
- It is mainly formed by the left atrium. Only a small part of the right atrium contributes to it.
- Four pulmonary veins open into the left atrium in the base.

- Oblique sinus of the pericardium lies behind the base of the heart.

The following structures of middle mediastinum lie behind it
1. Right and left bronchi.
2. Right pulmonary veins.

Posteriorly base of the heart is related to the following structures of posterior mediastinum:
1. Oesophagus.
2. Descending thoracic aorta.
3. Thoracic duct.
4. Azygos and hemiazygos veins.

APPLIED ANATOMY

Distended left atrium in mitral stenosis (narrowing of the mitral valve) might cause difficulty of swallowing because of its relation to the oesophagus.

Clinical base of the heart: Line connecting the auscultatory areas of pulmonary sound in the left second intercostal space and the aortic sound in the right second space is the clinical base of the heart.

Anterior Surface of the Heart

It is also called the sternocostal surface.

Boundaries

- It is separated from the diaphragmatic surface by the inferior border.
- Right border separates it from the base of the heart.
- Left border of the heart separates it from the left surface.

Following parts of the heart constitute this surface:
- Anterior surface of the right atrium and its auricle.
- Part of the left auricle.

- Anterior surface of the right ventricle (2/3rd of ventricular area).
- Anterior surface of the left ventricle (1/3rd of ventricular area).
- There are two grooves on this surface:
  - Anterior part of the right atrioventricular groove lies between the right atrium and the right ventricle and it contains the right coronary artery.
  - Anterior interventricular groove lies between the right ventricle and left ventricle. It contains the:
    - Anterior interventricular branch of left coronary artery.
    - Great cardiac vein.

Relations

- Covered by the pericardium and is related to the posterior surface of the body of the sternum.
- Anterior margins of both lungs and pleurae lie superficial to pericardium except on the left side, below the level of 4th costal cartilage where pericardium is directly related to the sternum due to the cardiac notch of the left lung.

Inferior Surface (Diaphragmatic Surface) of the Heart

It is also called "diaphragmatic surface" because it is related to diaphragm.

Boundaries

- It is separated from the sternocostal surface by the inferior border.
- It is separated from the base of the heart by the posterior part of the atrioventricular groove. This groove is also called "coronary sulcus".

Parts of the Heart forming this Surface

- Left ventricle forms the left 2/3rd of the surface.

- Right ventricle forms the right 1/3rd of the surface.
- Posterior interventricular groove lies between the right ventricle and left ventricle. This groove contains the anastomosis between the anterior and posterior inter-ventricular arteries and the middle cardiac vein.

Crux of the heart: It is the junction of the posterior interventricular groove with the posterior part of the atrioventricular groove.
Relations: Fibrous pericardium is adherent to the diaphragm. Diaphragm separates the pericardium from the fundus of the stomach and cardiac impression of the liver.

Left Surface of the Heart

It is formed by the left ventricle and at its upper end by the left auricle.

Relations

Pericardium and outside the pericardium the left phrenic nerve, and left pericardiaco-phrenic vessels are related.

Borders

Lower border:
- It is also called the inferior border.
- It separates the sternocostal surface form the diaphragmatic surface.
- Right marginal artery which is a branch of right coronary and right marginal vein which is a tributary of small cardiac vein lie along this border.

Right border:
- It is formed by the right atrium.
- It separates the base from the sternocostal surface.
- A shallow groove called sulcus terminalis lies along this border.

Relations

Right phrenic nerve and right pericardiaco-phrenic vessels lie between the pericardium and the mediastinal pleura.

Left border:
- It separates the sternocostal surface from the left surface of the heart.
- It extends from the left auricle to the apex of the heart. Greater part of it is formed by the left ventricle.

Relations

Left marginal artery. This may be accompanied by the left marginal vein which opens into the great cardiac vein.

RIGHT ATRIUM

External Features

- It is the venous chamber of the heart situated on its right side.
- It forms the right side of the sternocostal surface of the heart, right border of the heart and right 1/3rd of the base of the heart.
- Its upper end presents right auricle which covers the root of the ascending aorta and partly overlaps the infundibulum.
- Anterior part of the right atrioventricular groove separates it from the right ventricle and it contains the right coronary artery.

- Sulcus terminalis lies along the right border of the heart.

Relations

- *Anteriorly:* Pericardium, pleura and right lung.
- *Posteriorly and to the right:* Right pulmonary veins.
- *Posteriorly and to the left:* Left atrium separated by the interatrial septum.
- *Medially:* Root of the ascending aorta and pulmonary trunk.
- *Laterally:* Pericardium and right phrenic nerve and pericardiacophrenic vessels lie between the pericardium and the mediastinal pleura.

Interior of the Right Atrium

- Interior of the right atrium is divided into two parts by the crista terminalis (Fig. 4.16).
- Crista terminalis is a smooth muscular ridge which extends from the opening of superior vena cava superiorly to the opening of inferior vena cava inferiorly. It separates the posterior smooth part of right atrium from the rough and ridged anterior part.

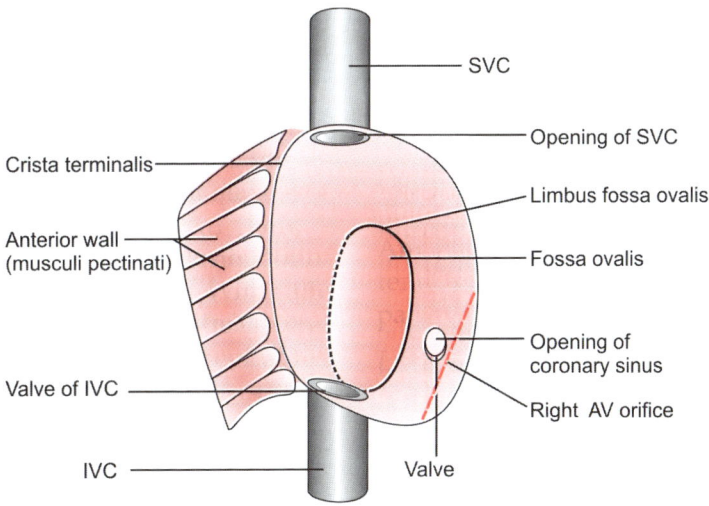

Fig. 4.16: Interior of right atrium

- Anterior part is rough because of musculi pectinati. These are parallel muscle ridges which extend from the crista terminalis to the right atrioventricular opening. This part is developed from the primitive atrium.
- Posterior part is smooth and is developed from the absorbed part of right horn of sinus venosus. It is called "sinus venarum". All veins open into sinus venarum except anterior cardiac veins which open into rough part (atrium proper).

Veins opening into the right atrium are:
1. Superior vena cava.
2. Inferior vena cava.
3. Coronary sinus.
4. Venae cordis minimae.
5. Anterior cardiac veins.
   - Opening of superior vena cava lies in the posterosuperior part of the sinus venarum. It does not possess a valve.
   - Opening of inferior vena cava lies in the posteroinferior part of the sinus venarum. It is guarded by a rudimentary valve.
   - Coronary sinus opens between the opening of inferior vena cava and right atrioventicular orifice. It is guarded by an incomplete (thebesian) valve.
   - Foramina venarum minimarum are the small foramina present in the interatrial septum. Venae cordis minimiae (minute veins from the heart) open into the right atrium through these foramina venarum minimarum.
   - Anterior cardiac veins open into the right atrium proper (anterior to crista terminalis) through separate openings.

The septal wall of the right atrium:
- It has fossa ovalis (a depression superior and left of the opening of inferior vena cava) and a prominent margin of the fossa ovalis called "limbus fossa ovalis".
- Fossa ovalis represents the septum primum of embryonic heart.
- Limbus fossa ovalis represents the free margin of the septum secundum.
- *Triangle of Koch:*
  - It is a triangular area bounded by the opening of coronary sinus, right atrioventricular opening and tendon of Todaro (subendocardial ridge).
  - AV node is situated in this triangle.

APPLIED ANATOMY

Right auricle contains the irregular network of musculi pectinati. This might contribute to the formation of blood clots here. If they slip into the circulation, it might result in fatal pulmonary embolism.

Developmental defects of the interatrial septum result in atrial septal defects like the patent foramen ovale.

Right Ventricle

- This is the chamber which pumps deoxygenated blood into the lungs.
- It forms the sternocostal surface, inferior border and diaphragmatic surface.
- It is separated from the right atrium by the anterior atrioventricular groove which contains the right coronary artery.
- It is separated from the left ventricle by the anterior interventricular groove which contains the anterior interventricular branch of the left coronary artery and the great cardiac vein.
- On the diaphragmatic surface, it is separated from the left ventricle by the posterior interventricular groove which contains three structures:

1. The terminal part of the anterior interventricular artery.

2. The posterior interventricular artery and their anastomosis.
3. Middle cardiac vein.

Interior of the Right Ventricle

It is divided into two parts:
- Inflowing part.
- Outflowing part.

Inflowing Part

- It is the ventricle proper. It is designed to receive blood from the right atrium through right atrioventricular orifice. It has rough muscular ridges called "trabeculae carneae".
- It develops from the primitive ventricle of the tubular heart.
- Trabeculae carneae are made up of ridges, bridges and papillary muscles.
  - The ridges are elevations of myocardium.
  - The bridges are attached at their ends and the middle part is free. Good example of a bridge is the "septomarginal trabecula" (moderator band) which connects the interventricular septum with the anterior wall of the right ventricle.
  - The papillary muscles are the conical muscular projections which are attached at one end and free at the other end (3 in number—anterior, posterior and septal)
- The inflowing part consists of tricuspid valve complex which is made up of the following parts:
  1. Right atrioventricular orifice.
  2. Fibrous ring of the tricuspid valve.
  3. Three cusps of the tricuspid valve.
  4. Chordae tendineae.
  5. Papillary muscles.

Right Atrioventricular Orifice

It usually admits three fingers. It is set at an angle of 45 degrees with the sagittal plane. It is surrounded by a fibrous ring made up of collagenous tissue.

Cusps of the Tricuspid Valve

- They are three in number. Each cusp is formed as a duplication of endocardium enclosing connective tissue. The atrial surface of the cusp is smooth while the ventricular surface is rough. Their attached margin is attached to the ring of the tricuspid orifice. The free margin and the ventricular surface of the cusps receive the attachment of chordae tendinae (Fig. 4.17).

Chordae Tendinae

- These are endothelial covered collagenous threads. They connect the apex of the papillary muscle with the free margin and the ventricular surface of the cusp.

Papillary Muscles

- They are conical muscular projections. Usually they are three in number in right ventricle—the anterior, septal and the posterior.
- The anterior papillary muscle is attached to the sternocostal surface of the ventricle.
- The posterior papillary muscle is attached to the inferior surface of the ventricle.
- The septal papillary muscle is attached to the interventricular septum.

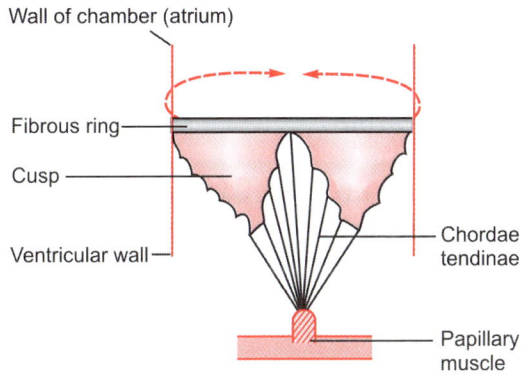

Fig. 4.17: Structure of atrioventricular valve

Note: Septomarginal trabecula: It connects the interventricular septum with the base of the anterior papillary muscle. It transmits the right branch of atrioventricular bundle.

Outflow Tract

- This part of the right ventricle is smooth.
- It is separated from the inflow tract by a smooth muscular ridge called "supraventricular crest". It is situated between the tricuspid and pulmonary orifices.
- The upper end of this part gives rise to the pulmonary trunk which is guarded by a "pulmonary valve". Pulmonary valve has three cusps.
- Outflow tract is called "conus arteriosus" or infundibulum.
- Smooth wall of the conus arteriosus increases the velocity of blood flow from the ventricle.
- The wall of the right ventricle is thinner than the wall of the left ventricle by three times. That is, the wall of the left ventricle is three times thicker than that of right ventricle. In cross section, wall of the right ventricle appears semilunar (cresentic).

CLINICAL ANATOMY

Developmental defects of the interventricular septum result in ventricular septal defects which may be isolated or may occur in collaboration with other defects as seen in cases of tetralogy of Fallot.

LEFT ATRIUM

- It receives oxygenated blood from the lung through pulmonary veins.
- Four pulmonary veins, two from each lung open into the left atrium.
- It forms the base of the heart.
- It forms the anterior wall of the oblique sinus of the pericardium.

- It has a conical muscular projection called "left auricle" which skirts the left margin of the pulmonary trunk.
- Anterior and to the right of the left atrium, right atrium is situated.
- It is connected to the left ventricle through bicuspid orifice.

Interior of the Left Atrium

- Musculi pectinati are found only in the region of left auricle.
- The remaining part of the interior is smooth. The smooth part is developed from the absorbed pulmonary veins.
- Only small anterior part including left auricle is developed from the left half of the primitive atrium.
- The septal wall of the left atrium presents a lunate impression which is formed by the septum secundum.
- The lower margin of the lunate fossa is bounded by a concave semilunar fold (concave upwards) which represents the upper margin of septum primum.
- Foramina venarum minimarum are found in the septal wall.

APPLIED ANATOMY

Thrombi (blood clots) may be formed in the left auricle. If they are dislodged into circulation, it might result in cerebral or renal embolism.

Left Ventricle

- It is the thickest chamber of the heart.
- It receives the oxygenated blood from the left atrium through the bicuspid orifice.
- It pumps the blood into ascending aorta.
- The contraction of the left ventricle generates the systolic blood pressure.
- Its wall is three times thicker than that of right ventricle.

- It forms the sternocostal surface, left surface, diaphragmatic surface and the apex of the heart.

Interior of the Left Ventricle

It is divided into two parts:
1. Inflow tract.
2. Outflow tract.

Inflow Tract

It is the left ventricle proper and is developed from the left part of the primitive ventricle. It consists of the following:
1. Trabeculae carneae.
2. Mitral valve complex.

Mitral valve complex has the following parts:
1. Left atrioventricular orifice.
2. Fibrous ring of the orifice.
3. Two cusps (leaflets) of the mitral valve.
4. Chordae tendineae.
5. Papillary muscles.

Left atrioventricular orifice admits the tips of two fingers. It connects the left atrium with the left ventricle. It is guarded by two cusps. Therefore, it is called as "bicuspid orifice" or "mitral valve".
- Cusps of the mitral valve are two in number:
  1. Anterior.
  2. Posterior (hence, bicuspid).
     - Anterior cusp is attached to the anteromedial part of the fibrous ring and it separates the aortic vestibule from the bicuspid orifice.
     - Posterior cusp is attached to postero-lateral part of fibrous ring.

There are two papillary muscles:
1. Anterior.
2. Posterior.
   - Anterior papillary muscle is attached to the sternocostal surface.
   - Posterior papillary muscle is attached to the diaphragmatic surface.

Chordae tendineae of both the muscles are attached to both the cusps of the mitral valve.

Outflow Tract

- It is smooth and is known as "aortic vestibule".
- It is mostly fibrous.
- The top of the vestibule has the aortic valve with three cusps.
- Ascending aorta begins here.
- Aortic valve opens during left ventricular systole and closes during the ventricular diastole.
- Bicuspid valve opens during ventricular diastole and closes during ventricular systole.

Note:

First heart sound: This is generated by the closure of the tricuspid and mitral valves.

Second heart sound: This is generated by the closure of the aortic and pulmonary valves.

Semilunar Valves

- Aortic and pulmonary valves are called semilunar valves. They are similar to each other (Fig. 4.18).
- Their cusps are semilunar in shape. Each valve has three cusps. The cusp forms a small pocket which is open superiorly away from the ventricular cavity. Opposite the cusps the vessels are slightly dilated to form aortic and pulmonary sinuses.

CLINICAL ANATOMY

Any of the valves mentioned may be affected by narrowing (stenosis) or incompetence (regurgitation). Stenosis causes impedance in passage of blood through the orifice while incompetence causes regurgitation of blood. Both stenosis and incompetence cause abnormal murmurs (sounds) on auscultation with a stethoscope.

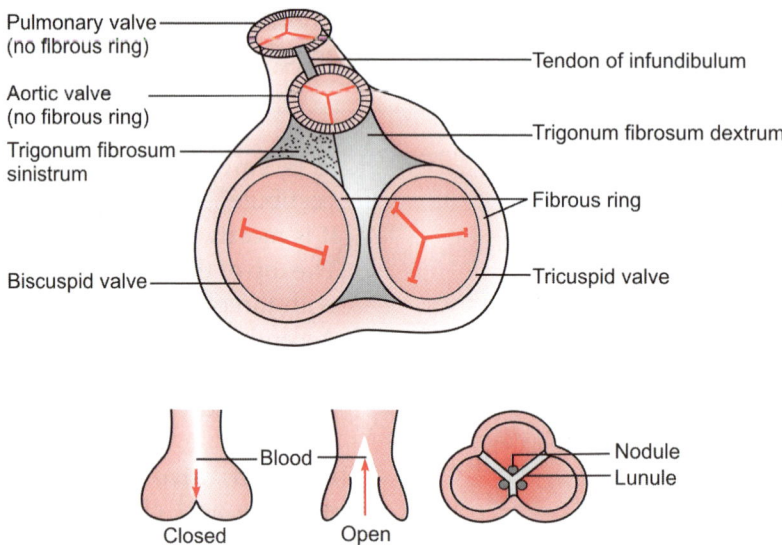

Fig. 4.18: Semilunar valves

- Depending on the valve involved we may have the following possibilities:

Mitral valve	Mitral stenosis	Mitral regurgitation
Tricuspid valve	Tricuspid stenosis	Tricuspid regurgitation
Aortic valve	Aortic stenosis	Aortic regurgitation
Pulmonary valve	Pulmonary stenosis	Pulmonary regurgitation

Surface Marking of the Heart

- Employing two points and joining them marks the upper border. The two points are as follows:
  1. A point at the lower border of the 2nd left costal cartilage about 1/2 inch from the sternal margin.
  2. A point at the upper border of the 3rd right costal cartilage about 1/2 inch from the sternal margin.

- Employing two points and joining them marks the lower border. The two points are as follows:

  1. A point at the lower border of the 6th right costal cartilage 2 cm from the sternal margin.
  2. A point at the apex of the heart in the left 5th intercostal space 9 cm from the midsternal line.

- The right border is marked by joining the right ends of the upper and lower borders with the maximum convexity at the level of 4th space (about 3.8 cm from the median plane).

- A convex line connecting the left ends of the upper and lower borders marks the left border.

Precordium is the area of the chest wall covering the heart.

Surface Marking of the Cardiac Valves

1. *Pulmonary valve:* Behind the 3rd left chondrosternal junction (3rd cartilage).
2. *Aortic valve:* Behind the left half of the sternum at the level of 3rd space.
3. *Mitral valve:* Behind the middle of the sternum at the level of 4th costal cartilage.

4. *Tricuspid valve:* Behind the right half of the sternum at the level of 4th space.

Auscultatory Areas of the Valves

All the valves are packed behind the level of sternum. Therefore, if a stethoscope is placed over the sternum, sounds of different valves are not clear. To hear the closure of valve clearly stethoscope is placed on the chest wall some distance from the valve in the direction of blood flow through it.

The auscultatory areas of different valves are as follows (Fig. 4.19):
1. *Pulmonary valve:* Second left intercostal space near the sternum.
2. *Aortic valve:* Second right cartilage or intercostal space near the sternum.
3. *Mitral valve:* Cardiac apex.
4. *Tricuspid valve:* Lower end of the sternum near left 5th intercostal space.

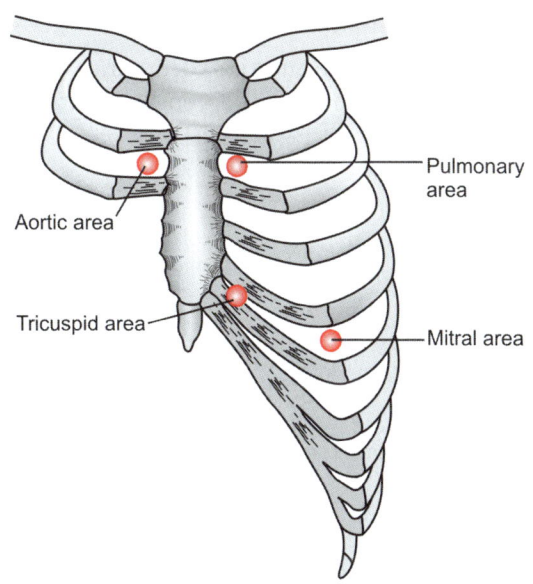

Fig. 4.19: Auscultatory areas for heart valves

Conducting System of the Heart

Specialised myocardial cells constitute the conducting system. They are specialised for the generation and conduction of cardiac impulse. The conducting system has the following parts (Fig. 4.20):
1. Sinuatrial node (SA node).
2. Atrioventricular node (AV node).
3. Atrioventricular bundle (AV bundle or bundle of His).
4. Right branch of AV bundle.
5. Left branch of AV bundle.
6. The Purkinje fibres.

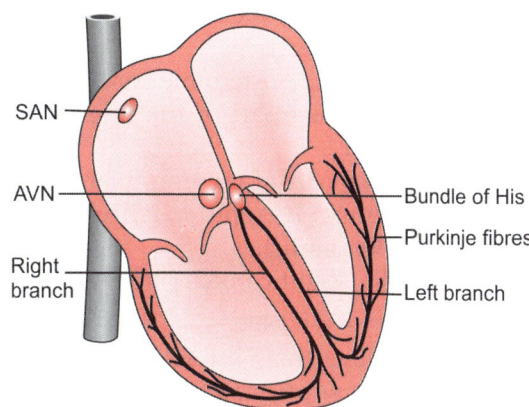

Fig. 4.20: Conducting system of the heart

SA Node

- This is situated at the upper end of the sulcus terminalis where the superior vena cava opens into the right atrium.
- It generates impulses at the rate of 70/min.
- It is known as the "pacemaker" of the heart.
- Right coronary artery supplies it by a SA nodal artery, but sometimes a branch of left coronary artery may supply it.
- Impulses travel through atrial wall to reach AV node.

AV Node

- It is situated in the triangle of Koch in the atrial septum just above the opening of coronary sinus.
- It is smaller than the SA node.
- It generates impulses at the rate of 60/min.
- An AV nodal artery, branch of posterior interventricular artery, usually supplies it. This posterior interventricular artery is usually a branch of right coronary artery; in a few cases it may be a branch of left coronary artery.

AV Bundle

- It is the only muscular connection between the atrium and the ventricle, otherwise the fibrous skeleton of the heart separates the atria from the ventricle.
- It runs along the posteroinferior border of the membranous part of the interventricular septum.
- At the upper part of the muscular part of the interventricular septum, it divides into right and left branches.
- *Blood supply:* Right coronary artery.

Right branch of AV bundle:
- It passes along the right side of the interventricular septum. Part of it passes through the septomarginal trabecula and reaches the anterior wall of right ventricle.
- It divides into terminal Purkinje fibres.
- *Blood supply:* Right coronary artery.

Left branch of AV bundle
- It descends on the left side of the interventricular septum.
- It supplies the left ventricle after dividing into teminal Purkinje fibres.
- *Blood supply:* Greater part of it is supplied by the anterior interventricular branch of left coronary. Part of it is supplied by right coronary artery.

Note: Whole of conducting system is usually supplied by right coronary artery except part of left branch of AV bundle which is supplied by left coronary artery.

Arterial Supply of the Heart

The heart is supplied by two coronary arteries:
1. Right coronary artery (Fig. 4.21).
2. Left coronary artery.

Note: Blood flows in coronary arteries during diastole of the heart.

Right Coronary Artery

- It arises from the anterior aortic sinus (after rotation of heart) of the ascending aorta (or

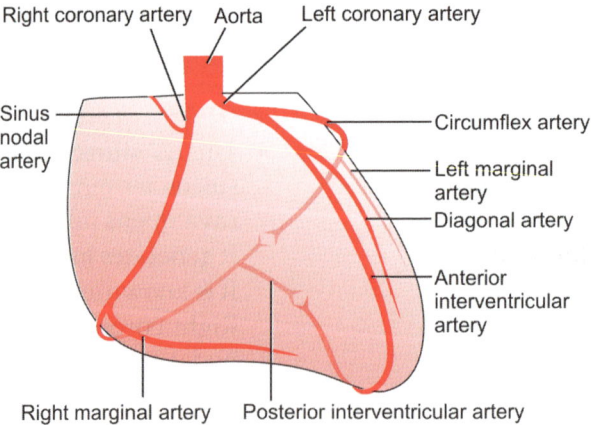

Right coronary artery   Aorta   Left coronary artery

Sinus nodal artery

Circumflex artery

Left marginal artery

Diagonal artery

Anterior interventricular artery

Right marginal artery   Posterior interventricular artery

Fig. 4.21: Arteries supplying the heart

right aortic sinus based on embryological origin before rotation).

- It runs downwards between the right auricle and the pulmonary trunk.
- It runs in the right anterior atrioventricular groove between the right atrium and right ventricle.
- It winds round the inferior border of the heart, passes upwards in the posterior part of the atrioventricular groove to reach the crux of the heart.

Branches

1. Branch to SA node.
2. Conus artery supplying the infundibulum (right conus artery).
3. Branches to right atrium.
4. Branches to right ventricle.
5. Marginal artery.
6. Posterior interventricular artery (it gives a branch to AV node).

Left Coronary Artery

- It arises from the left posterior aortic sinus (after rotation of heart) of the ascending aorta (or left aortic sinus based on embryological origin before rotation).
- It is wider branch and supplies larger volume of the myocardium.
- The trunk passes behind the pulmonary trunk and then appears between the pulmonary trunk and left auricle. Here it divides into two branches.
  1. Anterior interventricular artery.
  2. Circumflex artery.

Anterior interventricular artery descends along the anterior interventricular groove accompanied by great cardiac vein.

- It winds round the inferior border and continues on the diaphragmatic surface.
- It anastomoses with the posterior interventricular branch of right coronary artery along the posterior interventricular sulcus.

- It supplies both the ventricles and IV septum. It gives a diagonal artery.

Circumflex Artery

- It winds round the left border of the heart and runs in the posterior atrioventricular groove (coronary sulcus).
- Near the crux of the heart it anastomoses with the right coronary artery

Branches

- Anterior and posterior ventricular branches supply the adjacent sides of the left ventricle.
- Left marginal artery is a large branch which runs along the left border of the heart. Occassionally, circumflex artery gives a branch to SA node.

Note:
- Posterior interventricular artery sometimes arises from the circumflex artery. If posterior ventricular artery is a branch of left coronary artery, it is called left dominant arterial supply to the heart.
- If posterior ventricular artery is a branch of right coronary artery, it is called "right dominance".
- If posterior interventricular arteries arise from both right and left coronary, it is called "balanced arterial supply".

Summary of Blood Supply of the Heart

- Right atrium and ventricle (right half of heart) mainly by right coronary artery.
- Left atrium and ventricle (left half of heart) mainly by left coronary artery.
- Small part of each ventricle supplied by opposite coronary artery.
- Interventricular septum—anterior 2/3rd by left coronary artery and posterior 1/3rd by right coronary artery.
- Whole of conducting system (right coronary artery) except part of left branch of AV bundle (left coronary artery).

Venous Drainage of the Heart

- About 60% of venous blood of the heart drains into the right atrium through coronary sinus (Fig. 4.22).
- The remaining 40% of blood drains into different chambers of heart through venae cordis minimae and anterior cardiac veins.

Coronary Sinus

- It is a wide venous channel of about 2 to 3 cm in length.
- It is situated in the coronary sulcus (posterior part).
- It begins in the left part of the atrio-ventricular groove where it receives great cardiac vein.
- Near the crux it receives the middle cardiac vein.
- Middle cardiac vein accompanies the posterior interventricular artery in the posterior interventricular sulcus.
- At its right end it receives the small cardiac vein.

Tributaries of the Coronary Sinus

- Great cardiac vein (which receives left marginal vein before opening into the left end of the coronary sinus).
- Posterior vein of the left ventricle.
- Oblique vein of the left atrium.
- Middle cardiac vein.
- Small cardiac vein (which receives right marginal vein before opening into the right end of the coronary sinus).
- Coronary sinus opens into the right atrium.

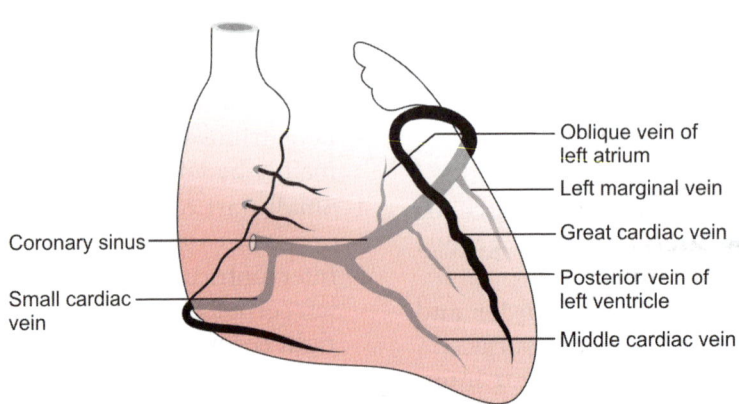

Fig. 4.22: Veins draining the heart

• Coronary sinus is developed from the left horn and body of the sinus venosus.

Nerve Supply of the Heart

Cardiac plexuses supply the heart. Cardiac plexuses are divided into two (Figs 4.23 to 4.25):

1. Superficial cardiac plexus.
2. Deep cardiac plexus.

Both sympathetic and parasympathetic contribute to the formation of cardiac plexus.

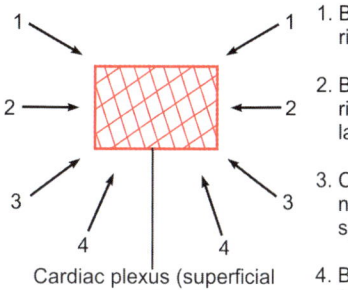

1. Branches from right and left vagus
2. Branches from right and left recurrent laryngeal nerves
3. Cardiac (branches) nerves from cervical sympathetic ganglia
4. Branches from upper four thoracic ganglia

Cardiac plexus (superficial and deep)

Fig. 4.25: Formation of cardiac plexus

Sympathetic Nerves

• Increase the heart rate and cardiac output, produce vasodilatation of the intramuscular branches of coronary arteries.
• They are derived from lateral horns of T1 to T5 segments of spinal cord.
• Pain fibres pass through sympathetic nerves and reach T1 to T5 segments through dorsal root ganglia.

Parasympathetic Fibers

• Reach the cardiac plexus through vagus nerves.
• Postganglionic neurons are situated in the cardiac plexus.
• They decrease the heart rate.

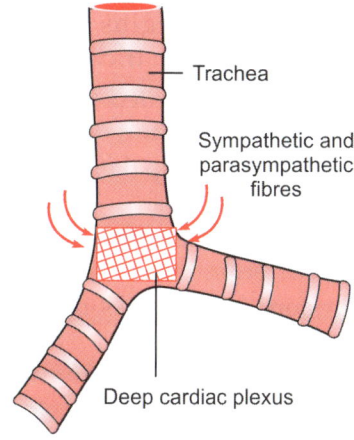

Trachea

Sympathetic and parasympathetic fibres

Deep cardiac plexus

Fig. 4.23: Deep cardiac plexus

Superficial Cardiac Plexus

• It is situated below the arch of aorta.
• It is formed by a branch of left superior cervical sympathetic ganglion (sympathetic) and an inferior cervical cardiac branch (lower of the 2) of left vagus nerve (parasympathetic).
• It gives branches to deep cardiac plexus and right coronary artery.

Deep Cardiac Plexus

• It is situated in front of the bifurcation of trachea.

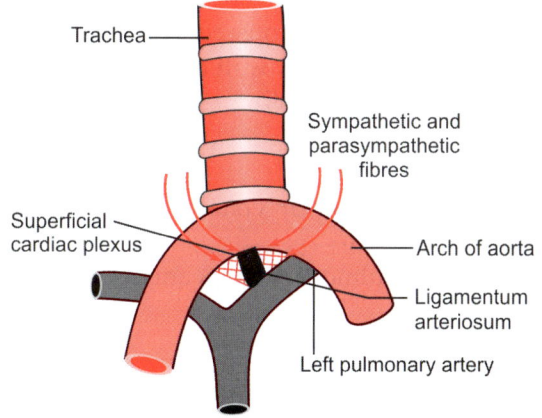

Trachea

Sympathetic and parasympathetic fibres

Superficial cardiac plexus

Arch of aorta

Ligamentum arteriosum

Left pulmonary artery

Fig. 4.24: Superficial cardiac plexus

- It is formed by all the cardiac branches (3) of cervical and upper thoracic ganglia of the sympathetic chains and the cardiac branches (2) of vagus of both sides except those which supply the superficial cardiac plexus.

- Right half supplies the right coronary artery and left coronary artery and left half supplies the left coronary artery.

Superior Vena Cava

- It drains the venous blood from the upper part of the body into the right atrium (Fig. 4.26).
- It has no valves.
- It begins by the union of right brachiocephalic vein with the left brachiocephalic vein behind the lower border of the first right costal cartilage.
- It pierces the fibrous pericardium behind the right second costal cartilage.
- Just before piercing the fibrous pericardium it receives azygos vein.
- It opens into the right atrium behind the third right costal cartilage.

Relations

- *Anterior:* Right internal thoracic vessels, anterior margin of the right lung and pleura.
- *Posterior* (behind): Root of the right lung.
- *Medially:* Ascending aorta, brachiocephalic artery.
- *Laterally:* Right phrenic nerve and pericardiophrenic vessels, right lung and pleura.

Tributaries

- Azygos vein arches over the root of the right lung and opens into the suprior vena cava.

- If superior vena cava is obstructed above the level of azygos vein, blood returns to the right atrium through collateral vessels reaching the azygos vein and IVC.
- If superior vena cava is obstructed below the level of azygos vein, blood has to return to the right atrium through inferior vena cava.

Ascending Aorta

- This large trunk begins in the aortic vestibule of the left ventricle.
- The beginning is guarded by aortic valve which has three cusps.
- At the level of each cusp there is a dilatation called aortic sinus.
- There are three aortic sinuses—one anterior and two posterior.
- Anterior aortic sinus gives right coronary artery.
- Left posterior aortic sinus gives origin to left coronary artery.
- Right posterior aortic sinus is often called "non-coronary sinus" as it does not give coronary artery.
- It is 5 cm in length.
- It lies inside the fibrous pericardium.
- It forms the anterior wall of the transverse sinus of the pericardium.

Relations

To the right: Superior vena cava and right atrium (Fig. 4.26).

To the left: Pulmonary trunk and left atrium.

Arch of Aorta

- It begins at the sternal angle at the level of lower border of 4th thoracic vertebra and terminates at the same level.

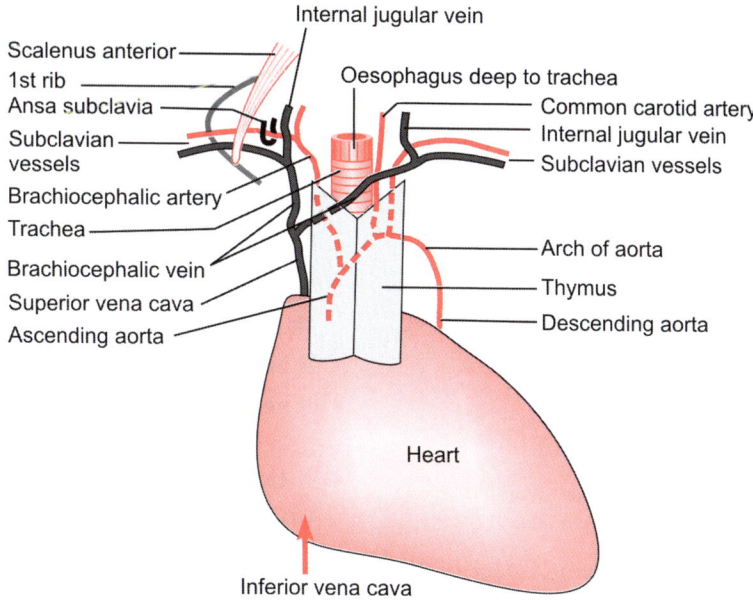

Fig. 4.26: Structures in superior mediastinum

- It is the continuation of ascending aorta and it continues as descending thoracic aorta (Fig. 4.26).
- It lies in the superior mediastinum

Relations

Anterior and to the left:
Four structures:
1. Left phrenic nerve.
2. Left vagus.
3. Left lung and pleura.
4. Left superior intercostal vein.

Posterior and to the right:
Four important structures:
1. Trachea with deep cardiac plexus.
2. Oesophagus.
3. Left recurrent laryngeal nerve.
4. Thoracic duct.

Superior:
Four structures:
1. Brachiocephalic.
2. Left common carotid.
3. Left subclavian.
4. Occasional thyroidea ima (all the above are the branches of arch of aorta).

Inferior:
Four structures:
1. Bifurcation of pulmonary trunk.
2. Left bronchus.
3. Ligamentum arteriosum with superficial cardiac plexus.
4. Left recurrent layngeal nerve.

Branches: Four (mentioned above under superior relations) namely brachiocephalic, left common carotid, left subclavian and occasional thyroidea ima artery.

COARCTATION OF AORTA

- It is the narrowing of arch of aorta mostly due to the extension of fibrosis of ligamentum arteriosum. An extensive collateral circulation is established between the branches of subclavian artery and descending thoracic aorta.
- The enlarged collateral vessels notch the ribs which is evident in X-rays.
- The shadow of arch of aorta seen in X-ray is called "aortic knuckle".

Descending Thoracic Aorta

- It is the continuation of the arch of aorta (Fig. 4.26).
- It begins at the level of lower border of 4th thoracic vertebra and continues as abdominal aorta at the level of 12th thoracic vertebra.
- It descends on the left side of the vertebral column with a slight inclination to the right.

Relations

- *Anterior:* Root of the left lung, pericardium and heart.
- *Posterior:* Vertebral column, hemiazygos veins.
- *To the right side:* Azygos vein, Thoracic duct, Right lung and pleura.
- To the left side: left lung and its pleura.

Note: Oesophagus is related to its right side in its upper part but it lies in front of aorta in the lower part.

Branches

- Nine paired posterior intercostal arteries for 3rd to 11th intercostal spaces.

- Right and left subcostal arteries.
- Two left bronchial arteries.
- Oesophageal branches.
- Pericardial branches.
- Mediastinal branches.
- Superior phrenic arteries to the diaphragm.

TRACHEA

- It is the tube which carries air to the lungs.
- Its wall is partly made up of cartilages, therefore, it is not completely collapsible.
- It is about 6 inches long.
- It lies both in the lower part of the neck and in superior mediastinum (Fig. 4.26).
- It begins at the lower end of the cricoid cartilage that corresponds to the level of 6th cervical vertebra.
- It terminates at the level of T5 vertebra (or lower border of T4).
- It divides into right and left principal bronchi at its bifurcation.
- Right bronchus is wide and is in line with the trachea while the left bronchus is at an angle and is narrow.
- It lies in the median plane except its terminal part which deviates slightly to the right side.
- In the living the bifurcation extends to a lower level (6th thoracic vertebral level).
- It has 16 to 20 C-shaped hyaline cartilaginous rings. They cover the tube anteriorly and the posterior part of the tube contains transversely arranged smooth muscle. It is called "trachealis". The trachealis muscle helps to alter the size of the lumen of trachea.

Relations of the Thoracic Part

Anterior contents of the superior mediastinum are related in front.

Anteriorly

- Manubrium sterni.
- *Two muscles:* Sternothyroid and sternohyoid.
- *Two veins:* Left brachiocephalic vein and inferior thyroid vein.
- *Two arteries:* Aortic arch and brachiocephalic artery.
- *Two other structures:* Remains of thymus and deep cardiac plexus.

Posteriorly

Two structures: Oesophagus and vertebral column.

Right side:
Four structures:
1. Right lung.
2. Right pleura.
3. Right vagus.
4. Azygos vein.

Left side:
Four structures:
1. Arch of aorta.
2. Left common carotid.
3. Left subclavian artery.
4. Left recurrent laryngeal nerve.
- *Arterial supply:* Inferior thyroid artery.
- Venous drainage into the left brachiocephalic vein.
- *Lymphatic drainage:* Drained into the pretracheal and paratracheal lymph nodes.
- *Nerve supply:*
  - Parasympathetic nerves come from recurrent laryngeal nerve which is a branch of vagus nerve.
  - Sympathetic nerves come from middle cervical sympathetic ganglia which reach trachea along the inferior thyroid artery.

OESOPHAGUS

- It is a muscular tube which carries food bolus to the stomach.
- It begins at the level of cricoid cartilage that corresponds to the level of C6 vertebra.
- It is 10 inches long.
- It runs downwards in the superior and posterior mediastinum and pierces the diaphragm at the level of T10 vertebra (Fig. 4.26).
- It opens into the stomach in the abdomen at the level of T11 vertebra.

Curvatures

- There are two lateral curvatures both to the left.
- One in the lower part of the neck which is directed towards the left.
- In the upper part of thorax it regains its median position but again deviates to the left near the lower end.
- It has anteroposterior curvatures corresponding to the anteroposterior curvature of the vertebral column in the cervicothoracic region.

Constrictions

It has four constrictions:
1. The first constriction is at its beginning and it is 6 inches from incisor teeth.
2. The second constriction corresponds to the crossing of arch of aorta and it lies about 9 inches from the incisor teeth.
3. The third constriction corresponds to the crossing of left bronchus in front of the oesophagus and it lies about 11 inches from the incisor teeth.
4. The fourth constriction corresponds to its passage through the diaphragm and it lies about 15 inches from incisor teeth.

These constrictions and their distance from the incisor teeth are very important clinically while passing tube into stomach.

Relations of the thoracic part of the oesophagus:

Anterior: Three important relations to be remembered are:

1. Trachea.
2. Left bronchus (which causes constriction of oesophagus).
3. Left atrium separated by the pericardium (The enlargement of the left atrium in mitral stenosis causes swallowing difficulty).

Posterior: Three important relations to be remembered are:

1. Right posterior intercostal arteries which cross from left to right behind the oesophagus.
2. Thoracic duct which crosses at the level of T5 vertebra from right to left side behind the oesophagus.
3. Terminal parts of the superior and inferior hemiazygos veins which cross from left to right to open into the azygos vein on the right side (of course vertebral column lies posterior to the oesophagus).

To the left: Three important relations to be remembered are:

1. Aortic arch which causes a constriction of the oesophagus.
2. Thoracic duct which lies on the left side of oesophagus in the superior mediastinum after crossing behind the oesophagus at the level of T5 vertebra.
3. The left recurrent laryngeal nerve which hooks around the arch of aorta and runs into the left side of the groove between the trachea and oesophagus (of course left lung and left pleura relation is evident).

To the right:

1. Right lung and pleura.
2. Azygos vein.

Arterial Supply

- Inferior thyroid artery supplies the cervical part.
- Oesophageal branches of thoracic aorta supply the thoracic part.
- Oesophageal branches of the left gastric artery supplies the abdominal part.

Venous Drainage

- Upper part of oesophagus drains into the brachiocephalic vein.
- Middle part drains into azygos veins.
- Lower end of the oesophagus drains into the left gastric vein.

APPLIED ANATOMY

- Left gastric vein is a tributary of the portal vein. Its tributaries communicate with the tributaries of the azygos veins in the wall of the lower end of the oesophagus. In portal hypertension, due to the back pressure, this communication enlarges causing oesophageal varices. These may burst into the lumen of the oesophagus resulting in haematemesis (vomiting of the blood).
- In left atrial enlargement oesophagus is compressed.
- In mediastinal syndrome, oesophagus is compressed.
- Oesophageal cancer causes difficulty in swallowing (dysphagia).

THORACIC DUCT

- It is the largest lymphatic vessel in the body (Fig. 4.8).
- It is 18 inches long.
- It has beaded appearance because of valves present in it.

- It receives lymph from both sides of the lower half of the body below the level of diaphragm, from the left half of the body above the level of the diaphragm.
- It begins in the abdomen at the upper end of the cisterna chyli (a lymphatic sac in the abdomen opposite upper lumbar vertebrae on the right side).
- It passes through the aortic opening at the level of T12 vertebra.
- It lies in the aortic opening between the aorta on the left side and azygos vein on the right side.
- It ascends in the posterior mediastinum on the right side till the level of T5 vertebra.
- It crosses from right to left side at the level of T5 vertebra.
- Then it ascends in the superior mediastinum on the left side of the oesophagus.
- It reaches the neck through the posterior part of the thoracic inlet and it opens into the junction of left internal jugular vein with the left subclavian vein.

Relations

At the aortic opening:
- *Anterior:* Median arcuate ligament of diaphragm.
- *Posterior:* Body of T12 vertebra.
- *Right:* Azygos vein.
- *Left:* Aorta.

In the posterior mediastinum:
- *Anterior:* Oesophagus lies in front of it.
- *Behind:*
  - Thoracic vertebrae.
  - Terminal parts of superior and inferior hemiazygos veins.
  - Right posterior intercostal arteries.
- *To the right:* Azygos vein.
- *To the left:* Descending thoracic aorta.

In the superior mediastinum:
- *To the right:* Oesophagus.
- *To the left:* Left lung and pleura.
- *Posterior:* Vertebral column.

Tributaries:
- Intercostal nodes.
- Posterior mediastinal lymph nodes.
- Before opening it receives subclavian lymph trunk from the left upper limb and left jugular lymph trunk from the left side of neck.
- Receives lymph from both sides of body below diaphragm and from left side of body above diaphragm.

THORACIC SYMPATHETIC TRUNK

- It is situated on either side of the vertebral column (Fig. 4.27).
- It is a ganglionated trunk (having ganglia).
- Superiorly, it is continuous with the cervical trunk and inferiorly, it is continuous with the lumbar trunk.
- Though we expect 12 thoracic sympathetic ganglia, one for each thoracic nerve, usually only 10 to 11 ganglia are seen because of fusion of ganglia.
- The thoracic trunk crosses in front of the neck of the first rib. Then the sympathetic chain lies in front of the heads of the ribs from 2nd rib to 10th rib and then in front of bodies of T11 and T12 vertebrae.
- It then passes behind the medial arcuate ligament of diaphragm and becomes continuous with the lumbar sympathetic trunk.
- The first thoracic ganglion is frequently fused with inferior cervical ganglion to form stellate ganglion.

Branches

Its branches are divided into lateral and medial branches.

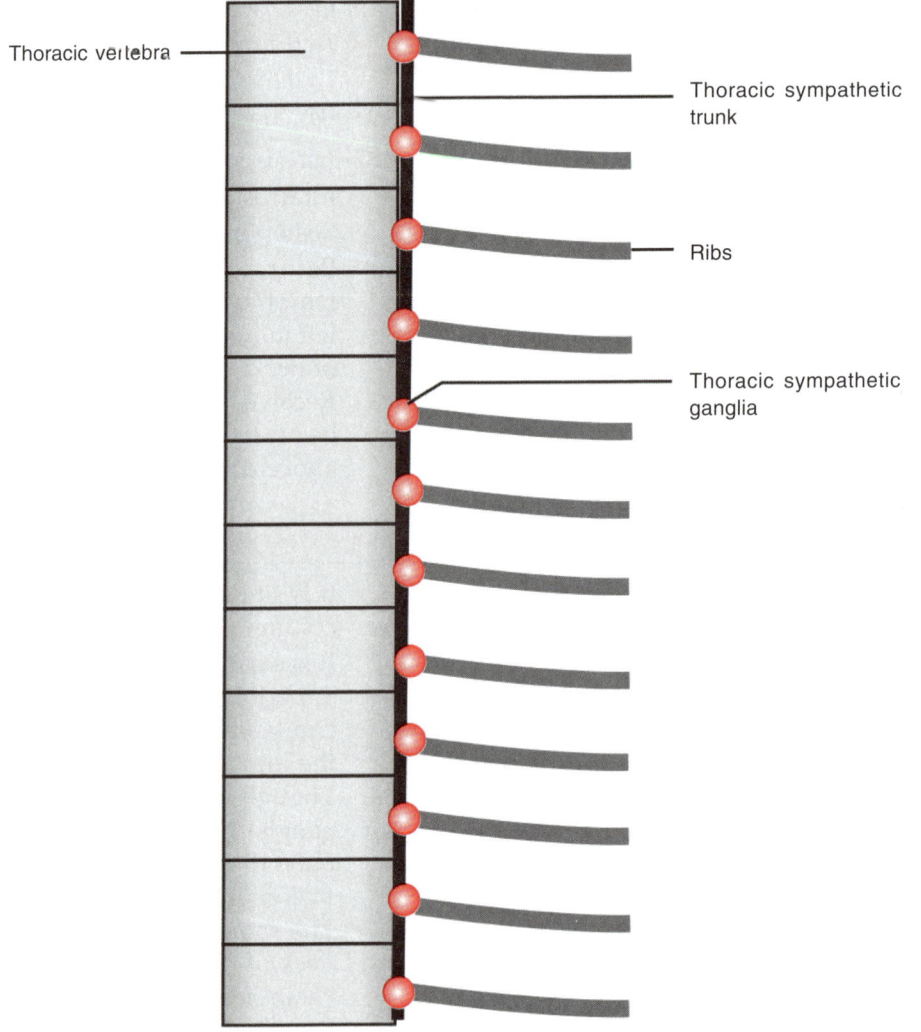

Fig. 4.27: Thoracic sympathetic trunk

- *Lateral branches* (for limbs and body wall): These branches join the corresponding spinal nerves through grey rami communicantes and are distributed along the spinal nerves. They receive white rami communicantes from the spinal nerve which are preganglionic fibres from the thoracic segments of the spinal cord.

- *Medial branches* (for viscera): Medial branches of the upper five ganglia supply structures in the thorax through plexuses.
  - Pulmonary branches to the pulmonary plexus.
  - Cardiac branches to the deep cardiac plexus.
  - Aortic branches to the aortic plexus.

– Oesophageal branches to the oeso-phageal plexus.

Medial branches from the lower seven ganglia form three splanchnic nerves which supply the visceral organs of the abdomen.

1. *Greater splanchnic nerve:* Formed by the branches of T5 to T9 ganglia.
2. *Lesser splanchnic nerve:* Formed by the branches of T10 and T11 ganglia.
3. *Least splanchnic nerve:* Formed by the branches of T12 ganglia.

Abdomen

5

Anterior Wall of the Abdomen

- Anterior wall of the abdomen extends from the costal margin to the pelvis (Fig. 5.1).
- Umbilicus is an important landmark on the anterior wall.
- However, the superior limit of the abdominal cavity is formed by the diaphragm which extends as high as 5th rib.

- Anterior wall is normally soft to palpate. It becomes rigid because of reflex contraction of muscles of the anterior abdominal wall when there is some pathology inside the abdominal cavity. This reflex contraction is called "guarding".

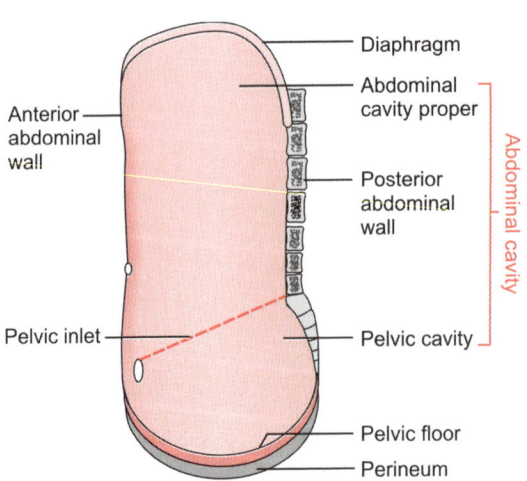

Fig. 5.1: Abdominopelvic cavity

- When a cold hand or object is kept on the anterior wall, it makes the abdominal wall muscles reflexly contract. That is the reason why abdomen is palpated very gently with the knees and hip being semiflexed. This position keeps the abdominal wall muscles relaxed.

- Whenever abdominal incisions are made, due care should be given to the Langer's lines. Langer's lines are usually horizontal in the anterior wall of the abdomen. Any incision perpendicular to the Langer's lines leaves a large scar. Sometimes, it may lead to the development of keloids. When the abdominal wall is distended the skin may form reddish streaks initially. These are especially marked in a pregnant woman, called linea gravidarum. They may permanently remain as white streaks called linea albicantes.

- Superficial fascia of the anterior wall of the abdomen has two layers in lower part:
  - Superficial fatty layer (Camper's fascia), deep membranous layer (Scarpa's fascia).

- What is liposuction?
  - It is the suction of fat from the superficial fatty layer.

- Deep membranous layer is called Colles' fascia in the perineum.
- There is no demonstrable deep fascia in the anterior wall of the abdomen (extremely thin according to some). If there were to be

thick deep fascia, then women would not have conceived and next meal of ours would not have been a welcome thing.

Nerve supply of the anterior abdominal wall: (skin and musculature)
- Skin below xiphoid process is supplied by the anterior cutaneous branches of T7.
- Skin around the umbilicus is supplied by the anterior cutaneous branches of T10.
- Skin around the pubic symphysis is supplied by the branches of L1.
- Therefore, totally seven nerves, lower five intercostals, subcostal and L1 through iliohypogastric and ilioinguinal nerves supply the anterior abdominal wall.
- Iliohypogastric is at a higher level and ilioinguinal nerve is below it.
- Iliohypogastric and ilioinguinal nerves have the same root value L1.
- These same nerves also supply the 4 large muscles of the anterior abdominal wall. But the skin is supplied by their anterior cutaneous branches (of all 7 nerves) and lateral cutaneous branches (of T10, 11).

Arterial supply of the anterior abdominal wall:
Important superficial arteries which come from the femoral artery are:
1. Superficial epigastric.
2. Superficial circumflex iliac.

Important deep arteries are the following:
1. Superior epigastric.
2. Musculophrenic branches.
3. Lower posterior intercostal arteries.
4. Deep circumflex iliac artery.
5. Inferior epigastric.

Venous drainage of the anterior abdominal wall:
Superficial veins can be divided into two streams:
1. Above the level of umbilicus which eventually drains into the superior vena cava.

2. Below the level of umbilicus which eventually drains into the inferior vena cava.
Therefore, the umbilicus is known as the plane of venous water-shed.

Therefore, the veins of the anterior wall are enlarged when the superior or inferior vena cavae are occluded. During this enlargement, a new channel opens up which is often found connecting the superficial epigastric vein to the lateral thoracic vein. This communicating vein is called the "thoracoepigastric vein".

Lymphatic drainage of the anterior abdominal wall:
In the case of lymphatic drainage also there is umbilical water shed. Superficial lymph vessels go in two directions.
1. Above the level of umbilicus, lymph vessels mainly drain into axillary (anterior) group of lymph nodes.
2. Below the level of umbilicus, lymph vessels drain into the superficial inguinal group of lymph nodes mainly.

CLINICAL ANATOMY

Umbilical vessel catheterization
- May be performed in a newborn.
- Umbilical vessels are present in the Wharton's jelly of the umbilical cord.
- Umbilical artery catheterization may be done up to 6 days after delivery.
- Umbilical vein catheterization may be done up to 7 days after delivery.
- Both the procedures enable resuscitation by administration of fluids or blood.

Quadrants of the anterior abdominal wall
- It is divided into four quadrants by the transumbilical and median plane (Fig. 5.3).
- They are right upper quadrant, left upper quadrant, right lower quadrant and left lower quadrant.

Nine regions of the anterior abdominal wall

Two vertical and two horizontal planes are employed:

- Vertical planes are: midclavicular planes (right and left).
- Horizontal planes are:
  1. Subcostal plane
  2. Transtubercular plane.

Nine regions are (Fig. 5.2):

1. Right hypochondrium.
2. Left hypochondrium.
3. Epigastric (all these lie superior to the subcostal plane).
4. Right lumbar.
5. Left lumbar.
6. Umbilical (all these lie between the subcostal and transtubercular planes).
7. Right iliac (inguinal).
8. Left iliac (inguinal).
9. Hypogastric (all these lie inferior to the transtubercular plane).

CLINICAL POINTS

- Pain arising out of the foregut-derived structures is referred to the epigastric region. Therefore, the pain of the stomach is referred to the epigastric region.

- Pain arising out of the midgut-derived structures is referred to the umbilical region. Therefore, the pain of the appendix is referred to this region.
- Pain arising out of the hindgut-derived structures is referred to the hypogastric region. Therefore, the pain of the sigmoid colon is referred to this region.

ABDOMINAL INCISIONS

- Surgical incisions are made in anterior abdominal wall to gain access to abdomen and its contents (Fig. 5.4).
- The need for these incisions has reduced in some cases with advent of newer surgical techniques like laparoscopy.
  a. In laparoscopy small incisions or holes can be made.
  b. Endoscopes with cameras are inserted and instruments are employed to perform surgeries.
  c. It overcomes many drawbacks of a large surgical incision.
  d. Laparoscopic cholecystectomy (removal of gallbladder) and appendectomy (removal of appendix) are widely practised.

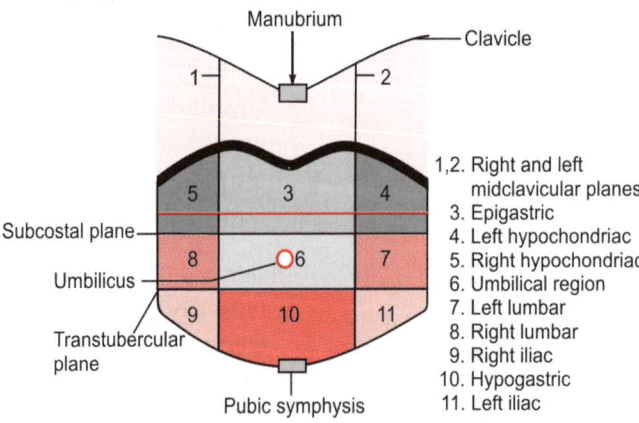

Fig. 5.2: Regions of anterior abdominal wall

Manubrium

Clavicle

Subcostal plane

Umbilicus

Transtubercular plane

Pubic symphysis

1,2. Right and left midclavicular planes
3. Epigastric
4. Left hypochondriac
5. Right hypochondriac
6. Umbilical region
7. Left lumbar
8. Right lumbar
9. Right iliac
10. Hypogastric
11. Left iliac

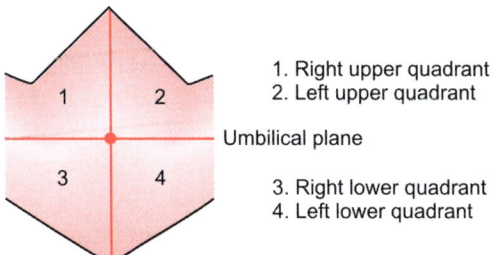

Fig. 5.3: Quadrants of anterior abdominal wall

1. Right upper quadrant
2. Left upper quadrant

Umbilical plane

3. Right lower quadrant
4. Left lower quadrant

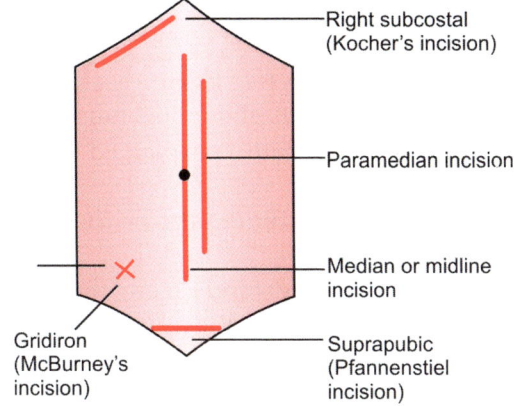

Right subcostal (Kocher's incision)

Paramedian incision

Median or midline incision

Gridiron (McBurney's incision)

Suprapubic (Pfannenstiel incision)

Fig. 5.4: Abdominal incisions

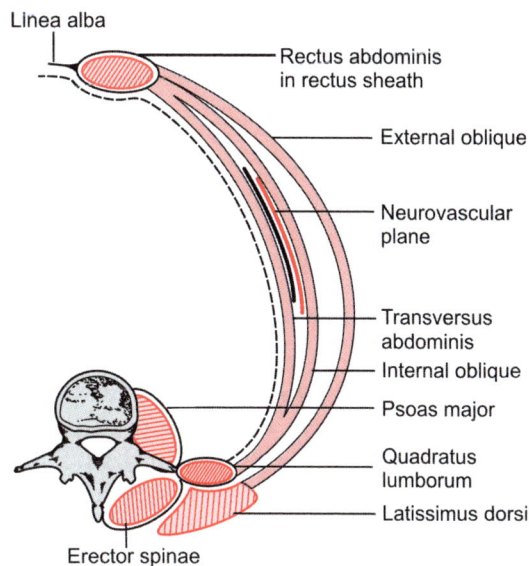

Linea alba

Rectus abdominis in rectus sheath

External oblique

Neurovascular plane

Transversus abdominis

Internal oblique

Psoas major

Quadratus lumborum

Latissimus dorsi

Erector spinae

Fig. 5.5: Muscles of anterior abdominal wall

Muscles of the anterior abdominal wall:
There are five muscles. Three flat muscles in the anterolateral part of the anterior abdominal wall are (Fig. 5.5):
1. External oblique abdominis.
2. Internal oblique abdominis.
3. Transversus abdominis.
    Two vertical muscles lie on the anterior aspect:
1. Rectus abdominis.
2. Pyramidalis.

External Oblique Abdominis

• It arises from 5th to 12th ribs.
• Fibers run downwards and medially and are inserted into the linea alba, pubic tubercle, anterior superior iliac spine and ventral part of the iliac crest. It forms the inguinal ligament between the pubic tubercle and anterior superior iliac spine (Fig. 5.6).
• Muscle fibers do not extend below the level of line connecting the anterior superior iliac spine to the umbilicus.
• *Nerve supply:* It is supplied by the lower 6 thoracic nerves.
• *Action:* While standing it acts at its origin and turns the trunk to the opposite side.
• It assists the opposite internus abdominis while rotating the trunk to the opposite side.

Internal Oblique Abdominis

• It arises from the anterior 2/3rd of iliac crest and lateral half of the inguinal ligament.
• It is expanded like a fan and is inserted into the lower ribs (10th to 12th), linea alba and lower fibers join the lower fibers of the transversus abdominis to form the conjoint tendon.

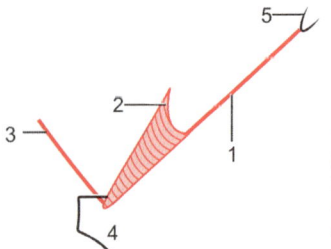

1. Inguinal ligament
2. Lacunar ligament
3. Reflected part
4. Pubic tubercle
5. Anterior superior iliac spine

Fig. 5.6: Parts of inguinal ligament (left side)

- *Action:* While standing, it acts at its insertion and turns the trunk to the same side. When both external and internal oblique muscles of the same side contract, the opposite rotation actions of these two muscles get cancelled and the trunk is bent to the same side. This is an example of synergic action.
- *Nerve supply:* Lower six thoracic nerves and L1 through ilioinguinal and iliohypogastric nerves.

Transversus Abdominis

- This muscle arises from inner aspect of costal cartilages (7th to 12th), from the thoracolumbar fascia and the inner lip of the iliac crest.
- It runs horizontally and is inserted into the linea alba and pubic crest. The lower fibers join the lower fibers of the internal oblique abdominis to form the conjoint tendon.
- *Nerve supply:* Lower six thoracic nerves and L1 through ilioinguinal and iliohypogastric nerves.
- *Action:* Its contraction increases the intraabdominal pressure and it protects the underlying viscera.

Note: When all three flat muscles contract, diaphragm relaxes. They relax when diaphragm contracts.

Neurovascular Plane

- This plane lies between the internal oblique abdominis and transversus abdominis muscles. This is comparable to the neurovascular plane of the intercostal spaces (Fig. 5.5).
- The neurovascular space of the anterior abdominal wall contains the lower intercostal nerves, lower intercostal arteries, iliohypogastric nerve, ilioinguinal nerve and deep circumflex iliac artery.

Rectus Sheath

- This is the connective tissue sheath which encloses the rectus abdominis muscle.
- Formation of sheath is explained at three levels (Fig. 5.7).
  - First level extends above the costal margin.
  - Second level extends from the costal margin to a point midway between the umbilicus and pubic symphysis.
  - Third level extends from the level of the point midway between the umbilicus and pubic symphysis to the lower end of the rectus abdominis.

First Level

- *Anteriorly:* The aponeurosis of external oblique abdominis.
- *Posteriorly:* It directly rests on the 5th, 6th and 7th costal cartilages and there is no aponeurosis here.

Second Level

- *Anteriorly:* It is covered by the aponeurosis of the external oblique and the anterior lamina of internal oblique muscle aponeurosis.
- *Posteriorly:* It is formed by the posterior lamina of the internal oblique aponeurosis and aponeurosis of the transversus abdominis.

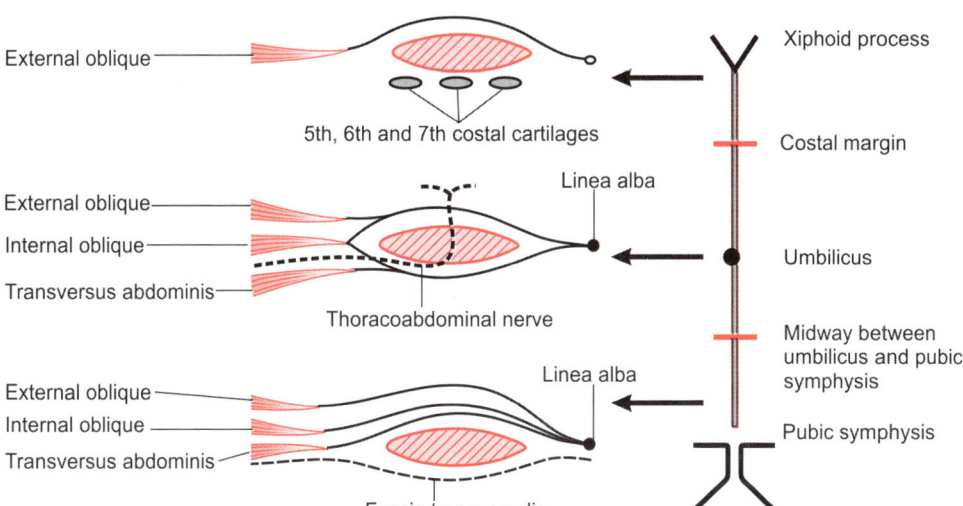

Fig. 5.7: Rectus sheath

Third Level
- *Anteriorly:* Aponeurosis of all 3 muscles.
- *Posteriorly:* Only fascia transversalis.

Contents
- 2 arteries (superior epigastric and inferior epigastric).
- 2 veins (superior epigastric and inferior epigastric).
- 2 muscles (rectus abdominis and pyramidalis).
- 6 nerves (terminal parts of lower six thoracic nerves).

Rectus Abdominis

- It arises below from the pubic crest and pubic symphysis.
- It is inserted into the 5th, 6th and 7th costal cartilages and xiphoid process.
- It has three tendinous intersections which bind the anterior surface of the muscle to the anterior wall of the rectus sheath.

- *Action:* It flexes the vertebral column. It helps to protect the anterior abdominal wall.
- *Nerve supply:* All the nerves which lie inside the rectus sheath supply it (lower six thoracic nerves).

Pyramidalis

- It arises with the rectus abdominis muscle from pubic crest.
- It lies in front of it and is inserted into the linea alba.
- It acts as a guide for the surgeon to identify the (midline) medial border of the rectus abdominis muscle.
- It is often absent.

CLINICAL POINTS

1. *Divarication of recti:* Due to the laxity of linea alba (may be due to previous surgical incisions or pregnancy), the two recti are widely separated by an interval and may predispose to hernia.

2. *Spigelian hernia:* Hernia just below the arcuate line, between rectus abdominis medially and linea semilunaris laterally. It lies within the muscles of the anterior abdominal wall and swelling may not be significant. Strangulation of herniated structures is very common in this type of hernia.

Action of all the main muscles of anterior abdominal wall:

1. Acts like micturition, defecation, parturition and vomiting by compressing abdominal contents.
2. Supports abdominal viscera.
3. Forced expiration.
4. Movements of trunk (flexion and rotation).

Linea Alba

- This is relatively avascular and non-nervous.
- This can easily be selected for incisions of abdominal surgery.
- The postoperative delay in healing is its drawback. It is because of its poor blood supply.
- Hernias may occur in linea alba superior to the umbilicus. These hernias are called the epigastric herniae.
- Any hernia through the umbilical ring (an opening in the linea alba) is called umbilical hernia.
- When two recti are separated by a considerable interval, it is called divarication of recti. It may predispose to hernia.

Hernia

Hernia is protrusion of a part of an organ or tissue through an abnormal opening.

Abdominal Herniae

Abdominal herniae occur through the abdominal wall. It has 3 parts:

- Sac derived from peritoneum which has a neck and a body.
- Contents of the sac.
- Coverings of the sac derived from the abdominal wall.

The important hernias include:

- Umbilical
  - Congenital (exomphalos): Due to failure in reduction of physiological hernia (midgut loop).
  - Acquired
    - ♦ *Infants:* Due to weakness in umbilical scar (occurs through umbilical scar).
    - ♦ *Adults (paraumbilical):* Occurs just above or below the umbilical scar through linea alba (not through umbilical scar).
- Epigastric: Occurs through linea alba between umbilicus and xiphoid process.
- Incisional: Follows postoperative weakness.
- Spigelian.
- Internal.
- Inguinal hernias.
  - Direct.   – Indirect.
- Femoral.
- Lumbar: Occurs through lumbar triangle of Petit; which is a weak area in the posterior abdominal wall bounded anteriorly by posterior border of external oblique, posteriorly by anterior border of latissimus dorsi muscle and below (base) by the iliac crest. Floor of the triangle is formed by internal oblique and transversus abdominis muscles.

Inguinal Region

- This is the weakest part of the anterior abdominal wall due to the bipedal posture of human being.
- It lies superior to the inguinal ligament.

Superficial Inguinal Ring

- It is a triangular opening in the aponeurosis of the external oblique abdominis muscle.
- It lies superolateral to the pubic tubercle.
- Spermatic cord and ilioinguinal nerve pass through it in male.
- Round ligament of uterus and ilioinguinal nerve pass through it in female.

Deep Inguinal Ring

- It is an oval opening in the transversalis fascia 1.25 cm superior to the middle point of the inguinal ligament.
- Spermatic cord begins here.
- Therefore, ductus deferens, artery to ductus deferens, testicular artery, pampiniform plexus of veins, sympathetic plexus of nerves and lymph vessels, pass through the spermatic cord.
- Inferior epigastric artery lies medial to the deep inguinal ring.

Inguinal Canal

- It is 4 cm in length (Fig. 5.8).
- It lies superior to the medial part of the inguinal ligament.
- It extends from the deep to the superficial inguinal ring.

Definition: It is an oblique musculofascial passage above the medial end of the inguinal ligament between the deep and superficial inguinal rings.

- Spermatic cord traverses it from the deep inguinal to the superficial inguinal ring.
- Ilioinguinal nerve lies between the internal oblique and transversus abdominis muscles and passes through the superficial inguinal ring.
- Ilioinguinal nerve does not pass through the deep inguinal ring.

Walls of the inguinal canal: It has a floor, anterior wall, posterior wall and a roof.

Floor is formed by the grooved upper surface of the medial part of the inguinal ligament.

Anterior Wall

- Entire extent of the anterior wall is formed by the aponeurosis of external oblique abdominis muscle.
- Lateral part of the anterior wall is reinforced by the origin of internal oblique muscle from the lateral half of the inguinal ligament.
- Therefore, the lateral part of the anterior wall is strong and medial part of the anterior wall is weak.

Posterior Wall of the Inguinal Canal

- Ilioinguinal nerve pierces this wall to enter the inguinal canal.
- Medial part is reinforced by the conjoint tendon.
- In its entire extent it is formed by the transversalis fascia.
- Therefore, the lateral part of the posterior wall is weak and medial part of the posterior wall is strong.
- Now visualize that the strong medial part of the posterior wall is placed opposite the weak medial part of the anterior wall.

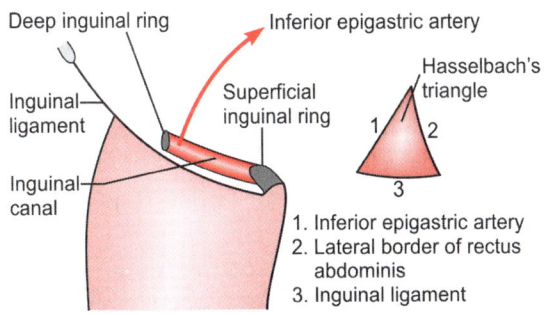

Deep inguinal ring — Inferior epigastric artery

Hasselbach's triangle

Inguinal ligament — Superficial inguinal ring

Inguinal canal

1. Inferior epigastric artery
2. Lateral border of rectus abdominis
3. Inguinal ligament

Fig. 5.8: Inguinal canal

- Similarly the weak lateral part of the posterior wall faces the strong lateral part of the anterior wall. This mechanism prevents the hernia normally.

Roof is formed by the arching fibers of the internal oblique muscle assisted by a few fibers of the transversus abdominis muscle.

Mechanism of prevention of hernia normally:

1. Flap valve mechanism where posterior wall is kept opposed to the anterior wall with increase in intra-abdominal pressure.
2. The fibers of the internal oblique which form the roof are drawn down like a shutter when this muscle contracts. Thereby it minimizes the width of the opening of inguinal canal. This mechanism is called "shutter mechanism" (roof approximated to floor).
3. When cremaster muscle contracts it pulls the spermatic cord up and thereby the testis, which closes the superficial inguinal ring like a ball. This mechanism is called "ball valve mechanism".

Inguinal Herniae

- Abnormal protrusion through inguinal canal or through its superficial ring is called inguinal hernia. This may occur due to the weakness of the inguinal region or may be congenital.
- Inguinal hernia is more common in males because of wider inguinal canal in male. This is due to the spermatic cord present in the male. Femoral hernia is more common in female because of wide femoral ring. This is due to the wider pelvis and smaller vessels.
- *There are two types of inguinal hernia:*
  1. Direct inguinal hernia.
  2. Indirect inguinal hernia.

Direct Inguinal Hernia

- It pierces the posterior wall directly and appears at the superficial inguinal ring.
- The neck of hernial sac lies medial to the inferior epigastric artery.

Indirect Inguinal Hernia

- It passes through the deep inguinal ring, inguinal canal and superficial inguinal ring.
- The neck of hernial sac lies lateral to the inferior epigastric artery.
- Indirect inguinal hernia may be congenital when the processus vaginalis persists or may be acquired.

Descent of Testis

- Testis develops in the lumbar region of the abdomen.
- It develops retroperitoneally.
- Lower end of the testis is connected to the gubernaculum which connects the testis to the wall of scrotum and passes through the site of future inguinal canal.
- A diverticulum of peritoneum called the processus vaginalis follows the gubernaculum in the inguinal canal through this part of the anterior abdominal wall.
- Processus vaginalis is completely obliterated except its terminal part which surrounds the testis as the tunica vaginalis testis.

- If testis does not descend then it is called "cryptorchidism" (crypto-hidden).
  Note: Cryptorchidism is often associated with tumor of testis.
- If testis descends to an abnormal location it is called "ectopic testis".
- If there is only one testis it is called "monorchism".
- The inflammation of testis is called "orchitis". Orchitis may occur following infection of mumps.

Spermatic Cord

- It extends from the deep inguinal ring to the testis. It is made up of the following structures (Fig. 5.9):
  1. Ductus deferens.
  2. Artery to ductus deferens.
  3. Testicular artery.
  4. Pampiniform plexus of veins.
  5. Lymph vessels of testis and epididymus.
  6. Testicular plexus of nerves.
- The nerves mainly come from T10 sympathetic segment. These autonomic fibers give that sickening feeling when testis is hit. Pain of the testis may be referred to the anterior abdominal wall.

Coverings of the spermatic cord:
- Innermost covering is the internal spermatic fascia derived from the transversalis fascia.
- The next layer is the cremasteric fascia and cremasteric muscle derived from the internal oblique abdominis muscle.
- The most superficial layer is given by the aponeurosis of the external oblique muscle of the abdomen. It is called the external spermatic fascia.

Note:
- Testicular artery is a branch of the abdominal aorta.
- Artery to dutus deferens is a branch of the superior/inferior vesical artery.
- Cremasteric artery is a branch of the inferior epigastric artery.

Testes

- They lie in the scrotum.
- Epididymis lies posterolateral to it.
- Testis is suspended by the spermatic cord.
- As testis descends from the abdomen it draws its artery along with it.
- Therefore, the testicular artery is a branch of the abdominal aorta.
- Pampiniform plexuses surround the ductus deferens till the deep inguinal ring. In the posterior abdominal wall one testicular vein is formed. The left testicular vein opens into the left renal vein while the right testicular vein opens into the inferior vena cava.
- Lymph vessels of testis hitch-hike the testicular artery. Therefore, lymph from the testis is drained into the lumbar lymph nodes.

- Cancer of the testis spreads to the lateral aortic lymph nodes via these lymph vessels.

You should be able to identify the following (Fig. 5.10):
- Parietal layer of tunica vaginalis.
- Cavity of tunica vaginalis.
- Visceral layer of tunica vaginalis.

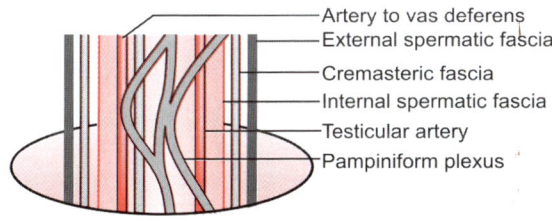

Fig. 5.9: Spermatic cord

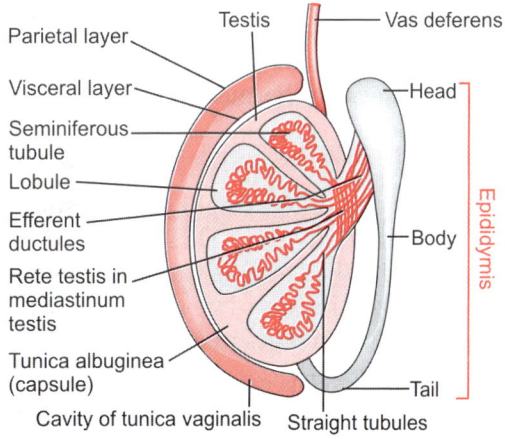

Fig. 5.10: Testis and epididymis

- Tunica albugenia (thick outer covering of the testis).
- Seminiferous tubules in lobules of testis.
- Rete testis, a communicating network of tubules along the posterior part of the testis.
- Efferent ductules of testis.
- Efferent ductules join to form the duct of epididymis in the head of epididymis.
- Head continues as body of the epididymis. Body of the epididymis is a highly coiled tube. It continues as the tail of the epididymis.
- On the top of testis, there is appendix of testis. This represents the upper end of the paramesonephric duct.
- On the top of epididymis, there is appendix of epididymis. This represents the upper end of the mesonephric duct.
- Visceral layer of tunica vaginalis tucks between the lateral part of the testis and epididymis and this small recess of cavity of tunica vaginalis is called the sinus of epididymis.

Note the following applied anatomy of the processus vaginalis:

- It may persist completely making way for the indirect congenital inguinal hernia.
- It may persist partially along the spermatic cord and might result in the hydrocele of the spermatic cord (encysted).
- In female it may persist in the inguinal canal as canal of Nuck. It might pave way for the indirect inguinal hernia.

Scrotum

- It is a bag of skin which houses testis in it (Fig. 5.11).
- There is no fat in its superficial fascia.
- It has tough crispy hairs and sebaceous glands which give characteristic smell.
- Sebaceous cysts are common in the skin of the scrotum.

Layers of the Scrotum

1. Skin.
2. Superficial fascia containing dartos muscle.
3. External spermatic fascia.
4. Cremasteric muscle and fascia.
5. Internal spermatic fascia.
6. Parietal layer of the tunica vaginalis.

Nerve Supply of the Scrotum

- Anterior part of the scrotum is supplied by L1 segment through ilioinguinal and genital branch of genitofemoral nerves.
- Posterior part of the scrotum is supplied by S3 segments by the posterior scrotal branches of pudendal nerve and posterior cutaneous nerve of thigh.
- Therefore, when the scrotum is supposed to be anesthetized, the anesthetic solution is injected at a higher level to include the L1 segment.

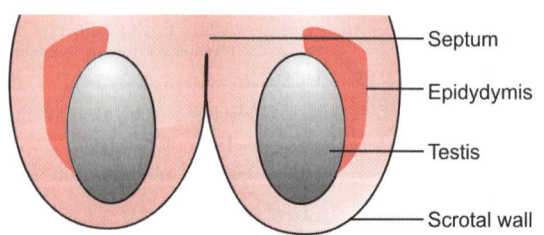

Fig. 5.11: Scrotum

Blood Supply of the Scrotum

- It is by the superficial and deep external pudendal branches of the femoral artery and the posterior scrotal branches of the internal pudendal artery.
- Veins accompany the corresponding arteries.

Lymphatic Drainage

- Lymph from the scrotum terminates in the superficial inguinal lymph nodes.

- Therefore, cancer of the scrotum metastasizes to the superficial inguinal lymph nodes while testicular tumors spread to lumbar lymph nodes in the abdomen.

Cremasteric Reflex

- By stroking the upper medial side of the thigh, the testis is retracted upwards.
- This is called the cremasteric reflex. The afferent limb of the reflex is through the ilioinguinal nerve. The efferent limb passes through the genital branch of genitofemoral nerve which innervates the cremaster muscle. This reflex demonstrates the integrity of L1 segment.

Penis

- It is male copulatory organ.
- It consists of root, body and glans penis.
- Penis is made of 3 cylindrical masses of erectile tissue—2 corpora cavernosa and 1 corpus spongiosum encased in fibrous tissue covering (Fig. 5.12).
- *Arterial supply:* Dorsal and deep artery of penis, artery of the bulb - branches of internal pudendal artery.
- *Veins:* Superficial and deep dorsal vein.
- Lymphatics from glans drain into deep inguinal node of cloquet while the rest of the penis drains into superficial inguinal lymph nodes.

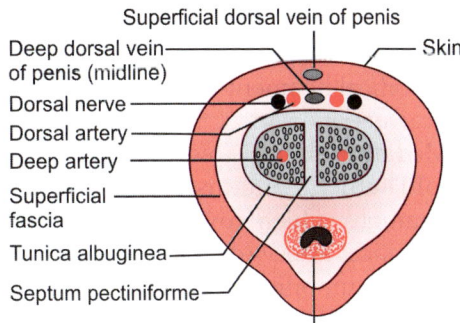

Fig. 5.12: Penis

- *Nerve supply:* Sensory from dorsal nerve of penis and ilioinguinal nerve. Sympathetic from L1 mainly mediates ejaculation and parasympathetic from S2, 3 and 4 mainly mediates erection.

- Erection is a vascular phenomenon caused by engorgement of the cavernous tissue with blood. Failure of erection results in impotency.

- Circumcision is a religious practice involving surgical excision of the prepuce.

Inner Side of the Anterior Abdominal Wall

- It presents one median fold and two folds on either side in the lower part below the level of umbilicus (Fig. 5.13).

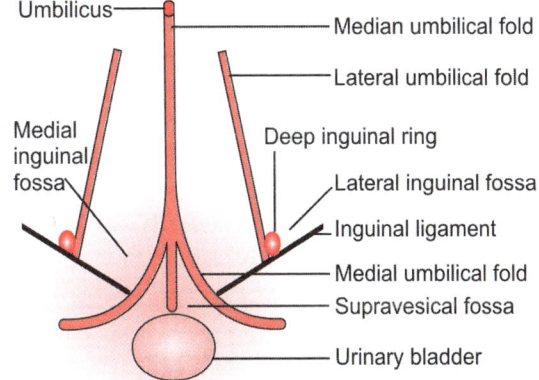

Fig. 5.13: Inner side of anterior abdominal wall

1. Median fold is called the median umbilical fold and contains median umbilical ligament which represents the urachus of embryo.
2. Medial umbilical fold is the peritoneal fold which contains lateral umbilical ligament which covers the obliterated umbilical artery (one on each side).
3. Lateral umbilical fold is the peritoneal fold which covers the inferior epigastric artery (one on each side).

- Therefore, only the lateral umbilical fold is vascular.
- There is no medial umbilical ligament.
- The space of the anterior abdominal wall between the median umbilical fold and medial umbilical fold is called the "supravesical fossa" as it lies above the urinary bladder.
- The space between the medial and lateral umbilical folds is called the medial inguinal fossa.

> Direct inguinal hernia traverses the supravesical or medial inguinal fossa.

- The space lateral to the lateral umbilical fold is called the lateral inguinal fossa.

> Indirect inguinal hernial sac passes through this fossa.

Hesselbach's Triangle

- This triangle is bounded by the rectus abdominis muscle medially, inferior epigastric vessels laterally and medial part of the inguinal ligament inferiorly.
- Direct inguinal hernial sac passes through this triangle.
- It is divided by obliterated umbilical artery into supravesical fossa medially and medial inguinal fossa laterally.

Peritoneum

- It is a thin transparent serous membrane which lines the abdominal wall and the viscera (Fig. 5.14).

- It consists of squamous epithelium (mesothelium) lying over a thin layer of connective tissue.
- It reduces friction and helps the motility of abdominal organs.
- It is divided into two layers.
- The outer parietal layer which lines the abdominal body wall.
- The inner visceral layer which lines the outer surfaces of the viscera.
- The potential cavity present between the parietal and visceral layers is the peritoneal cavity.
- It contains a thin film of fluid called peritoneal fluid.

Parietal Layer of the Peritoneum

- It is the outer layer of peritoneum which lines the body wall.
- It is developed from the somatopleuric mesoderm.
- It is supplied by the following somatic nerves:
  1. Phrenic nerve
  2. Lower intercostal nerves
  3. Subcostal nerve
     - It is supplied by the somatic blood vessels which supply the body wall.

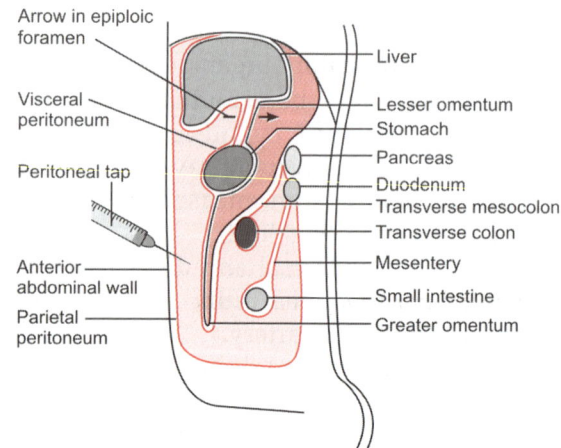

Fig. 5.14: Peritoneal cavity

– It is sensitive to touch and cutting (all cutaneous sensations).

– It has rich innervation and that is the reason why large incisions in abdominal operations are very painful. The latest endoscopic devices help reduce the trauma to the peritoneum and thereby making the operation relatively pain-free.

– When parietal peritoneum is inflamed, it usually results in "rebound tenderness".

Visceral Peritoneum

- This is the peritoneum which lines the outer surfaces of the organs of the abdomen. It is almost inseparably blended with the outer surface of the viscera. This layer is termed serosa in histology sections.
- Visceral peritoneum is derived from the splanchnopleuric mesoderm.
- It is supplied by the autonomic nerves.
- It is not sensitive to touch, heat, cold and cuts.
- It is sensitive to distention that is stretch.

Peritoneal Cavity

- The potential space between the parietal and visceral layers is the peritoneal cavity (Fig. 5.14).
- It is a single continuous space. It can be studied under 2 parts: greater sac and lesser sac.
- The sac present behind the anterior abdominal wall is the greater sac. When the parietal peritoneum is opened, the visceral peritoneum lining the viscera is seen as the outer shining layer covering the viscera.

Greater Sac

The peritoneal cavity is a potential space between the parietal and visceral layers of peritoneum. Greater sac constitutes the major region of this peritoneal cavity. Its small diverticulum is the lesser sac. The two communicate by way of epiploic foramen (Fig. 5.14).

Lesser Sac

- It is a diverticulum of the greater sac.
- It communicates with the greater sac at the epiploic foramen (Fig. 5.14).
- Its anterior wall is formed by the liver, lesser omentum, posterior surface of the stomach and anterior two layers of the greater omentum.
- It has a superior recess which is limited superiorly by the diaphragm.
- Its inferior recess extends into the greater omentum.
- Splenic recess extends to the left side towards the spleen.
- It separates the structures which form the stomach bed from the stomach.
- It is called "omental bursa".

Following structures lie behind the lesser sac:
1. Body of the pancreas.
2. Splenic artery.
3. Left kidney.
4. Left suprarenal gland.
5. Celiac trunk surrounded by the celiac plexus of nerves and its branches.
6. Crura of diaphragm.

Pancreatic pseudocyst: Since pancreas forms the immediate posterior relation of the lesser sac. Any pathological exudates from the pancreas tend to collect in the lesser sac forming a pancreatic pseudocyst.

Lesser sac development in brief:
- This is formed due to the rotation of the stomach to the right side.
- To start with the stomach is connected with the anterior abdominal wall by the ventral mesogastrium and with posterior abdominal

wall by dorsal mesogastrium in the early stages of the development of foregut.

- Ventral and dorsal mesogastrium are parts of ventral and dorsal mesentery respectively.
- Liver develops in the ventral mesogastrium, thereby ventral mesogastrium is divided into two parts.
- The part between the liver and the anterior abdominal wall becomes the falciform ligament while the part between the stomach and the liver becomes the lesser omentum. Stomach rotates towards the right side, thereby; anteroposteriorly running lesser omentum becomes transverse. There is no ventral peritoneal fold of peritoneum for the midgut and hindgut as it is resorbed. This leaves a free margin of the ventral mesogastrium at the level of 1st part of duodenum. After rotation, this free margin forms the anterior wall of the epiploic foramen.
- Lesser omentum is developed from the ventral mesogastrium and greater omentum is developed from the dorsal mesogastrium.

Lesser Omentum

- It is developed from that part of the ventral mesogastrium which lies between the stomach and the liver (Fig. 5.14).
- It is a fold of peritoneum which connects the stomach and first part of the duodenum with the liver.
- It is divided into two parts.
  1. Hepatogastric ligament.
  2. Hepatoduodenal ligament.

Attachments

- Superiorly it is attached to the fissure for ligamentum venosum and the margins of porta hepatis. This attachment is in the form of a hockey stick.
- Inferiorly it is attached to the lesser curvature of the stomach and the first part of the duodenum.
- It describes a free margin which contains the hepatic artery, bile duct and portal vein.
- The free margin forms the anterior boundary of the epiploic foramen.

Greater Omentum

- It develops from the dorsal mesogastrium.
- It is attached to the greater curvature of the stomach (Fig. 5.14).
- It is made up of four layers and theoretically lesser sac lies between its anterior two and posterior two layers.
- Right and left gastroepiploic vessels lie between the anterior two layers of the greater omentum about one inch away from the greater curvature.
- It covers the front of the transverse colon.

- It lies in front of the small intestine largely covering the infracolic compartment of the greater sac.
- It stores fat.
- It moves to the location of inflammation and restricts its spread.
- It has macrophages.
- It is called the policeman of the abdomen.

Internal Hernia

Any abnormal protrusion of viscus through the epiploic foramen into lesser sac forms an internal hernia. While reducing this hernia, no part of wall of epiploic foramen can be cut. Therefore, surgeon punctures the wall of herniated gut, releases the pressure and then reduces it to its normal position.

Epiploic Foramen

- It lies at the level T12 vertebra.
- It connects the greater sac with the lesser sac (Fig. 5.14).

Its boundaries are:

- *Anterior:* Free margin of lesser omentum which contains the hepatic artery proper, bile duct and portal vein.
- *Posterior:* Inferior vena cava covered by the peritoneum.
- *Superior:* Caudate process of the liver.
- *Inferior:* First part of the duodenum (gastroduodenal artery, bile duct, portal vein and inferior vena cava lie behind the first part of the duodenum).

Remember epiploic foramen is between 2 large veins (portal in front and IVC behind).

Mesentery

- It is the fold of peritoneum which suspends the small intestine (Fig. 5.15).
- It is attached to the posterior wall of the abdomen.

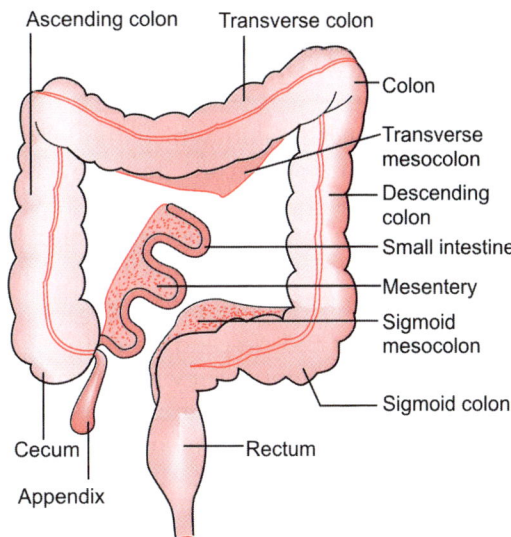

Fig. 5.15: Mesentery, transverse mesocolon and sigmoid mesocolon

- Its posterior attachment is 6 inches in length (root of mesentery).
- Its free margin contains the coils of jejunum and ileum. The length of its free border is approximately 6 meters.
- The average breadth of the mesentery is 6 inches.

It contains the following:

1. Jejunal and ileal vessels of superior mesenteric vessels.
2. Accompanying lymph vessels and lymph nodes.
3. Nerve plexuses.
4. Connective tissue.
5. Coils of jejunum and ileum.

Note: Superior mesenteric vessels are present in root of mesentery.

The root of mesentery crosses:

- 3rd part of duodenum.
- Abdominal aorta.
- IVC.
- Right psoas major.
- Right gonadal vessels.
- Right ureter.

Transverse Mesocolon

1. This is attached to the anterior border of the body of the pancreas transversely.
2. It is a fold of peritoneum which divides the greater sac into supracolic and infracolic compartments.
3. It contains the middle colic artery and its branches, corresponding veins, nerves and lymphatics of transverse colon.

Note: Ascending and descending colon as a rule, have no mesentery. They are retroperitoneal structures. But one important point is to be noted here. To start with both ascending and descending colons had mesocolon during development. Later after rotation it disappears by zygosis and it makes the ascending and descending colons retroperitoneal and relatively immobile.

Mesoappendix and Appendix

- Appendix is a worm-like diverticulum arising from posteromedial aspect of cecum (Fig. 5.16).
- It is about 10 cm long.
- Appendix has a fold of peritoneum called mesoappendix. It contains apendicular vessels, nerves, lymphatics and lymph node (Fig. 5.23).
- Appendicular artery is a branch of ileocolic artery.

- Inflammation of appendix might result in the occlusion of the appendicular artery and thereby causing gangrene of the appendix. Bursting of inflamed appendix is one of the most common causes of peritonitis.
- The pain of appendicitis corresponds to the junction of lateral one-third with the middle third of the spinoumbilical line on right side: McBurney's point. (Spinoumbilical line connects the anterior superior iliac

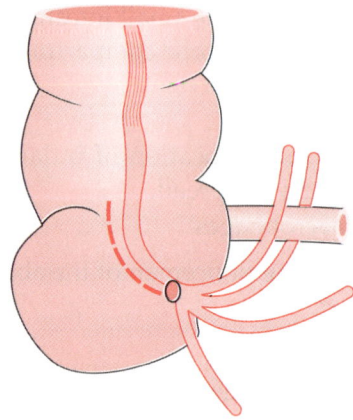

Fig. 5.16: Position of appendix (different possibilities)

spine with the umbilicus). There is tenderness over McBurney's point.

Sigmoid Mesocolon

- It is inverted V-shaped.
- It encloses the sigmoid colon (Fig. 5.15).
- The apex of "V" overlies the bifurcation of left common iliac artery and the left ureter.
- It has two limbs, the right and left. The left limb overlies the left external iliac artery and the right limb extends to the front of the S3 vertebra.

Note:

In the pelvis: There is rectovesical pouch in male. This is the most dependent space of the greater sac in the pelvis.

In female: There is rectouterine pouch between the rectum and uterus. The other pouch is uterovesical pouch which lies anterior to the rectouterine pouch.

Peritoneal Recesses or Pouches

Subphrenic recesses: (subphrenic spaces)
- Since they are all below the diaphragm they are called subphrenic spaces (Fig. 5.17).
- They may be divided into pocket-like recesses between the diaphragm and the liver (suprahepatic) and below the liver (subhepatic).

The suprahepatic spaces are two in number:
1. Right suprahepatic space.
2. Left suprahepatic space.

The subhepatic spaces are two in number:
1. Right subhepatic space.
2. Left subhepatic space.
- The 2 suprahepatic spaces are separated from each other by the falciform ligament.
- Right suprahepatic space is continuous with the right subhepatic space.
- The right subhepatic recess is a deep one and it lies between the liver and right kidney.

It is also known as the hepatorenal pouch or Morrison's pouch. Peritoneal fluid tends to collect here in the supine position as it is the most dependent part in that position.

- Left subhepatic space is the lesser sac. It is connected with the right subhepatic space through the epiploic foramen.

Fluid collected in the right subhepatic space drains towards the pelvis along the right paracolic gutter which lies on the right side of the ascending colon.

Note: Similarly fluid collected on the left side of the supracolic compartment drains into pelvis through the left paracolic gutter.

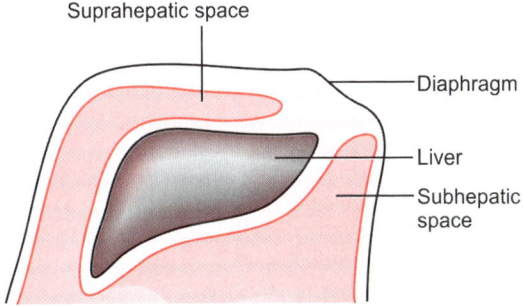

Suprahepatic space

Diaphragm

Liver

Subhepatic space

Fig. 5.17: Suprahepatic and subhepatic spaces

Duodenal Recesses

Occur in relation to 4th part of duodenum where the fourth part of the duodenum ascends and abruptly bends down to form the duodenojejunal junction. They include:
- Superior duodenal recess.
- Inferior duodenal recess.
- Paraduodenal recess.
- Retroduodenal recess.

Paraduodenal Recess

There is a possibility of internal hernia here. What is important to note here is the presence of inferior mesenteric vessels along the recess. Care should be taken to identify these vessels first before reducing any internal hernia here to avoid injuring them.

LIGAMENTS

Falciform Ligament

It is a sickle-shaped fold of peritoneum which connects the anterior abdominal wall to the liver. The round ligament (ligamentum teres) of the liver which is the obliterated remains of the left umbilical vein, lies along free margin of falciform ligament, from the fissure for the ligamentum teres to the umbilicus. It is accompanied by the paraumbilical veins within the fold of falciform ligament. These paraumbilical veins connect the (veins of the liver) portal vein with the systemic veins of the anterior abdominal wall around the umbilicus.

Therefore, in portal hypertension, the back pressure in the portal vein dilates the paraumbilical veins and eventual dilatation of veins around the umbilicus is like a hood of a snake. This enlargement is called "caput medusae".

Gastrosplenic Ligament

- It is a double layer of peritoneum which connects the spleen with the upper part of the greater curvature of the stomach.

- It contains the short gastric vessels, accompanying lymph vessels, connective tissue and gastrosplenic lymph nodes.

Lienorenal Ligament

- It connects the front of the left kidney with the hilum of the spleen.
- It contains the tail of the pancreas, splenic vessels and the accompanying lymph vessels and nodes (pancreaticosplenic).

Stomach

Following are the parts of the stomach:
- Fundus.
- Body.
- Pyloric part:

  ↓

  Pyloric antrum
  Pylorus

  ↓

  Pyloric sphincter and pyloric canal

- It has two curvatures, two surfaces and two ends (Fig. 5.18).

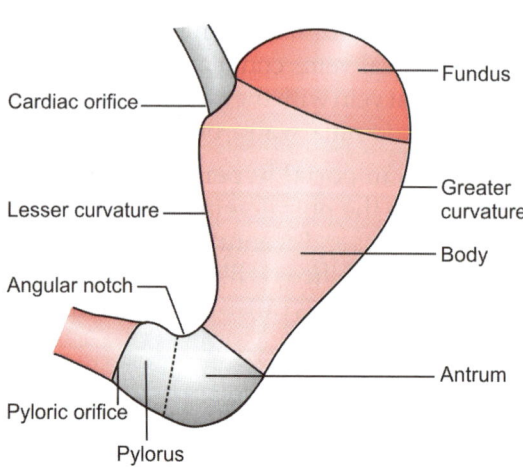

Fig. 5.18: Parts of stomach

Two curvatures are:
- *Lesser curvature:*
  - It is a short curve along the right border of the stomach.
  - Lesser omentum is attached to it.
  - Left gastric vessels and right gastric vessels and branches of vagi nerves lie between the two layers of lesser omentum.
- *Greater curvature:*
  - It is three to four times longer than the lesser curvature.
  - Greater omentum is attached to the greater curvature.
  - Left gastro-omental vessels, right gastro-omental vessels lie between the two layers of greater omentum.

Its two surfaces are anterosuperior and postero-inferior:
- Anterosuperior surface is related to the following:
  - Anterior abdominal wall.
  - Diaphragm.
  - Left lobe of liver (Mnemonic: American Dull Lady).
- Posteroinferior surface is related to the following structures. All of them are separated from the stomach by the lesser sac except the spleen which is separated by the greater sac.
  - Transverse mesocolon.
  - Left suprarenal gland.
  - Splenic artery.
  - Spleen.
  - Diaphragm.
  - Pancreas.
  - Left kidney.
  - Splenic flexure of colon.

(Mnemonic: Three Sweets, Domino Pizza and Kentucky Chicken)

It has two ends: Cardiac, the upper end and pyloric, the lower end.

- Stomach begins at the level of left 7th costal cartilage which lies at the level of T11 vertebra (cardiac orifice).
- It terminates half inch to the right of median plane on the transpyloric plane (L1) at the pyloric orifice.

Note: The fundus reaches the level of left 5th intercostal space.

Blood Supply of the Stomach (Fig. 5.20)

- Left gastric artery—a branch of celiac trunk.
- Right gastric artery—a branch of common hepatic artery.
- Short gastric arteries (5–7)—branches of splenic artery.
- Left gastro-omental artery—a branch of splenic artery.
- Right gastro-omental artery—a branch of gastroduodenal artery.

Venous Drainage

- Left gastric and right gastric veins drain into the portal vein.
- Short gastric and left gastro-omental veins drain into the splenic vein.
- Right gastro-omental vein opens into the superior mesenteric vein.

Lymphatic Drainage (Fig. 5.20)

- Stomach is divided into upper 2/3rd and lower 1/3rd.
- The upper 2/3rd is again divided into right half and left half.
- The lower 1/3rd is divided into right and left unequal parts.
- Right half of upper 2/3rd is drained into left gastric lymph nodes.
- Left half of upper 2/3rd is drained into pancreaticosplenic group of lymph nodes and left gastro epiploic nodes.

- Right part of lower 1/3rd is drained into pyloric group of lymph nodes.
- Left part of the lower 1/3rd is drained into right gastro-omental group of lymph nodes placed along the right gastro-omental vessels.
- All the above said nodes are drained into the celiac group of lymph nodes.
- Celiac nodes drain into the cisterna chyli which continues as thoracic duct.
- Thoracic duct opens into the angle at the junction of left subclavian vein with the left internal jugular vein.

- Cancer of the stomach is one of the major killers. Cancer cells pass through the thoracic duct and may overflow at its opening into junction of left subclavian and left IJV and infect the surrounding left supraclavicular lymph nodes. These are sentinel (sentinel means to guard) nodes which herald the possibility of cancer of the stomach. These nodes are called Virchow's nodes. Therefore, any enlarged nodes at the root of the neck on the left side should force a physician to do further investigations on the stomach.

Nerve Supply of the Stomach

- It is supplied by the parasympathetic and sympathetic nerves.
- Parasympathetic nerves come from anterior and posterior gastric nerves.
  - Anterior gastric nerve is the continuation of the left vagus.
  - Posterior gastric nerve is the continuation of the right vagus (Fig. 5.19).
  - Anterior gastric nerve gives hepatic branch and pyloric branch which reach their destinations by passing between the two layers of the lesser omentum and it also supplies the stomach (anterior gastric branches).

Anterior vagal trunk

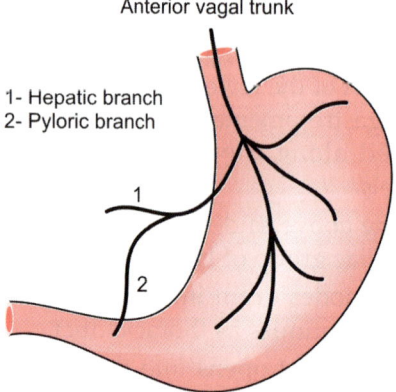

1- Hepatic branch
2- Pyloric branch

Posterior vagal trunk (not shown)

Fig. 5.19: Nerve supply of stomach

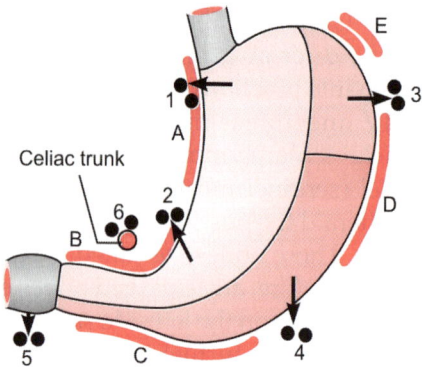

Celiac trunk

1. Left gastric nodes, 2. Right gastric nodes,
3. Left gastroepiploic nodes, 4. Right gastroepiploic nodes,
5. Pyloric nodes, 6. Celiac nodes

A. Left gastric artery, B. Right gastric artery,
C. Right gastroepiploic artery, D. Left gastroepiploic artery,
E. Short gastric arteries

Fig. 5.20: Lymphatic drainage and blood supply of stomach

- Posterior gastric nerve supplies the stomach (posterior gastric branches) and gives branches to celiac plexus.
- Sympathetic fibers of T5–T9 segments come through greater splanchnic nerves.
  - They contribute to the celiac plexus. Branches of celiac plexus reach the stomach wrapping around the branches of the celiac artery.

Clinical Anatomy

- Peptic ulcer in the stomach is called gastric ulcer and similarly the peptic ulcer in duodenum is called duodenal ulcer.
  - Vagi are responsible for the acid secretion in the stomach.
  - Therefore, if there is gastric ulcer, the part of the stomach ulcerated is removed (gastrectomy) and it is followed by the vagotomy.
  - These days highly selective vagotomies (parietal cell vagotomy) are performed. This means only that part of the vagus which is actually responsible for the secretion in the area involved is resected.
  - Most ulcers are due to an infection of a specific bacterium called *Helicobacter pylori.*
- Gastrectomy is the removal of the stomach. It may be total gastrectomy or partial gastrectomy.
- Posterior gastric ulcer may erode through the posterior wall of the stomach into the pancreas resulting in referred pain to the back. Erosion of splenic artery is very common in posterior gastric ulcers because of the proximity of the artery to this wall.
- *Congenital hypertrophic pyloric stenosis:* It is due to the hypertrophy of the pyloric sphincter and genetic factors appear to be involved in this. There will be copius nonbiliary vomiting.
- Pyrosis is the heartburn. It is seen in gastroesophageal reflux disorder (GERD). It is also present in the hiatal hernia.
- Hiatal hernia occurs due to a weakening of the diaphragm in the region of the esophageal hiatus resulting in the widening of the esophageal hiatus. Hiatal hernia which occurs in individuals past middle age is caused by the hernia of stomach into the thorax through the esophageal hiatus.

- *Congenital diaphragmatic hernia:* Hernia of stomach and intestines through a posterolateral defect in diaphragm (foramen of Bochdalek). It is seen in infants and the mortality rate is high because of left lung hypoplasia.

Following clinical conditions can cause heartburn:
1. GERD.
2. Hiatal hernia.
3. Esophagitis.
4. Gastric ulcer.

Endoscopes

Instrument used to see the interior of a hollow viscus using an illuminated tube fitted with a camera. Depending on the hollow viscus viewed it may be:
- Esophagoscope (for oesophagus).
- Gastroscope (for stomach).
- Sigmoidoscope (for sigmoid colon).
- Cystoscope (for urinary bladder), etc.

Duodenum

- It is the proximal part of the small intestine.
- It is shaped like "U" placed sidewards (Fig. 5.21).
- It is called duodenum because it is of the width of 12 fingers (10 inches).
- It is divided into four parts.

First part of the duodenum (superior part): two inches long
- Its first inch is covered by the peritoneum. Therefore, it is movable. In barium meal X-rays the 1st part is seen as a triangular shadow and it is called "duodenal cap".
- Lesser omentum is attached to this part superiorly.
- Greater omentum is attached to this part inferiorly.
- The second inch of the first part of the duodenum is retroperitoneal and does not move.

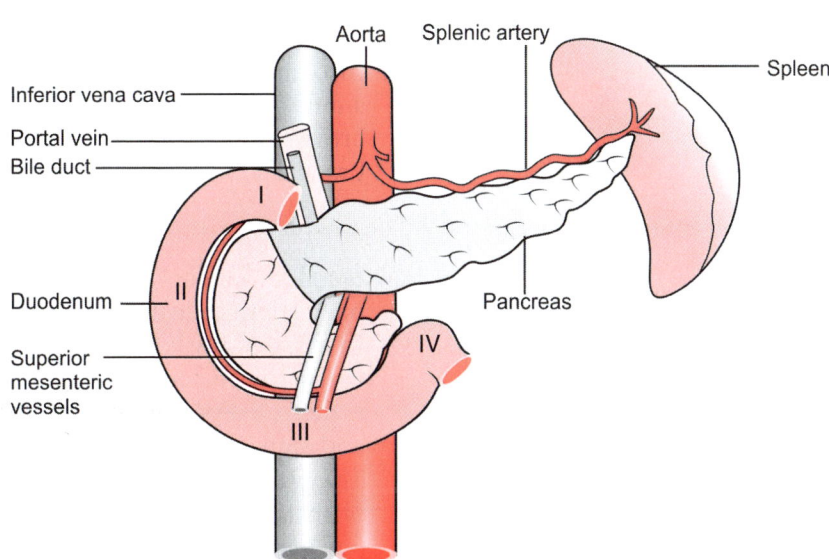

Fig. 5.21: Duodenum and its parts

Relations:
- *Anterior:* Body of the gallbladder and quadrate lobe of the liver.
- *Posterior:* Gastroduodenal artery, bile duct, portal vein and inferior vena cava.
- *Superior:* Epiploic foramen.
- *Inferior:* Head and neck of pancreas.

Second part of the duodenum (descending part):
- It extends from the superior duodenal flexure at the level of L1 vertebra to the inferior duodenal flexure at the level of L3 vertebra.
- It is three inches long.
- Two ducts open into it on the postero-medial wall.
- Hepatopancreatic ampulla opens on the top of major duodenal papilla about 8 to 10 cm distal to the pylorus. This is the common opening of the bile duct and major pancreatic duct.
- Accessory pancreatic duct opens on the top of minor duodenal papilla which is about 2 to 3 cm proximal to the opening of the major duodenal papilla.

Relations:
- *Medial:* Head of the pancreas.
- *Lateral:* Right colic flexure.
- *Anterior:* Transverse mesocolon, transverse colon, coils of jejunum.
- *Posterior:*
  a. Medial part of the anterior surface of the right kidney.
  b. Pelvis of the right ureter.
  c. Right psoas major.
  d. Right renal vessels.

Third part of the duodenum (horizontal part):
- It is roughly 4 inches long.
- It lies at the level of L3 vertebra.

Relations:
- *Anterior:* Root of the mesentery, superior mesenteric artery and vein.

- *Posterior:* Right ureter, right gonadal vessels, inferior vena cava, origin of the inferior mesenteric artery and abdominal aorta.
- *Superior:* Head and uncinate process of pancreas.
- *Inferior:* Coils of small intestine.

Fourth part of the duodenum (ascending part)
- Shortest part: One inch long.
- It continues as the jejunum at the duodenojejunal junction which lies to the left of L2 vertebra.

Relations:
- *Superior:* Body of the pancreas.
- *Inferior:* Coils of small intestine.
- *Posterior:* Left psoas major and left renal vessels.
- *Anterior:* Stomach and transverse mesocolon.

Blood Supply

- Supplied by the anterior and posterior pancreaticoduodenal arterial arches.
- Superior pancreaticoduodenal artery is a branch of the gastroduodenal artery.
- Inferior pancreaticoduodenal artery is a branch of superior mesenteric artery.
- Superior pancreaticoduodenal artery divides into anterior and posterior branches; similarly the inferior pancreatico-duodenal artery divides into anterior and posterior branches.

APPLIED ANATOMY

- Duodenal ulcers are common in the first part. They erode the gastroduodenal artery. In duodenal ulcer pain is referred to the epigastric region. But if duodenal rupture is there, the pain is all around the abdomen and signs of peritonitis set in.
- The pyloric orifice (junction of duodenum with the stomach) is identified by the surgeon by finding the prepyloric vein of Mayo which lies anterior to the pylorus.

- Gallstones may block the top of the hepatopancreatic ampulla and it may lead to pancreatitis.
- In paraduodenal hernia, care is taken not to injure the inferior mesenteric vessels and ascending branch of left colic artery.

Mesentery

- It is the fold of peritoneum which connects the small intestine with the posterior abdominal wall.
- It has two borders, a free border and an attached border which is called its root. The root is attached to the posterior abdominal wall.
- Its root is 6 inches long.
- Its free margin is 6 meters long.
- Its average breadth is 6 inches.
- It begins on the left side of the L2 vertebra and ends in front of the right sacroiliac joint.
- The root of the mesentery is obliquely attached to the posterior abdominal wall. It crosses the horizontal part of the duodenum, aorta, inferior vena cava, right gonadal vessels, right ureter and right psoas major.

Ileal Diverticulum (Meckel's diverticulum)

- It is seen in 2% of cases.
- It lies about 2 feet proximal to iliocecal junction and it may be 2 inches long.
- It may cause intussusception and intestinal obstruction.
- It is the remnant of the proximal part of the vitellointestinal duct.
- It may become inflamed and may produce pain similar to appendicitis.
- Peptic ulcer may occur in this diverticulum.

Large Intestine

Following are the parts of the large intestine:
- Cecum and appendix.
- Ascending colon.
- Transverse colon.
- Descending colon.
- Sigmoid colon.
- Rectum.
- Anal canal.

Table 5.1: Differences between the jejunum and ileum	
Jejunum	*Ileum*
It has wider lumen.	The lumen is not so wide.
Wall is thicker (2 tubes are felt on palpation similar to the feeling of shirt sleeve and coat sleeve together).	Wall is relatively thin (1 tube is felt similar to the feeling of shirt sleeve only).
Plenty of plicae circularis (circular folds).	Very few plicae circularis.
Less fat in the mesentery; confined along the root. When light is allowed to pass through the mesentery it gives the resemblance of windows between vasa recta (Fig. 5.22).	More fat in the mesentery; uniformly distributed and light does not easily pass through this because of fat.
Only 1 or 2 tiers of arterial arcades.	3–6 tiers of arterial arcades (Fig. 5.22).
Long vasa recta.	Short vasa recta (Fig. 5.22).
Solitary lymphatic nodules are fewer and Peyer's patches are absent.	Solitary lymphatic nodules are more and Peyer's patches are present.

Table 5.2: Differences between the small and large intestines	
Large intestine	*Small intestine*
It has greater distensible capacity.	It cannot be distended so much.
It has tenia coli.	It has no tenia coli.
It has appendices epiploicae.	No appendices epiploicae.
It has sacculations (haustrations).	No sacculations.
It has no plicae circularis.	Plicae circularis present in jejunum.
Marginal artery connects all the vessels.	There is no marginal artery.

Cecum

- It is the proximal dilated part of the large intestine (Fig. 5.23).
- Its breadth is more than its height.
- It is large in herbivores.
- It lies in the right iliac fossa below the level of transtubercular plane.

Anterior Relations

- Anterior abdominal wall.
- Coils of the small intestine.

Posterior Relations

- Right psoas major.
- Iliacus.
- Femoral nerve.
- Lateral cutaneous nerve of the thigh.

- In its interior there is ileocecal valve which has two lips.
- Appendix opens into the cecum 2 to 3 cm inferior to the ileocecal valve.
- *Blood supply:*
  - It is supplied by the anterior and posterior branches of ileocolic artery.
  - Ileocolic vein drains the venous blood into the superior mesenteric vein.
- Lymph vessels of the cecum are drained into the ileocolic lymph nodes along the ileocolic artery in the mesentery of the ileum and from there they are drained into the superior mesenteric lymph nodes.

Ascending Colon

- It extends from the level of transtubercular plane to the right colic flexure (Fig. 5.15).
- It has no mesentery.

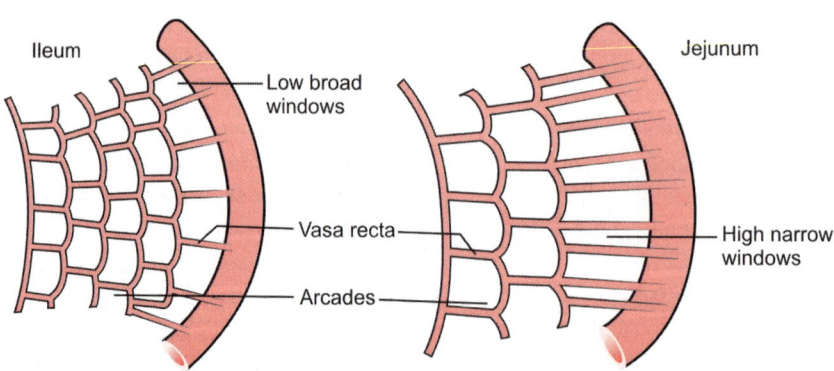

Fig. 5.22: Arterial arcades, vasa recta and windows

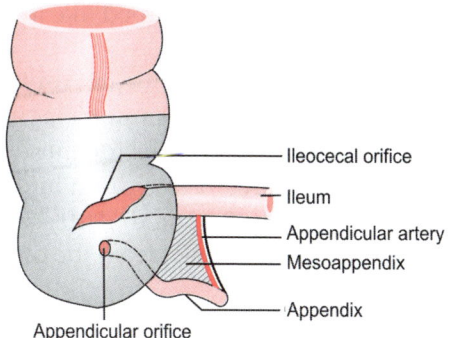

Fig. 5.23: Cecum and appendix

- Ileocecal orifice
- Ileum
- Appendicular artery
- Mesoappendix
- Appendix
- Appendicular orifice

Anterior Relations

- Anterior abdominal wall.
- Greater omentum.
- Coils of small intestine.

Posterior Relations

- Quadratus lumborum muscle.
- Ilioinguinal nerve.
- Iliohypogastric nerve.
- Subcostal nerve.
- Lower part of the front of the right kidney.
- *Blood supply:*
  - It is supplied by the right colic branches of the superior mesenteric artery and the branches of the ileocolic artery which is the continuation of the superior mesenteric artery.
- *Nerve supply:* Both sympathetic and parasympathetic come from the celiac and superior mesenteric plexus. Parasympathetic fibers are contributed by the vagus nerve through the above said plexus.
- Lymph vessels of the ascending colon are drained into the paracolic and epicolic lymph nodes and from them they pass to the superior mesenteric lymph nodes.

Paracolic gutter: On the lateral side of the ascending colon there is right paracolic gutter. This is important as the fluid collected in the hepatorenal recess is gravitated down through this into the pelvis.

Transverse Colon

- It is the largest and most mobile part of the large intestine (Fig. 5.15).
- It is about 45 cm in length.
- It extends from the right colic flexure to the left colic flexure.
- It forms a loop which may extend as low as pelvis inferiorly.
- It is suspended to posterior abdominal wall by the transverse mesocolon.
- The transverse mesocolon is fused to the posterior wall of the greater omentum in later life.
- It is mainly supplied by the branches of middle colic artery. This is a branch of the superior mesenteric artery. It is also supplied by the branches of right colic artery on the right side and the branches of the left colic artery on the left side. The junction of the right two-thirds with the left one-third of the transverse colon indicates the junction of the midgut with the hindgut. That is the reason why both midgut and hindgut arteries supply this.
- Veins of the transverse colon are drained into the superior mesenteric vein.
- Lymph vessels drain into the superior mesenteric lymph nodes.
- *Nerve supply:* Superior mesenteric plexus transmit both sympathetic and parasympathetic fibers (vagus) to the right two-thirds of the transverse colon. The left one third of the transverse colon is supplied by the inferior mesenteric plexus which carries both sympathetic fibers and parasympathetic fibers. The parasympathetic fibers to this plexus come from S2, 3 and 4 through hypogastric plexus.

Note: Transverse mesocolon is attached to the head of the pancreas and body of the pancreas. Transverse colon and its mesocolon with greater omentum separate the greater sac of the peritoneum into the supracolic and infracolic compartments.

Descending Colon

- It extends from the left colic flexure to the left pelvic brim (Fig. 5.15).
- It is retroperitoneal.

Anterior Relations

- Anterior abdominal wall.
- Greater omentum.
- Small intestine coils.

Posterior Relations

- Lower part of the anterior surface of the left kidney.
- Subcostal nerve and vessels.
- Iliohypogastric nerve.
- Ilioinguinal nerve.
- Left iliacus.
- Lateral cutaneous nerve of thigh.
- Femoral nerve.
- Left psoas major.
- *Blood supply:*
  - It is supplied by the branches of the left colic branches of the inferior mesenteric arteries.
  - Veins drain into the inferior mesenteric vein.
- *Lymphatic drainage:* It is drained into the inferior mesenteric group of lymph nodes.
- *Nerve supply:*
  - It is supplied by the branches of inferior mesenteric plexus.
  - Sympathetic fibers come from the inferior mesenteric plexus and the parasympathetic fibers come from the hypogastric plexus (S2, 3 and 4 parasympathetic).

Note: S2, 3, 4 parasympathetic fibers constitute pelvic splanchnic nerves or Nervi erigentes.

Sigmoid Colon

- It has sigmoid mesocolon (Fig. 5.15).

- Sigmoid mesocolon is shaped like inverted "V".
- The apex of "V" overlies the left ureter and termination of the left common iliac artery.
- Sigmoid branches of inferior mesenteric artery supplies this. Veins drain into IMV.
- Nerve supply is the same as descending colon as it is also derived from the hindgut.

CLINICAL ANATOMY

- *Diverticulitis:*
  - Diverticula are the evaginations of mucous membrane into the thickness of the wall of the intestine. Infection of diverticula leads to diverticulitis. It is very common in the sigmoid colon as the pressure is very high there. Diarrhea and pain abdomen are the main symptoms. Though less common it may occur in small intestine also.

Note: Tenia coli begin at the junction of the appendix with the cecum and extends upto the junction of the sigmoid colon with the rectum. No appendices epiploicae in the appendix and rectum.

Liver

- Aids in many metabolic activities.
- How is it maintained in its normal anatomical position?
  - Intra-abdominal pressure.
  - Opening of hepatic veins into IVC.
  - Peritoneal ligaments and peritoneal folds do not offer as much support, but aid in it.
- Situated in the right hypochondrium and epigastrium.
- Normally, liver cannot be palpated, it is within the costal margin.
- *Weight:* 1.5 kg, the largest organ in the body; 1/40th of body weight in adults; in newborn, 1/20th of body weight.

- Covered by connective tissue capsule (Glisson's capsule) and the visceral peritoneum around the liver.
- Paraumbilical veins and ligamentum teres are in the free margin of falciform ligament (Fig. 5.27).
- Liver is directly related to the diaphragm.
- *Surfaces related to diaphragm:*
  - Anterior.
  - Posterior.
  - Superior.
  - Lateral.
- Bare area-triangular region with no peritoneum covering it, on posterior surface of right lobe (Fig. 5.24).
  - Directly related to diaphragm, veins of liver belonging to the portal system communicate with veins of diaphragm which are systemic.
  - This is one of the portosystemic anastomosis sites.
  - Boundaries of bare area:
    - Base is formed by groove of IVC.
    - *Superior:* Upper layer of coronary ligament.

- *Inferior:* Lower layer of coronary ligament.
- *Right side:* Right triangular ligament.
- *Caudate lobe:*
  - Forms anterior wall of superior recess of lesser sac.
  - Limited by diaphragm superiorly.
  - The epiploic foramen lies inferior to the caudate process of caudate lobe.
- Inferior/visceral surface is related to stomach, 1st part of duodenum, lesser omentum, gallbladder, right colic flexure, right kidney and right suprarenal. It shows:
  - Quadrate lobe
    - Quadrate in shape, closer to inferior border.
    - It has clear cut-out boundaries.
    - Fissure for ligamentum teres lies to the left side and fossa for gallbladder lies to its right side.
    - Superiorly it is bounded by the porta hepatis.
    - Anteriorly it ends in the inferior border.
- *Porta hepatis:*
  - It is a transverse slit between caudate (posteriorly) and quadrate lobes (Fig. 5.24).

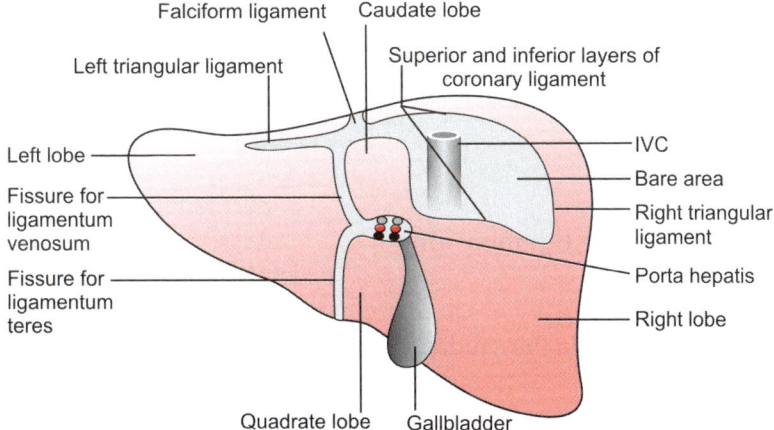

Fig. 5.24: Posterior view of liver

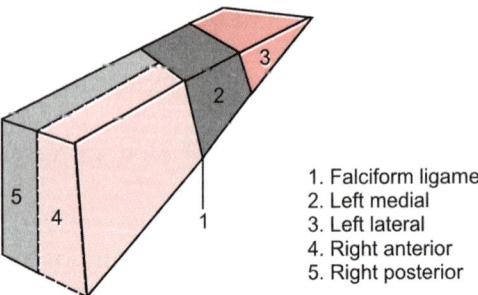

1. Falciform ligament
2. Left medial
3. Left lateral
4. Right anterior
5. Right posterior

Fig. 5.25: Sectors of liver

– Contains structures that enter and leave liver.
– It is surrounded by free edge of lesser omentum.
– Arrangement of structures at porta hepatis is as follows:
  ♦ Most anterior—hepatic ducts.
  ♦ Most posterior—portal vein.
  ♦ In the middle—hepatic artery.
• Right and left lobes are separtated by:
  – Fissure for ligamentum teres (inferior surface).
  – Fissure for ligamentum venosum (posterior surface).
  – Ductus venosus which was connecting the left umbilical vein with the inferior vena cava in the fetal circulation becomes ligamentum venosum after birth.
• Caudate lobe
  – Forms the anterior wall of superior recess of lesser omentum.
  – *Boundaries:*
    ♦ *Right side:* IVC.
    ♦ *Left side:* Fissure for ligamentum venosum.
    ♦ *Anterior:* Porta hepatis.
  – Connects with right lobe via the caudate process.
  – *The caudate process:*
    ♦ Separates the IVC posteriorly and the portal vein anteriorly.

  ♦ Forms the superior boundary of the epiploic foramen.
• Left and right hepatic ducts merge to form the common hepatic duct.
• Common hepatic duct receives the cystic duct and becomes the bile duct.
• Structural relations to liver:
  – Left lobe:
    ♦ Groove for oesophagus.
    ♦ Stomach related.
  – Right lobe:
    ♦ Related to right kidney.
    ♦ Morrison's pouch (between the kidney and liver).
    ♦ Right suprarenal lies just behind the inferior vena cava.
• Following structures are related to the quadrate lobe.
  – Transverse colon.
  – Pylorus.
  – First part of duodenum.

• Right lateral surface of the liver (along mid-axillary line).
  – Important for taking liver biopsies.
  – 7th to 11th ribs are related and separated by diaphragm.
  – The area can be divided into 3 parts in mid-axillary line:
    ♦ *Upper 1/3rd:* Related to right lung, right pleura and diaphragm.
    ♦ *Middle 1/3rd:* Costodiaphragmatic recess (no lung because its lower limit is at 8th rib).
    ♦ *Lower 1/3rd:* Diaphragm (no costodiaphragmatic recess because lower limit of pleura is at 10th rib).
  – Therefore, pierce in right 10th intercostal space in midaxillary line.
  – Ask patient to hold breath in expiration.
• *Physiological lobes of the liver:*
  – *Left physiological:* Supplied by left branch of hepatic artery and left branch of portal vein.

– *Right physiological:* Supplied by right branch of hepatic artery and right branch of portal vein.

CLINICAL ANATOMY

- *Liver biopsy:* It is done in the right 10th intercostal space. Person is supposed to hold the breath in full expiration. It reduces the costodiaphragmatic recess.
- *Liver rupture:* It is common because of the large size and because it is fixed in position. A fractured rib may tear through the diaphragm and puncture the liver. Rupture of liver causes considerable hemorrhage and pain in the right hypochondriac region.
- *Cirrhosis of liver:* It blocks the blood circulation through the liver. It is the main cause of portal hypertension. In the cirrhosis of liver the following three symptoms are found.
  – Caput medusae.
  – Esophageal varices.
  – Hemorrhoids.
- Lobectomy refers to removal of a lobe of liver.
- Segmentectomy refers to removal of the involved segment only. Intersegmental hepatic veins serve as a guide (Fig. 5.26).
- Liver transplantation becomes necessary in cases of extensive liver damage when the patient's liver is replaced with a healthy liver from a donor.

Extrahepatic Biliary Apparatus

- *It is made up of the following structures (Fig. 5.28):*
  – Right and left hepatic ducts.
  – Common hepatic duct.
  – Gallbladder.
  – Cystic duct.
  – Bile duct.
- Cystohepatic triangle (Calot's triangle)
  – It is bounded medially by the common hepatic duct and laterally by the cystic duct. The base is formed by the undersurface of liver (Fig. 5.28).
  – Cystic artery crosses the triangle. Right hepatic artery may also cross the triangle. This is a guide to the operating surgeon.
- Right and left hepatic ducts join to form the common hepatic duct.
- Common hepatic duct is 3 cm long.
- *Gallbladder:*
  – A pear-shaped sac.
  – Stores and concentrates bile.
  – It has a capacity of about 30–50 ml.
  – It has three parts:
    ♦ Fundus.
    ♦ Body.
    ♦ Neck.
  – It is 3 inches long.
  – Fundus lies opposite the tip of right 9th costal cartilage which corresponds to the

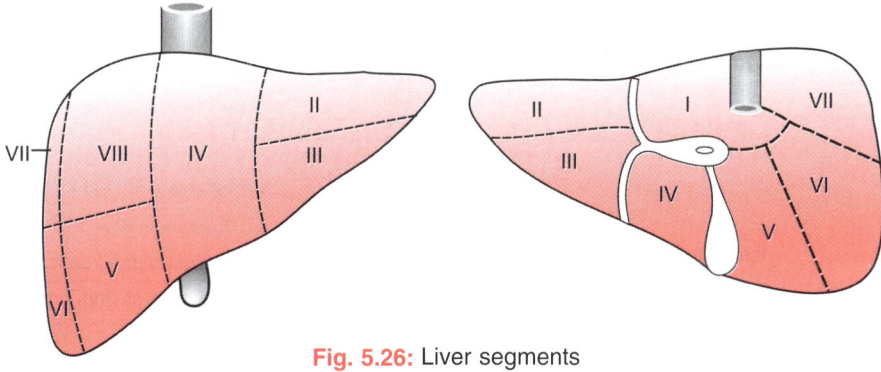

Fig. 5.26: Liver segments

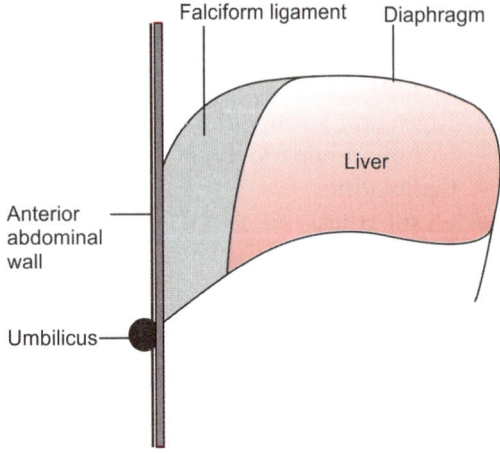

Fig. 5.27: Falciform ligament

junction of linea semilunaris with the right costal margin.
- Body lies over the fossa for the gallbladder.

- The body of the gallbladder is directly superior to the first part of the duodenum.
- Neck is continuous with the cystic duct. Neck shows a diverticulum called the Hartmann's pouch.
- Mucosa of the cystic duct has a spiral valve of Heister.
- Cystic artery is a branch of the right hepatic artery.
- Cystic vein opens into the right branch of portal vein.
- Veins from the body of the gallbladder may open directly into the liver.
- Lymph is drained into the cystic lymph node which is located in the Calot's triangle. Finally lymph goes to the celiac lymph nodes.
- *Nerve supply:* Celiac plexus.
- Cholecystokinin contracts the GB on arrival of the fatty food from the stomach.

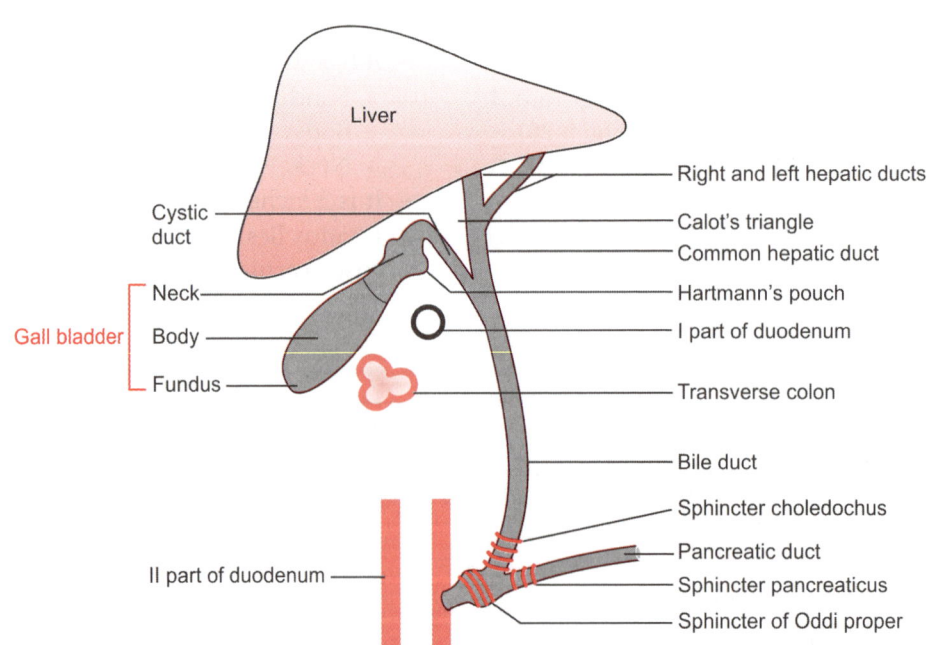

Fig. 5.28: Extrahepatic biliary apparatus

- *Bile duct:*
  - It is 3 inches long.
  - It begins by the union of common hepatic duct with the cystic duct.
  - It lies in the free margin of the lesser omentum.
  - It lies behind the first part of duodenum.
  - It lies behind the head of the pancreas and opens into the second part of the duodenum on the top of major duodenal papilla. This opening is about 8 to 10 cm away from the pyloroduodenal junction. The opening is on the posteromedial wall of the second part of the duodenum.
  - Sphincter choledochus is present at the terminal part of bile duct.
  - Sphincter ampullae or sphincter oddi proper is present at the hepatopancreatic ampulla.

CLINICAL ANATOMY

- Hepatopancreatic ampulla is a common site of gall stone impaction. It results in biliary colic which is pain in the epigastric region.
- Pain of the gallbladder is referred to the epigastric region in the early stages as it is developed from the foregut.
- Visceral pain due to distension is referred to the right hypochondriac region and is poorly localized.
- *Cholecystitis* is inflammation of gallbladder. Murphy's sign is positive.
- *Murphy's sign:* Patient is asked to take deep breath while physician keeps his finger pressed at the tip of right 9th costal cartilage. Patient suddenly checks his breath because of sharp pain.
- In cancer of the head of the pancreas, the bile duct is obstructed which results in jaundice.
- *Cholelithiasis* is presence of gallstones in the gallbladder.
- *Cholecystectomy* is removal of gallbladder.

Spleen

- It is a lymphoid organ present in the left hypochondrium.
- Remember all the odd numbers from 1 to 11.
  - It is 1 inch thick.   1
  - It is 3 inches wide.   3
  - It is 5 inches long.   5
  - It weighs 7 ounces.   7
  - It lies between 9th and 11th ribs   9 and 11
- It has two surfaces, two borders and two ends.
- *Two surfaces:* Visceral surface and diaphragmatic surface.
- *Two borders:* Superior border and inferior border.
- *Two ends:* Anterior end and posterior end.
- It lies in the long axis of the 10th rib.
- It has two ligaments attached to the margins of the hilum (Fig. 5.29):
  - Gastrosplenic ligament.
  - Lienorenal ligament.
- Gastrosplenic ligament connects the spleen with the upper end of the greater curvature of the stomach. It contains the short gastric vessels and accompanying lymph vessels.
- Lienorenal ligament connects the spleen with the left kidney. It contains the tail of the pancreas, splenic artery, splenic vein and accompanying lymph vessels and nerves.
- Spleen rests on the phrenicocolic ligament.
- Superior border is sharp and has notches. Posterior end is pointed and anterior end is broad.
- Diaphragmatic surface is related to the diaphragm, 9–11th ribs, intervening intercostal spaces and costodiaphragmatic recess of pleura.
- Visceral surface is related to the following structures (Fig. 5.29):
  - Stomach separated by the greater sac.

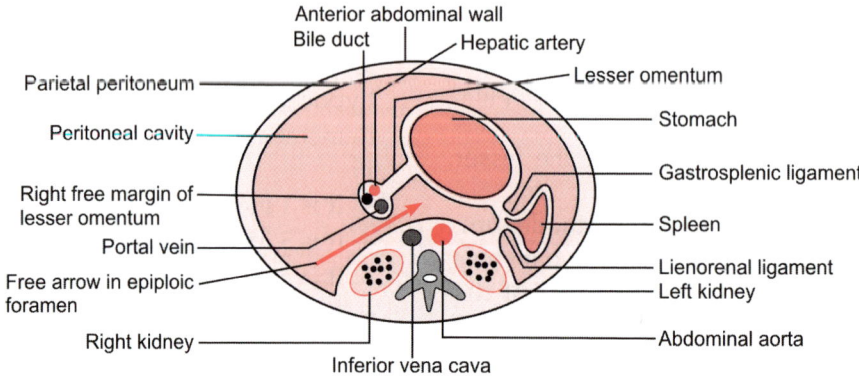

Fig. 5.29: Ligaments of spleen

– Left kidney.
– Tail of the pancreas.
– Left colic flexure.

- When spleen is ruptured, it cannot be sutured, therefore, removal is preferred. The operation is called splenectomy. While performing splenectomy, one has to be careful in preserving the tail of the pancreas. As the tail of the pancreas contains more beta cells, there is a possibility of developing iatrogenic diabetes following inadvertent removal of tail of the pancreas with the spleen.

- When spleen is ruptured, blood collected deep to the diaphragm irritates the phrenic nerve. The pain is referred to the left shoulder as the left shoulder is supplied by the supraclavicular nerves which have the same root value as the phrenic nerve. This sign is known as "Kehr's sign".

- Removal of spleen is indicated in certain blood disorders. In those cases accessory spleens should be identified if any and be removed. Accessory spleens are present as small nodules of splenic tissue in the lienorenal ligament, gastrosplenic ligament or greater omentum.

- Splenomegaly is a condition where spleen is enormously enlarged. It may extend as far as the right iliac fossa. Normally spleen is not palpable as it lies deep to the left costal margin. Nevertheless, the enlarged spleen can easily be felt. When there is a mass inferior to the left costal margin, this might have come from the stomach, left kidney or spleen. Splenic enlargement can always be identified if notches of superior border are felt on palpation.

- Spleen moves with respiration as it is intimately related to the diaphragm. If spleen has to be punctured, as in the case of splenic biopsy or splenoportography (visualizing portal vein by injecting dye into spleen), the patient is asked to hold his breath in exhaled position. This maneuver keeps the costodiaphragmatic recess at a higher level and spleen can be safely punctured in the 10th intercostal space in the left midaxillary plane.

- Spleen is not very essential for life. However, latest research shows that absence of spleen has immunological problems. That is the reason; the spleen is not removed unless it is extremely necessary to do so.

Portal Vein

- It is formed behind the neck of the pancreas by the union of superior mesenteric vein with the splenic vein.
- It is 3 inches long (about 8 cm).
- It lies behind the first part of the duodenum.
- It is one of the contents of the free margin of the lesser omentum (Fig. 5.29).
- It divides into right and left branches.
- Each branch supplies the corresponding functional physiological lobe of the liver.
- Tributaries of the portal vein:
  - Superior mesenteric vein.
  - Splenic vein.
  - Superior pancreaticoduodenal vein.
  - Right gastric vein.
  - Left gastric vein.
  - Cystic vein drains into its right branch.
  - Paraumbilical veins are connected to the left branch of the portal vein.

In portal hypertension, the following portcaval (portosystemic) veins open up.
1. Anastomosis between the tributaries of the left gastric vein and the tributaries of the azygos system in the wall of the lower end of the oesophagus. In portal hypertension these anastomotic veins enlarge in the wall of the oesophagus (esophageal varices) and later burst into the lumen of the oesophagus resulting in hematemesis.
2. Anastomosis between the paraumbilical vein and the systemic veins of the anterior abdominal wall around the umbilicus. In portal hypertension, this anastomosis gets enlarged and dilated veins form "caput medusae" around the umbilicus.
3. Anastomoses between the superior rectal vein (which eventually drains into the portal vein) and inferior rectal vein which drains into the internal iliac vein which eventually drains into the inferior vena cava. In portal hypertension this anasto-

mosis gets dilated resulting in hemorrhoids and bleeding per anus.
4. There is another portosystemic anastomosis between the veins of the ascending and descending colons (portal) and veins of the posterior abdominal wall (systemic).
5. There is also another portosystemic anastomosis between the veins of liver (portal radicles) and veins of diaphragm in the bare area of the liver.

Pancreas

- This endocrine and exocrine organ lies transversely on the posterior abdominal wall at the level of L1, 2 vertebra.
- It is retroperitoneal. Only the end of the tail of the pancreas is in the lienorenal ligament.
- It has the following parts:
  - Head, neck, body and tail.
- Head of the pancreas lies within the concavity of the duodenum (Fig. 5.21).
  - Head has anterior and posterior surfaces.
  - Anterior surface of the head is related to the transverse mesocolon, transverse colon.
  - Posterior surface of the head is related to the inferior vena cava, left renal vein, right renal artery and right renal vein. It is also related to the bile duct; which remains actually embedded in the substance often.
  - Superiorly is the first part of the duodenum.
  - To the right side lies the second part of the duodenum.
  - Inferiorly lies the horizontal part of the duodenum.
  - The lower part of the head extends as a hook-shaped process behind the superior mesenteric vessels called the uncinate process.
  - In the groove between the head of the pancreas and the duodenum there are

anterior and posterior pancreatico-duodenal vascular arches.

- *Neck of the pancreas:* Anteriorly there is pylorus and posteriorly splenic vein and superior mesenteric veins join to form the portal vein.
- *Body of the pancreas:*
  - Transverse mesocolon is attached to the anterior border of the body of the pancreas.
  - Anterior surface of the body of the pancreas is related to the stomach separated by the lesser sac.
  - Posterior surface of the body of the pancreas is related to the abdominal aorta, the origin of the superior mesenteric artery, left psoas major, left kidney, left suprarenal gland. The splenic vein lies behind the body of the pancreas.
  - Superior border of the pancreas has an elevation called "tuber omentale". Celiac artery lies just superior to the tuber omentale and common hepatic artery lies to the right side of the tuber omentale. Splenic artery is related to the superior border to the left of the tuber omentale. Splenic artery is tortuous and very conspicuous artery lying along the upper border of the pancreas and it supplies pancreatic branches.
- *Tail of the pancreas:*
  - It lies within the lienorenal ligament. It is accompanied by the splenic vessels and accompanying lymph vessels in the ligament. Tip of the tail is related to the hilum of the spleen.
- *Ducts of the pancreas:*
  - The major pancreatic duct is shaped like a herring fish bone. It receives smaller ducts at right angles. It turns inferiorly in the head and pierces the wall of the duodenum where it receives the bile duct. Both bile duct and main pancreatic ducts have independent sphincters. Later both the ducts join and form a common hepatopancreatic ampulla. Sphincter of bile duct is prominent and seen commonly; other sphincters around pancreatic duct and at ampulla are less common. This ampulla opens on the top of major duodenal papilla which lies on the posteromedial wall of duodenum about 8 to 10 cm away from the pyloro-duodenal junction.
  - Accessory pancreatic duct opens onto the top of the minor duodenal papilla which is about 2 cm proximal to the major duodenal papilla on the postero-medial wall of the duodenum.

APPLIED ANATOMY

- Cancer of the head of the pancreas compresses the bile duct and it results in obstructive type of jaundice.
- Sphincter of oddi is the sphincter of the hepatopancreatic ampulla. When it is thrown into spasm or obstructed, bile regurgitates into the pancreatic duct resulting in pancreatitis.
- Pain of the pancreas is referred to the back. Pancreatitis may cause pancreatic pseudocyst in the lesser sac.
- During removal of pancreas, small part of the head along the duodenum is retained to assure blood supply to the duodenum.
- One has to be careful in not removing the tail of the pancreas during splenectomy operations.

RECTUM

- Part of the large intestine (Fig. 5.15).
- Lies between sigmoid colon and the anal canal.
- Begins at the level of the S3 vertebra.
- Has a complete longitudinal muscle layer instead of tenia coli (thick in front and behind).

- Does not have haustra, appendices epiploicae or mesentery.
- Inner surface has 3–4 transverse folds.
- Proximal 1/3rd is covered by peritoneum on the anterior and lateral sides.
- Middle 1/3rd is covered by peritoneum only on the anterior surface.
- Distal 1/3rd has no peritoneal covering.
- 12 cms long.
- Not straight but has curvatures.
- Starts from the end of sigmoid colon at S3 level.
- Lower part of the rectum is dilated and called rectal ampulla.
- Ends at the anorectal junction at the level of coccyx where it pierces the pelvic diaphragm.
- Anorectal flexure (perineal flexure) is an important mechanism for fecal continence.

Curvatures

Anteroposterior

1. Sacral flexure follows the concavity of the sacrum and coccyx and
2. Perineal flexure which is caused by the puborectal sling. Perineal flexure lies 2–3 cm in front and slightly below the tip of the coccyx.
3. Lateral curvatures: 2 curvatures to the right and 1 to the left.
   Rectum begins and ends at the midline.

Relations of the Rectum

- In females separated from the posterior fornix of the vagina by rectouterine pouch of Douglas. The pouch of Douglas lies 5.5 cm above the anal orifice.
- In males separated from the bladder by rectovesical pouch. The rectovesical septum (Denonvilliers fascia) is closely associated

with the seminal vesicles and prostate. Rectovesical pouch lies at a distance of 7.5 cm above the anal orifice.
- In both sexes separated from the lower 3 pieces of sacrum by the median sacral vessels and lower end of the sympathetic chain.
- On the sides pararectal fossa, piriformis and levator ani.

Transverse Folds of Rectum

- Valves of Houston.
- They are usually 3 (sometimes 4).
- Two are on the left side (superior and inferior folds) and one on the right (middle fold).
- Include mucosa, submucosa, circular muscle.
- The folds are permanent.
- Are more obvious when the rectum is distended.

Blood Supply of the Rectum

Arterial Supply

- Mainly the superior rectal artery (inferior mesenteric).
- Middle and inferior rectal arteries (internal iliac).
- Median sacral artery.

Venous Drainage

- Mainly superior rectal vein.
- Middle and inferior rectal veins.
- Portal caval anastomosis.
- Internal hemorrhoids are due to varicosity of submucous venous plexus (internal). Venous columns at 3 o'clock, 7 o'clock and 11 o'clock positions in submucosa are involved. They are painless.

Lymphatic Drainage of Rectum

- From superior half-along superior rectal vessels → pararectal nodes → inferior mesenteric lumbar nodes.
- From inferior half → internal iliac nodes.

Nerve Supply

- Hypogastric plexus (sympathetic + para-sympathetic).
- Pelvic splanchnic nerve (parasympathetic fibres).

CLINICAL ANATOMY

Per Rectal Examination

- Done by a gloved finger passed through the anus.
- Prostate and seminal vesicles in males.
- Cervix of uterus in females.
- Perineal body.
- In both sexes, pelvic surfaces of the sacrum and coccyx.
- Ischial spines and tuberosities.
- Enlarged internal iliac nodes.
- Pathological thickening of ureters.
- Swellings in the ischiorectal fossa and pouch of Douglas.

  Proctoscope and sigmoidoscopes may be passed and biopsies are taken. Curvatures of the rectum must be borne in mind while inserting the sigmoidoscope. Rectal folds are useful landmarks.

  Rectal prolapse may occur because supports of rectum (puborectal sling of levator ani) are weakened.

Anal Canal

- Is continuous with the rectum at the pelvic diaphragm.
- At anorectal junction the anal canal bends posteriorly (the perineal flexure) because of the forward pull of the puborectalis muscle.
- Opens externally at the anus.

- Its anterior wall is shorter than the posterior wall.
- Anteriorly it is related to the perineal body, urethra and bulb of penis in males.
- In females, it is related to the perineal body and lower part of vagina.
- Posteriorly it is connected to the coccyx by the anococcygeal ligament.
- Laterally it is related to the ischirectal fossa and its contents.
- Its beginning is 2–3 cm in front of the tip of the coccyx.
- Is kept closed by internal and external anal sphincter except during defecation.
- *External anal sphincter*
  - Is composed of three adjacent rings of skeletal muscle (Fig. 5.31).
    - Subcutaneous.
    - Superficial.
    - Deep parts.
  - Surrounds the entire length of the anal canal.
  - Is controlled voluntarily by the inferior rectal nerve from the pudendal nerve which is part of sacral plexus and perineal branch of 4th sacral nerve.

- *Internal anal sphincter*
  - Thickened ring of circular smooth muscle. Surrounds the upper part of the anal canal terminating at the level of the white line (of Hilton).
  - Is controlled reflexly and involuntarily by:
    - Parasympathetic system promoting relaxation.
    - Sympathetic system promoting contraction.

- *Interior of the anal canal (Fig. 5.30)*
  - *Anal columns*
    - 5 to 10 longitudinal columns of mucosa in the upper part of the anal canal. Columns limited below by anal valves at the pectinate line.

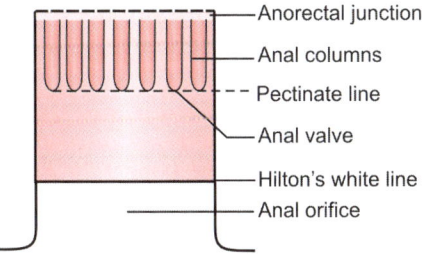

Fig. 5.30: Interior of anal canal

- *Anal valves*
  - ♦ Crescentric folds of mucosa (site of anal membrane) join the lower ends of adjacent anal columns.
- *Anal sinuses*
  - ♦ Pocket-like recesses above the anal valves.
- Pectinate line
  - ♦ Is the serrated line at the level of the anal valves.
- Marks the junction between
  - ♦ 1-embryonic hindgut lined by endoderm and
  - ♦ 2-the proctodeum lined by ectoderm.
- Marks the transition from
  - ♦ The simple columnar epithelium of the gut tube to the stratified squamous epithelium of the skin.

- Marks the divide between
  - ♦ Visceral and somatic nerve supply, venous drainage, lymphatic drainage, and arterial supply.
- Pecten
  - ♦ It is the area between the pectinate line and Hilton's line.
  - ♦ It is lined by stratified squamous nonkeratinized epithelium.
  - ♦ It has no sweat or sebaceous glands or hair follicles.
  - ♦ Numerous nerve endings are present in this area.
- White line
  - ♦ Is also known as the Hilton's line.
  - ♦ Lies below the pectinate line.
  - ♦ Marks the palpable intersphincteric groove separating the lower border of the internal anal sphincter and the subcutaneous part of the external anal sphincter.

- Internal hemorrhoids occur above the pectinate line.
  - ♦ Are relatively insensitive to pain because they are supplied by visceral afferent fibers.
  - ♦ Internal rectal venous plexus are responsible.
  - ♦ Are covered by rectal mucosa.

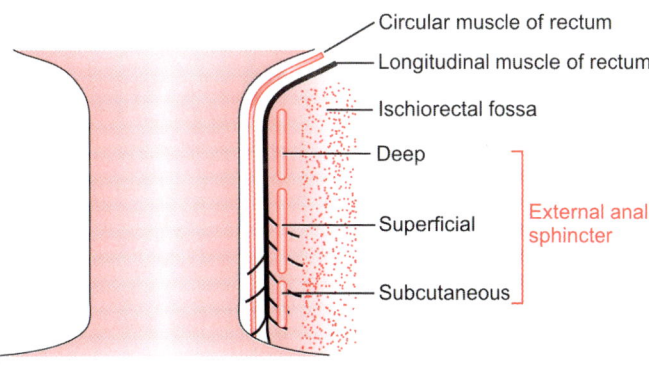

Fig. 5.31: Anal sphincters

– External hemorrhoids occur below the pectinate line.
  ♦ Are very sensitive to pain because they are supplied by somatic afferent fibers.
  ♦ External rectal venous plexus are responsible.
  ♦ Are covered by skin.

Blood Supply

• *Arterial supply:*
  – Inferior rectal arteries-branches of the internal pudendal arteries below pectinate line.
  – Superior rectal arteries supply the anal canal above the pectinate line.
• *Venous drainage:*
  – Above the pectinate line, drain into the superior rectal vein and thus reach the portal system. There are no valves.
  – Below the pectinate line, drain into the inferior rectal veins and thus reach the venacaval system.

  – Thus there is a connection between the portal and the systemic veins, site of portocaval anastomosis.
  – Reverse blood flow due to portal obstruction leads to varicosities of veins which bulge and form the haemorrhoids.

• *Lymphatic drainage:*
  – Above the pectinate line, internal iliac lymph nodes.
  – Below the pectinate line, superficial inguinal lymph nodes.

Nerve Supply

• Above the pectinate line, by the autonomic nerves:
  – Sympathetic—L1 and 2 (hypogastric plexus).
  – Parasympathetic—S2, 3 and 4.
  – Pain insensitive.

• Below the pectinate line, by the Inferior rectal nerves. Pain sensitive.

• *Anal fissures:* It is an elongated ulcer extending from tear of anal valves. Usually the result of chronic constipation and subsequent injury to mucosa by fecal matter.
• *Perianal abscess* may be subcutaneous, submucous or ischiorectal.
• *Anal fistula:*
  – Spread of infection from an abscess may lead to formation of anal fistula (open at both ends) or anal sinus (open at only one end).
  – Fistula extends from lumen to skin surface.
  – It can be high level or low level fistula.

Kidneys

• They are paired excretory organs placed on the posterior abdominal wall (Fig. 5.32).
• They are retroperitoneal structures.

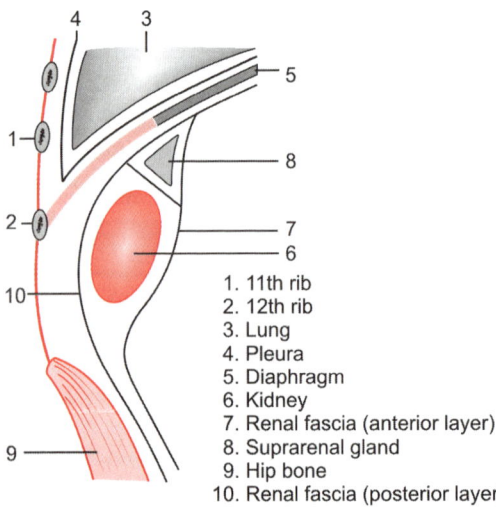

1. 11th rib
2. 12th rib
3. Lung
4. Pleura
5. Diaphragm
6. Kidney
7. Renal fascia (anterior layer)
8. Suprarenal gland
9. Hip bone
10. Renal fascia (posterior layer)

Fig. 5.32: Relations and coverings of kidney

- They move about 3 cm downwards during inspiration.

Surface Anatomy

Anteriorly kidneys can be roughly marked by considering the following facts:

1. Transpyloric plane crosses the upper border of the hilum of the right kidney and lower border of the hilum of the left kidney.
2. The upper pole is one inch away from median plane (4 cm above hilum).
3. Hilum is two inches away from the median plane just medial to tip of 9th costal cartilage.
4. Lower pole is three inches away from the median plane (4 cm below hilum).

Measurements of kidney: Remember 1, 2 and 4. It is one inch thick, two inches breadth and four inches long.

Surface marking on the posterior wall:

1. Mark a horizontal line at the level of T11 spine. Mark two points on that. The first point 2.5 cm from the midline and the second point 9 cm from the midline.
2. Mark a horizontal line at the level of L3 spine. Mark two points on that. The first point 2.5 cm from the midline and the second point 9 cm from the midline.
3. Join medial two points by a vertical line.
4. Join the lateral two points by a vertical line.
5. The parallelogram marked is called "Morris' parallelogram".
6. Kidney lies within this parallelogram.
7. As a rule left kidney is slightly higher than the right kidney.

Renal Angle

It is the angle between the last rib and erector spinae muscle. The tenderness in this angle is generally attributed to kidney.

As a basic mental drill let us name all the structures that we meet if we approach the kidney from the back.

1. Skin.
2. Superficial fascia.
3. Deep fascia with the posterior layer of the thoracolumbar fascia (attached to the spines of lumbar vertebrae.
4. Erector spinae muscle
5. Middle layer of thoracolumbar fascia (attached to the tips of transverse processes of lumbar vertebrae).
6. Quadratus lumborum muscle.
7. Anterior layer of thoracolumbar fascia (attached to the anterior surface of the transverse processes of the lumbar vertebrae).
8. Pararenal fat.
9. Renal fascia.
10. Perirenal fat.
11. Renal capsule (which immediately surrounds the kidney).

Renal Fascia

- It covers the kidney and suprarenal gland and sends septa between the kidney and suprarenal (Fig. 5.32). The anterior and posterior layers covering the anterior and

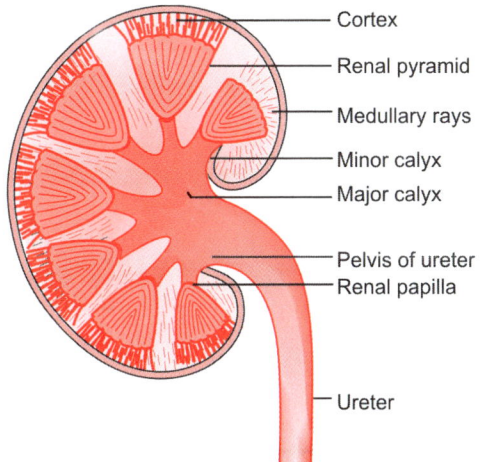

Cortex

Renal pyramid

Medullary rays

Minor calyx

Major calyx

Pelvis of ureter

Renal papilla

Ureter

Fig. 5.33: Structure of kidney

posterior surfaces of the kidney respectively are fused laterally and superiorly but not inferiorly.

This is the reason why kidneys sink downwards when fat is suddenly depleted in an individual. This movement of the kidney is called 'nephroptosis". Following nephroptosis, the ureter kinks.
- Nephropexy is the operation which fixes the kidney to the posterior abdominal wall.

- *Note:* Medially anterior and posterior layers of renal fascia are connected by a septum.

APPLIED ANATOMY

These days, renal transplantation is a very common operation in an individual whose both kidneys have failed. Harvested kidneys are transplanted to the iliac fossa and the renal vessels are connected to the external iliac vessels and the ureter is connected to the urinary bladder.

Anterior relations of the right kidney:
It is related to the following structures.
1. Right suprarenal gland.
2. Second part of duodenum.
3. Right lobe of liver (separated by the Morrison's pouch).
4. Right colic flexure.
5. Coils of small intestine.

Anterior relations of the left kidney:
1. Left suprarenal gland (along its upper and medial border).
2. Spleen.
3. Stomach (separated by the lesser sac).
4. Tail of the pancreas.
5. Coils of the small intestine.
6. Left colic flexure.

Posterior relations of the kidneys:
- *Note:* The only difference between the left and right kidney is: Left kidney is related

to the 11th and 12th ribs while the right kidney is related to the 12th rib only.
- The other relations common to both the kidneys are as follows:

Four muscles:
1. Diaphragm.
2. Psoas major.
3. Quadratus lumborum.
4. Aponeurosis of origin of transversus abdominis.

Three nerves:
1. Subcostal.
2. Ilio hypogastric.
3. Ilioinguinal.

Two arcuate ligaments:
1. Medial arcuate ligament (fibrous arch anterior to the psoas major).
2. Lateral arcuate ligament (fibrous arch anterior to the quadratus lumborum).

One artery:
- Subcostal artery.

Hilum of the Kidney

Hilum is the entry to the kidney present on the concave medial border. Structures present in the hilum are (Fig. 5.34):
1. Renal vein.
2. Renal artery.

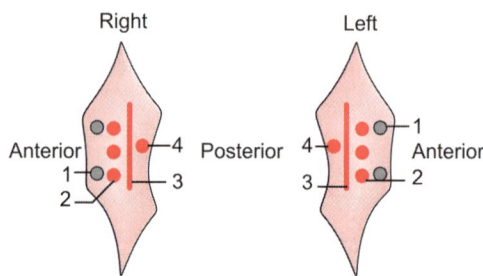

1. Renal vein, 2. Anterior rami of renal artery, 3. Ureter, 4. Posterior rami of renal artery

Fig. 5.34: Hilum of kidneys

3. Pelvis of ureter.
4. Renal plexus of nerves.
5. Lymph vessels.
6. Connective tissue.

Structures are arranged in this order at hilum from front to back: (VAD)

- Renal vein.
- Renal artery.
- Ureter lying most posterior.

Renal Veins

- The right renal vein is short and lies behind the second part of duodenum and head of the pancreas and opens into the inferior vena cava. It lies in front of the right renal artery. It has no other tributaries except the ones from the right kidney.

- The left renal vein is long. It receives left suprarenal vein from above and left gonadal vein from below. It lies behind the body of the pancreas. It lies sandwitched between the superior mesenteric artery and abdominal aorta.

Brief note on the development:

- Kidneys develop in the pelvic region and ascend later due to growth of the embryo's body below the kidneys.

- During ascent, they take branches from the nearby arteries. As ascent continues; it gets new vessels from the arteries nearby and the old ones disappear.

If they fail to disappear, they remain as accessory renal arteries. They are very common in the kidney. They supply a separate area in the kidney and are end arteries.

- If kidney fails to ascend, it remains as a pelvic kidney.

- One kidney may ascend normally and the other may remain as a pelvic kidney.

- During ascent, if the lower ends of the two kidneys fuse together, the ascent of this fused mass is prevented from the stem of the inferior mesenteric artery. Such kidneys resemble a horse shoe and, therefore, they are called "horse shoe kidneys".

- Secretory part is developed from the metanephric mass and the collecting part is developed from the ureteric diverticulum. Failure of the fusion of 2 parts might result in the polycystic kidney where majority of secretory parts remain unconnected with their respective collecting parts.

Renal calculi: Stones form in renal calices.

Ureter

- It is the muscular tube which conducts the urine to the urinary bladder from the kidney.

- Its dilated upper end is called the pelvis of the ureter. Renal sinus is the space just beyond the hilum in the kidney (Fig. 5.33).

- It is 10 inches (25 cm) long.

- Its upper half lies in the abdomen and lower half lies in the pelvis.

- It lies anterior to the corresponding psoas major muscle and genitofemoral nerve. It crosses the bifurcation of the corresponding common iliac artery and enters the pelvis.

Anterior Relations of the Right Ureter

1. Third part of the duodenum.
2. Right gonadal vessels.
3. Right colic and ileocolic vessels.
4. Ileum (terminal part).
5. Root of the mesentery.

Anterior Relations of the Left Ureter

1. Left colic vessels.
2. Left gonadal vessels.
3. Sigmoid colon.
4. Sigmoid mesocolon.

Remember: The inferior mesenteric vein lies medial to left ureter.

Blood Supply of Ureter

It receives branches from the nearby arteries:
1. Renal.
2. Gonadal.
3. Abdominal aorta.
4. Common and internal iliac.
5. Inferior vesical artery and uterine artery in the pelvis.
   - There is a vertical anastomosis connecting all these branches in the wall of the ureter.

Nerve Supply of the Ureter

It is supplied by T11 to L2 segments. These are sympathetic nerves. They also carry pain sensation. That is the reason why pain of ureteric colic is referred from the loin to the groin. Parasympathetic supply is by vagus and S2-4 nerves.

Constrictions of Ureter

- The first constriction is at the pelviureteric junction.
- The second constriction lies at the level of pelvic brim.
- The third constriction appears where ureter lies obliquely in the wall of urinary bladder.

These constrictions are easily seen in special X-rays where radiopaque material is injected prior to taking X-ray (descending pyelogram).

1. The first constriction lies at the level of transverse process of L2.
2. The second constriction lies opposite the sacroiliac joint.
3. The third constriction lies at the level of ischial spine.

CLINICAL ANATOMY

Ureteric colic is an excruciating pain arising out of spasmodic contraction of ureter usually originated because of impacted stones (hardened minerals). They tend to get lodged at the three constrictions of ureter.

Ureters may be injured at the site where they are crossed by the uterine artery, close to the cervix, in hysterectomy surgeries.

Suprarenal Glands

- Suprarenal glands lie superior to the corresponding kidney (Fig. 5.32).
- They lie within the renal fascia but there is septum of renal fascia which separates the kidney from the suprarenal.

That makes removal of kidney easy as suprarenal can be safely left behind.

- They are endocrine glands having cortex and medulla.
- The cortex secretes the mineralocorticoids, glucocorticoids and sex hormones.
- The medulla secretes the catecholamines.
- The suprarenal cortex is essential for life.

The Right Suprarenal Gland

- It is triangular in shape.
- *Anterior relations:* Inferior vena cava medially and right lobe of liver laterally.
- *Posterior relations:* Diaphragm (right crus).
- It has only one vein issued from its hilum. This right suprarenal vein opens into the inferior vena cava.
- There are three groups of arteries which supply the right suprarenal gland.
  1. The superior suprarenal comes from the right inferior phrenic artery.
  2. The middle suprarenal comes from the abdominal aorta.
  3. The inferior suprarenal comes from the right renal artery.

The Left Suprarenal Gland

- It is semilunar in shape.
- *Posterior relation:* Diaphragm (left crus).
- *Anterior relations:* From above downwards, they are:
    - Stomach (cardiac end).
    - Splenic artery.
    - Body of the pancreas.
- Left suprarenal vein opens into the left renal vein.
- There are three groups of arteries in the left just like the right suprarenal gland.

The space between the two suprarenals is about 2 inches long and it contains the following structures from right to left:
1. Right crus of diaphragm.
2. Right celiac ganglion.
3. Celiac trunk.
4. Left celiac ganglion.
5. Left crus of diaphragm.

Abdominal Aorta

- It is the continuation of the thoracic aorta.
- It begins at the level of T12 vertebra and terminates at the level of L4 vertebra.
- It passes through the aortic opening accompanied by the azygos vein and thoracic duct.
- It lies between the right and left crura above.

Anterior Relations

1. Celiac plexus of nerves.
2. Superior mesenteric plexus of nerves.
3. Body of the pancreas.
4. Left renal vein.
5. Uncinate process of pancreas.
6. Horizontal part of the duodenum.
7. Inferior mesenteric plexus of nerves.
8. Peritoneum.

Posterior Relations

1. Left psoas major.
2. Bodies of lumbar vertebrae.

Branches (Fig. 5.35)

Unpaired ventral branches:
1. Celiac trunk.
2. Superior mesenteric artery.
3. Inferior mesenteric artery.
Unpaired dorsal branch:
1. Median sacral artery.
Paired dorsal branches:
1. Four lumbar arteries.
Paired lateral branches:
1. Inferior phrenic arteries.
2. Middle suprarenal arteries.
3. Renal arteries.
4. Gonadal arteries.

Two terminal branches: common iliac arteries.

CLINICAL ANATOMY

Abdominal aortic aneurysm is an abnormal enlargement of the aorta due to weakness of its wall. It carries a risk of rupture which is a surgical emergency. Hence, it should be repaired.

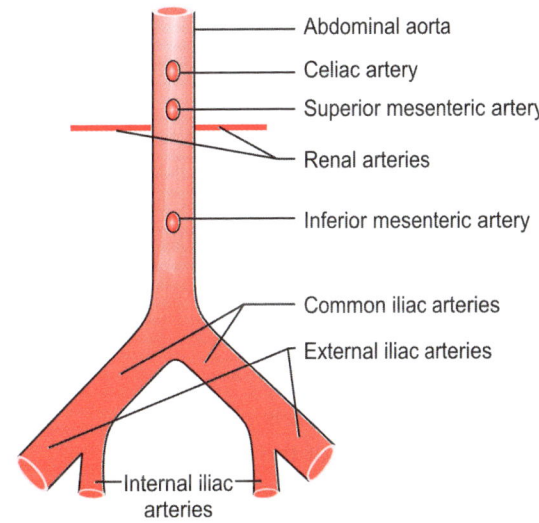

Fig. 5.35: Abdominal aorta and its branches

Table 5.3: Arteries of the gut

	Celiac trunk	Superior mesenteric artery	Inferior mesenteric artery
Territory supplied	Foregut—lower end of oesophagus, stomach, duodenum proximal to bile duct opening, liver, extrahepatic biliary apparatus, spleen, major portion of pancreas	Midgut—gastrointestinal tract from the level of opening of bile duct into duodenum till the junction of right 2/3rd and left 1/3rd of transverse colon and small portion of pancreas	Hindgut—from junction of right 2/3rd and left 1/3rd of transverse colon till the anal canal (up to the level of anal valves)
Level of origin from abdominal aorta	T12	L1	L3
Branches	Left gastric, common hepatic, splenic	Inferior pancreaticoduodenal, middle colic, right colic, ileocolic, jejunal and ileal	Left colic, sigmoid, superior rectal

Arteries of the Gut (Table 5.3)

Marginal Artery of Drummond

Forms an arterial arcade along the concavity of colon (Fig. 5.36). It is formed between branches of superior and inferior mesenteric artery supplying the colon. Colon is supplied by vasa recta arising from this artery.

Inferior Vena Cava

- It is formed at the level of L5 by the union of two common iliac veins.
- It enters thorax by piercing the diaphragm at the level of T8 vertebra (Fig. 5.37). It is accompanied by branches of the right phrenic nerve in this opening.

Anterior Relations

1. Peritoneum.
2. Root of the mesentery.
3. Right gonadal vessels.
4. Horizontal part of the duodenum.
5. Head of the pancreas.
6. Epiploic foramen.
7. Liver.

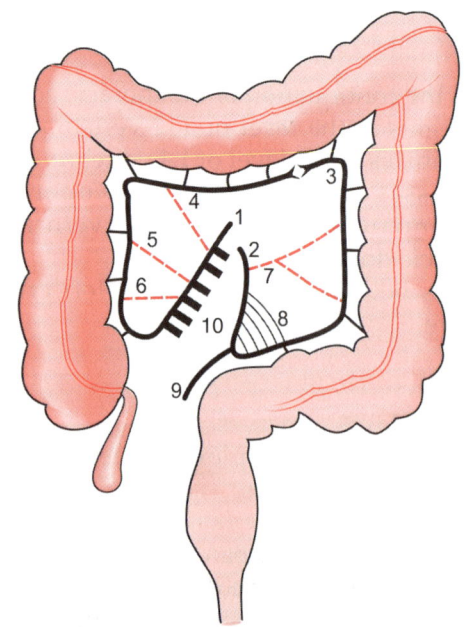

1. Superior mesenteric artery, 2. Inferior mesenteric artery,
3. Marginal artery of Drummond, 4. Middle colic artery,
5. Right colic artery, 6. Ileocolic artery, 7. Left colic artery
8. Sigmoid artery, 9. Superior rectal artery,
10. Jejunal and ileal branches

Fig. 5.36: Marginal artery of Drummond

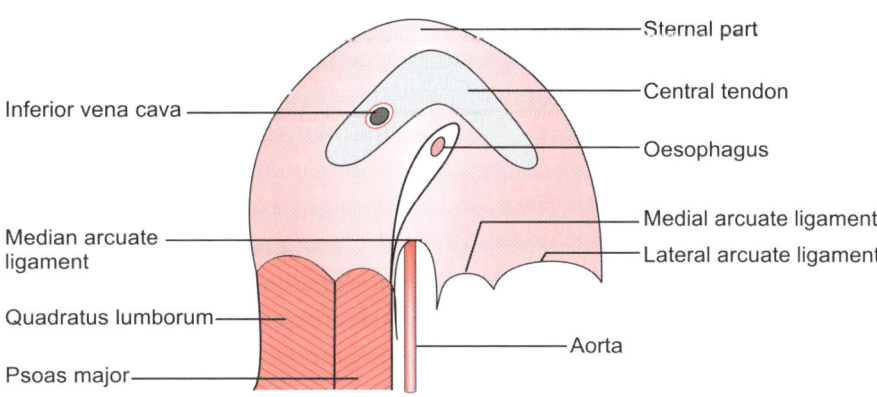

Fig. 5.37: Diaphragm

Posterior Relations

1. Right psoas major.
2. Right suprarenal gland.
3. Right crus of diaphragm.

Tributaries

1. Two common iliac veins.
2. Right gonadal vein.
3. Right and left renal veins.
4. Right suprarenal vein.
5. Right inferior phrenic vein (occasionally left inferior phrenic vein also).
6. Hepatic veins.
7. Third and fourth lumbar veins.

Lumbar Plexus

• It is formed by the union of ventral rami of L1 - L4 in the substance of the muscle psoas major.

It gives the following branches:
1. Iliohypogastric nerve (L1).
2. Ilioinguinal nerve (L1).
3. Genitofemoral nerve (L1 and 2).
4. Femoral nerve (dorsal divisions of ventral rami of L2, 3 and 4).
5. Lateral cutaneous nerve of thigh (dorsal divisions of ventral rami of L2 and 3).
6. Obturator nerve (ventral divisions of ventral rami of L2, 3 and 4).

7. Lumbosacral trunk (L4 and 5) crosses the ala of sacrum and joins the sacral plexus.

Diaphragm

• It is the muscular partition between thorax and abdomen (Fig. 5.37).
• It arises from the right and left crura, inner aspect of the lower costal cartilages and their ribs, back of the xiphoid process.
• Inserted into the central tendon of diaphragm.
• *Nerve supply:*
  – It is supplied by the phrenic nerve. The phrenic nerve is motor to the muscle and sensory to the central part of the diaphragm. Lower intercostal nerves are sensory to the peripheral part of the diaphragm.

Therefore, irritation of the central part results in the referred pain to the corresponding shoulder. The involvement of the peripheral part results in the pain being referred to the region of costal margin.

• Openings in the diaphragm:
  1. *Opening of the inferior vena cava:*
     – It lies at the level of T8 verterbra.

– Inferior vena cava and right phrenic nerve branches pass through it.

– It lies within the central tendon of diaphragm.

2. *Oesophageal opening:*

– It lies at the level of T10 vertebra.

– It lies within the loop of the right crus of the diaphragm.

– Oesophagus, right and left vagi, esophageal branches of left gastric artery, accompanying veins and lymph vessels pass through this opening.

3. *Aortic opening:*

– Boundaries are:

a. *Anterior:* Median arcuate ligament.

b. On either side, the corresponding crus of the diaphragm.

c. *Posterior:* The body of 12th thoracic vertebra.

– It is at the level of T12 vertebra.

– Structures passing through this opening are:

a. Abdominal aorta.

b. Thoracic duct.

c. Azygos vein.

CLINICAL ANATOMY

Diaphragmatic hernias: Developmental defects or gaps in the diaphragm lead to herniation of abdominal contents into the thorax resulting in diaphragmatic hernia.

Injury to phrenic nerve results in paralysis of ipsilateral side of diaphragm.

External Iliac Artery

• It is the terminal branch of the common iliac artery at the level of sacroiliac joint (Fig. 5.35).

• It is accompanied by the external iliac vein and external iliac group of lymph nodes.

• It gives two branches:

1. Inferior epigastric artery.

2. Deep circumflex iliac artey.

• It continues as the femoral artery behind the inguinal ligament.

• It is crossed on the right side by the following:

1. Right ovarian artery (in females).

2. Right ductus deferens (in males).

3. Terminal ileum.

4. Sometimes appendix.

• It is crossed on the left side by the following:

1. Left ovarian artery (in females).

2. Left ductus deferens (in males).

3. Sigmoid colon.

4. Coils of small intestine.

Lymph Nodes of the Posterior Abdominal Wall

• Lymph vessels from the lower limb open into the inguinal lymph nodes.

• Inguinal lymph nodes continue as the external iliac nodes around the external iliac vessels. These vessels receive all the lymph from the lower limb and the deeper part of the anterior abdominal wall.

• Lymph from the pelvis mainly drains into the internal iliac lymph nodes.

• Internal and external lymph nodes open into the common iliac nodes around the common iliac vessels.

• These will continue as the lumbar (aortic) lymph nodes in the region of the lumbar vertebrae around abdominal aorta.

• The lumbar or aortic nodes are divided into preaortic, lateral aortic and retroaortic groups.

i. Preaortic located around origins of celiac, superior mesenteric and inferior mesenteric artery (ventral branches of aorta) in front of aorta drain lymph along the above mentioned branches from the territory supplied by them. All the lymph from the gastrointestinal tract is drained into the celiac, superior mesenteric and inferior mesenteric nodes. Lymph from these three groups of nodes join to form intestinal lymph trunks. These entire nodes lie anterior to the aorta, therefore, they are also collectively termed as preaortic nodes.

ii. Para-aortic nodes are called lateral aortic nodes, situated on sides of abdominal aorta. It recieves lymph corresponding to territories supplied by lateral and dorsal branches of abdominal aorta (kidneys, suprarenals, gonads, posterior abdominal wall). It also recieves lymph from pelvis and lower limbs.

iii. Retroaortic are extension of lateral aortic.

- Two lumbar trunks from lateral aortic and intestinal trunks from preaortic open into the dilated lymph sac called "cisterna chyli".
- Cisterna chyli lies at the level of L1 and L2 vertebrae.
- It continues as the thoracic duct (Fig. 5.38).

Muscles of Posterior Abdominal Wall (Table 5.4)

PERINEUM

- It is the lower end of the trunk, between the thighs.

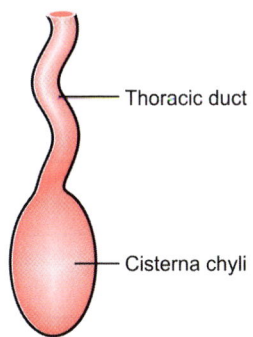

Fig. 5.38: Cisterna chyli

- It lies below the inferior pelvic aperture or pelvic outlet.
- It is clearly seen only in the lithotomy position.

Boundaries

Diamond-shaped.
Outlet of the pelvis forms its bony boundaries:
- Anteriorly: Pubic symphysis.
- Anterolaterally: Ischiopubic rami.
- Laterally: Ischial tuberosities.
- Posterolaterally: Sacrotuberous ligaments.
- Posteriorly: Tip of Coccyx.

Subdivisions

The diamond-shaped area can be subdivided into 2 triangles by an imaginary line connecting the ischial tuberosities into:

	Table 5.4: Muscles of the posterior abdominal wall	
Muscle	*Psoas major*	*Quadratus lumborum*
Origin	Transverse process of all 5 lumbar vertebrae, sides of vertebral bodies of T12–L5 and intervertebral discs between them	Iliolumbar ligament and posterior part of inner lip of iliac crest
Insertion	Lesser trochanter of femur	Lumbar transverse processes and medial half of 12th rib
Nerve supply	Lumbar plexus	Ventral rami of T12–L4
Action	Flexes thigh and trunk	Extension and lateral flexion of vertebral column fixes 12th rib during inspiration so that contraction of diaphragm is more effective.

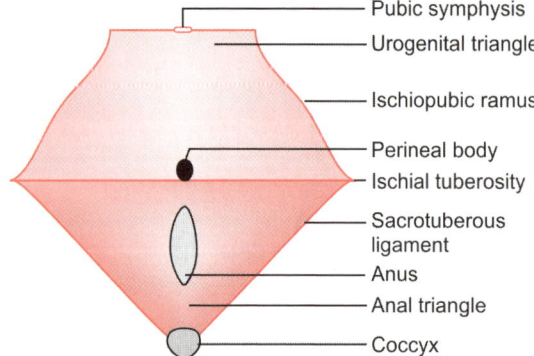

Fig. 5.39: Urogenital and anal triangles

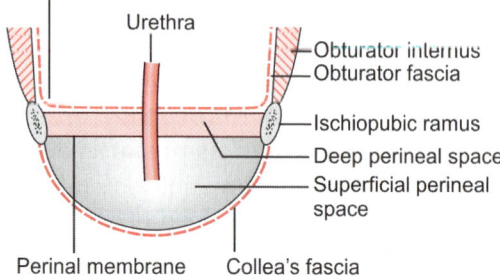

Fig. 5.40: Superficial and deep perineal space

- Anterior urogenital triangle consisting of external parts of the urinary and genital systems (Fig. 5.39).
- Posterior anal triangle consisting of the anal canal and ischiorectal fossa (Fig. 5.39).

Urogenital Triangle

Boundaries

- Pubic symphysis in front.
- Ischiopubic rami on the sides.
- Imaginary line joining the ischial tuberosities—behind.
- It has two pouches or spaces—superficial and deep perineal pouches (Fig. 5.40).
- Superficial fascia of the urogenital triangle consists of two layers:
  - Superficial (inferior) fatty layer
  - Deep (superior) membranous layer (Colles' fascia).
- Fatty layer is absent over the scrotum (replaced by Dartos muscle) and penis in males. In females, it is continuous with the fascia camper in the anterior abdominal wall.
- Membranous layer (Colles' fascia) lies below the perineal membrane. Superficial perineal pouch lies between the perineal membrane and membranous layer. Posteriorly, the membranous layer is attached to the posterior border of the perineal membrane. Laterally, is attached to the ischiopubic rami. Anteriorly, is continuous with the deep membranous layer of the superficial fascia of the anterior abdominal wall.

- Extravasated urine due to rupture of the membranous urethra below perineal membrane collects in the superficial perineal pouch. It cannot spread behind or laterally, but can ascend into the anterior abdominal wall between the fascia scarpa and the external oblique muscle. It cannot descend to the thigh because the fascia scarpa is attached to the fascia lata of the thigh along the Holden's line (a line about 1 cm below the inguinal ligament).
- Rupture above perineal membrane causes urine to spread upwards into extraperitoneal space; around bladder and prostate, into anterior abdominal wall in a different path. It is in a deeper plane and does not enter superficial perineal pouch.

Perineal Membrane

(Triangular ligament or inferior fascia of the urogenital diaphragm)

- It is a triangular fibrous sheet.

- It provides attachment for muscles there.
- In the anatomical position, it is horizontally placed and has superior and inferior surfaces.
- It lies superior to the Colles' fascia (membranous layer of the superficial fascia of the perineum).
- It is attached laterally to the ischiopubic rami.
- Posteriorly, it fuses with the Colles' fascia below, and the superior fascia of the urogenital diaphragm above.
- Perineal body lies in the middle of its posterior border.
- Anterior border of the perineal membrane is free and thickened to form the transverse perineal ligament.
- Deep dorsal vein of the penis or clitoris passes in the gap between the ligament and the inferior pubic angle to join the prostatic or vesical plexus respectively. It is accompanied by dorsal nerve of penis or clitoris.
- The inferior surface of the perineal membrane forms the roof of the superficial perineal pouch. The superior surface forms the floor or the deep perineal pouch.

Structures piercing the perineal membrane:
1. Urethra, in the middle, 2.5 cm behind the pubic angle.
2. Arteries to the bulb.
3. Deep arteries of the penis or clitoris.
4. Dorsal arteries of the penis or clitoris.
5. Posterior scrotal or labial nerves and vessels.
6. Ducts of the bulbourethral glands (in the male).
7. Vagina (in the female) just behind the urethra.

Superficial Perineal Pouch

Boundaries

- *Roof:* Perineal membrane.
- *Floor:* Colles' fascia.
- *Lateral:* Ischiopubic rami.

- *Posterior:* Closed, because the perineal membrane and the Colles' fascia fuse.
- *Anterior:* Open, continues into the anterior abdominal wall deep to the fascia scarpa.

Contents

In the male:
1. Spongy urethra.
2. Root of the penis: Two crura and a bulb.
3. Three pairs of muscles: Ischiocavernosus, bulbospongiosus and transverse perinei superficialis.
4. Arteries and nerves.
   a. Posterior scrotal vessels and nerves.
   b. Transverse perineal arteries.
   c. Perineal branch of posterior cutaneous nerve of thigh.

In the female:
1. Urethra.
2. Vagina (behind the urethra).
3. Bulbs of the vestibule.
4. Greater vestibular glands (Bartholin's glands).
5. Crura of the clitoris.
6. Three pairs of muscles: Ischiocavernosus, bulbospongiosus and transverse perinei superficialis.
7. Posterior labial vessels and nerves.
8. Perineal branch of posterior cutaneous nerve of thigh.

Deep Perineal Pouch

Boundaries

- *Roof:* Superior fascia of the UG diaphragm.
- *Floor:* Perineal membrane.
- *Lateral:* Ischiopubic rami.
- *Posterior:* Closed, because the perineal membrane and the superior fascia of UG diaphragm fuse.
- *Anterior:* Closed, because the perineal membrane and the superior fascia of UG diaphragm fuse.

- *Note:* The deep perineal pouch is closed on all sides.

Contents

1. Membranous part of the urethra.
2. *Muscles:* Transverse perinei profundus, sphincter urethrae.
3. *Vessels and nerves:* Deep artery of penis or clitoris. Dorsal artery of penis or clitoris. Arteries to the bulb (penis/vestibule). Dorsal nerve of penis or clitoris.
4. Bulbourethral (Cowper's) glands in the male.
5. Vagina in the female.

Urogenital Diaphragm

The deep transversus perinei and sphincter urethrae muscle, superior fascia of the UG diaphragm and perineal membrane (inferior fascia of UG diaphragm) together form the UG diaphragm.

Sphincter Urethrae

External urethral sphincter

- It surrounds the membranous urethra in male and both urethra and vagina in females.

- *Origin:* From the transverse perineal ligament and pudendal canal.
- *Insertion:* Continues with the opposite side by passing around the urethra and some fibers inserted into perineal body.
- *Nerve supply:* Perineal branch of the pudendal nerve.
- *Action:* External sphincter for the urethra. It is voluntary.

ANAL TRIANGLE

- Bounded in front by the imaginary line drawn connecting the ischial tuberosities, on either side by the sacrotuberous ligaments and behind by the tip of coccyx.
- It contains the lower end of the anal canal in the midline, and the ischiorectal fossa on either side of the anal canal.

ISCHIORECTAL FOSSA

- *Pair of spaces:* One on either side of the lower end of the anal canal. Hence, ischioanal fossa is the more appropriate name (Fig. 5.41).

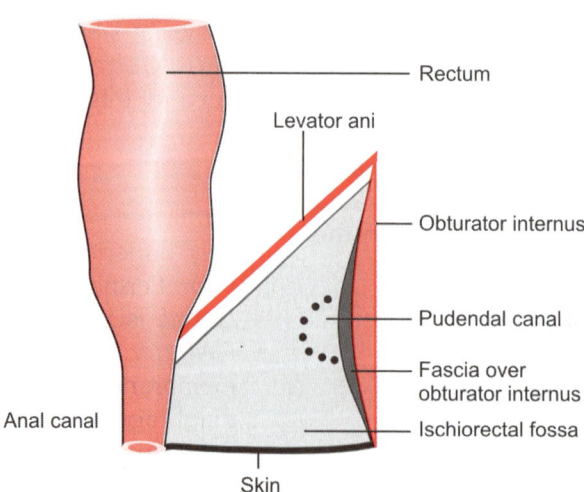

Fig. 5.41: Ischiorectal fossa

- The two fossae communicate with each other behind the anal canal.
- *Shape:* Wedge-shaped.
- *Boundaries:*
  - *Laterally:* Obturator internus, obturator fascia (fascia covering obturator internus), pudendal canal (Alcock's canal) with its contents.
  - *Medially:* Medial wall sloping downwards and medially. Formed by Levator ani, sphincter ani externus (in the lower part).
  - *Posteriorly:* Sacrotuberous ligament, lower border of gluteus maximus.
  - *Anteriorly:* Forms an anterior recess which extends till the pubic bones above perineal membrane
  - *Below:* Bounded by skin and superficial fascia.

- *Hiatus of Schwalbe* is a gap seen sometimes between the defective origin of the levator ani and obturator fascia. Ischiorectal hernia may occur in such cases.

- Lunate fascia is a dome-shaped fascia in the ischiorectal fossa. It starts from the pudendal canal laterally and fuses with the anal fascia covering external anal sphincter medially.

Contents of the ischiorectal fossa:
- Ischiorectal pad of fat. The pads of two sides support the anal canal.
- Inferior rectal vessels and nerves which cross from lateral to the medial wall to supply the sphincter ani externus and perianal skin
- Perineal branch of the 4th sacral nerve which supplies the sphincter ani externus.

- Prolapse of the rectum may occur because of loss of the pad of fat due to debilitating diseases like diarrhea in children.

- *Ischiorectal abscess:* Ischiorectal fat is susceptible to infections due to poor blood supply and nearness to the anal canal. The abscess may open into the anal canal or rectum internally, or on the perianal skin-ischiorectal sinus (open at only one end). If the pus opens on both ends, it is called ischiorectal fistula or fistula-in-ano.
- Ischiorectal hernia occurs through the hiatus of Schwalbe.

Pudendal Canal

- It runs in the lateral wall of the ischiorectal fossa (Fig. 5.41).
- It is about 3 cm long and 3 cm above the lower end of ischial tuberosity.
- It begins posteriorly at the lesser sciatic notch and ends anteriorly in the deep perineal pouch.
- The canal is formed by the splitting of the obturator fascia (according to some, between the obturator fascia laterally and the lunate fascia medially).
- *Contents:*
  1. Pudendal nerve and its branches.
  2. Internal pudendal vessels and its branches.

Pudendal nerve block is performed by injecting an anaesthetic at the point where pudendal nerve crosses the ischial spine, to produce analgesia during child-birth.

Pudendal Nerve

- *Origin:* From the sacral plexus.
- *Root value:* Ventral rami of S2, S3 and S4.
- It is the main nerve supply to the perineum.
- It enters the perineum through the lesser sciatic foramen along with the internal pudendal artery and runs forwards in the pudendal canal on the lateral wall of the ischiorectal fossa.

- Its branches are distributed to the anal triangle, urogenital triangle, scrotum or labium majus, penis or clitoris.
- *Branches:*
  - Inferior rectal nerve.
  - Perineal nerve.
  - Dorsal nerve of the penis or clitoris.
- Inferior rectal nerve runs medially in the ischiorectal fossa to supply sphincter ani externus and perianal skin.
- Perineal nerve divides into superficial and deep branches.
  - Deep branch supplies the muscles of the perineal pouches, sphincter ani externus and the levator ani.
  - Superficial branches run as posterior scrotal or labial nerves to supply posterior parts of the skin of scrotum or labium majus.
- Dorsal nerve of the penis or clitoris supplies glans penis, prepuce and skin of the penis or clitoris.

Pudendal nerve block.

Internal Pudendal Artery

Origin

From the anterior division of the internal iliac artery.

- Is the principal blood supply to the perineum.
- Enters the perineum through the lesser sciatic foramen adjacent to the ischial spine.
- Lies in the pudendal canal on the lateral wall of the ischiorectal fossa.
- Is accompanied in its course by the pudendal nerve.

Branches

- Inferior rectal artery.

- Perineal artery gives transverse perineal and posterior scrotal or labial artery.
- Artery of the bulb of the penis or clitoris.
- Deep artery of the penis or clitoris (a terminal branch) runs in the corpus cavernosum.
- Dorsal artery of the penis or clitoris (a terminal branch).

Venous Drainage of the Perineum

- Veins corresponding to the branches of the internal pudendal artery mostly follow the internal pudendal vein to the internal iliac vein.

Deep dorsal vein of the penis or clitoris:

- Is unpaired.
- It lies in the midline of the penis or clitoris between the paired dorsal arteries.
- It enters the pelvis through the gap between transverse perineal ligament and the arcuate pubic ligament.
  - In the male, it drains into the prostatic venous plexus.
  - In the female, it drains into the vesical venous plexus (tributaries of the internal iliac veins).

Lymphatic Drainage of the Perineum

- Mostly to the superficial inguinal nodes along the external pudendal vessels, includes drainage of the lower part of the anal canal and vagina.
- To the internal iliac nodes along the internal pudendal vessels for the deep perineal space
  - Membranous urethra.
  - Part of the vagina.
- From the glans of the penis lymph drains into the deep inguinal lymph node of cloquet. From the rest of penis it drains into superficial inguinal nodes.

Perineal Body

(Centrum tendineum perinei)

- It is a central fibromuscular node (Fig. 5.39).

- It is situated between the anus behind and the bulb of the penis in the male and the vagina in the female, in front.
- It forms a very important support for the pelvic floor and pelvic visceral organs.
- Muscles converging on it are:
  - Bulbospongiosus.
  - Sphincter ani externus.
  - Transverse perinei superficialis and profundus.
  - Levator ani.
  - Smooth muscles from the wall of the rectum and anal canal.
- Fibrous components converging on it are:
  - Perineal membrane.
  - Colles' fascia.
  - Superior fascia of UG diaphragm.
  - Rectovesical (rectovaginal) fascia (septum).

THE PELVIS

Bony Pelvis
- Hip bones (2).
- Sacrum.
- Coccyx

Ligaments
- Sacrotuberous.
- Sacrospinous.

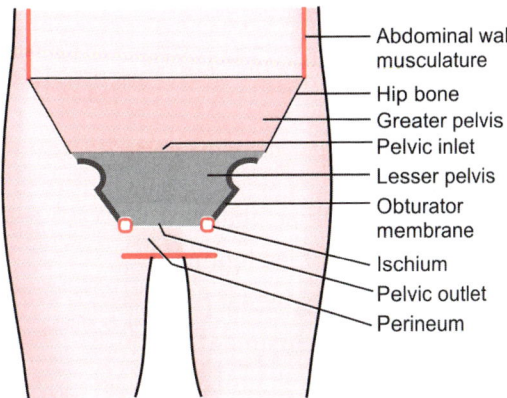

Fig. 5.42: Pelvis

Anatomical Position
- Anterior superior iliac spines and pubic tubercles lie in the same coronal plane.
- Tip of coccyx and the upper margin of the pubic symphysis lie in the same horizontal plane.

The pelvis consists of two subdivisions:
- False or greater pelvis.
- True or lesser pelvis.

Pelvic inlet or pelvic brim separates the two parts.

Greater Pelvis
- Above the pelvic brim.
- Forms the lowest part of the abdominal cavity.

Lesser Pelvis
- Below the pelvic brim.
- Above opens into the abdominal cavity.
- Below closed by the pelvic diaphragm.

Joints of the Pelvis
Lumbosacral Joint

Occurs between L5 and S1.

Sacroiliac Joint

- Synovial joint.
- Its irregular surface allowing for little movement.
- Is reinforced by interosseous sacroiliac ligament.
  - Dorsal sacroiliac ligament.
  - Ventral sacroiliac ligament.
  - Iliolumbar ligament.
  - Sacrospinous ligament.
  - Sacrotuberous ligament.

Sacrococcygeal joint: Occurs between S5 and C1.

Pubic Symphysis

- Secondary cartilaginous joint (symphysis).
- Supported by
  - Superior pubic ligament.
  - Arcuate pubic ligament.
- Negligible movement except in the later stage of pregnancy when movement is increased (hormonal effect).

Pelvic Inlet

Pelvic inlet is formed by:

- The promontory and anterior border of ala of the sacrum, the arcuate lines of ilium, pecten pubis, pubic crest and superior margin of pubic symphysis.

True Pelvis

- *Bony wall is formed by:*
  - Sacrum and coccyx behind.
  - Pelvic surfaces of the hip bones in front and sides.
- *Muscles:*
  - Piriformis (posteriorly).
  - Obturator internus and obturator fascia (laterally).
  - Levator ani and coccygeus (pelvic diaphragm) form the floor.

Pelvic Outlet

- Diamond-shaped area is bounded by:
  - Tip of coccyx.
  - Sacrotuberous ligament.
  - Ischial tuberosities.
  - Ischiopubic rami.
  - Pubic symphysis.
- Outlet closed by pelvic diaphragm.

Sexual Differences in the Bony Pelvis (Table 5.5)

Diameters of the Pelvis

Anteroposterior, oblique and transverse diameters (Fig. 5.43B).

Inlet of the pelvis:
- A-P diameter: 10 cm.

Table 5.5: Sexual differences in bony pelvis		
Feature	*Male pelvis*	*Female pelvis*
Pelvic inlet	Heart-shaped	Oval or rounded
Subpubic angle (Fig. 5.43C)	< 70°	> 80°
Sacrum	Longer and narrow	Shorter and wide
Ischiopubic rami	Significantly everted	Not much everted
Obturator foramen	Oval	Triangular
Greater pelvis	Deep	Shallow
Lesser pelvis	Narrow and deep	Wide and shallow
Pelvic outlet	Relatively small	Relatively large
Acetabulum	Larger	Smaller

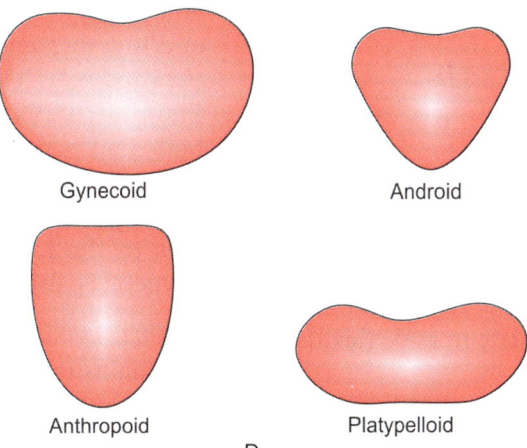

Plane of pelvic inlet — Posterior wall

Axis of pelvic cavity

Anterior wall

Pelvic outlet

A

Posterior

3   3

2

1

Anterior

B

1. Anteroposterior diameter
2. Transverse diameter
3. Oblique diameter

Female

Short segment of a broad cone

Wide pubic angle

Male

Long segment of a narrow cone

Pubic arch

Narrow pubic angle

C

Gynecoid

Android

Anthropoid

Platypelloid

D

Fig. 5.43: A. Plane of pelvic inlet and outlet, B. Diameters of pelvis, C. Differences between male and female pelvis, D. Shapes of pelvis based on pelvic inlet

- Oblique diameter: 11 cm.
- Transverse diameter: 12 cm.

Pelvic cavity:
- All diameters: 11 cm.

Pelvic outlet:
- A-P diameter: 12 cm.
- Oblique diameter: 11 cm.
- Transverse diameter: 10 cm.

The maximum diameters:
- Pelvic inlet: Transverse.
- Pelvic outlet: Anteroposterior.

Thus, during childbirth, the head must rotate 90 degrees between the pelvic inlet and outlet.

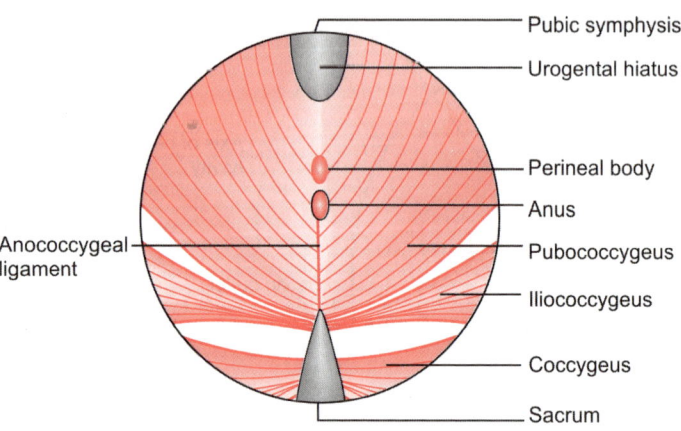

Fig. 5.44: Pelvic diaphragm

Pelvic Diaphragm

- Forms the floor of the pelvis.
- Supports the pelvic organs.
- Incomplete anteriorly for passage of the urethra + vagina.
- Forms the medial wall of the ischiorectal fossa.
- Functions as a unit to raise the pelvic floor.
- Covered by the superior and inferior fascia of the pelvic diaphragm.

Consists of two muscles (Fig. 5.44):
1. Levator ani (anteriorly)
   a. Pubococcygeus.
   b. Iliococcygeus.
2. Coccygeus (ischiococcygeus) (posteriorly).

Pubococcygeus part of the levator ani:
- Anterior component surrounds
  – The base of the prostate in male (levator prostate muscle).
  – Lower end of the vagina in the female (pubovaginalis muscle).
  – Anchors to the perineal body.
- Middle component—puborectalis muscle
  – Forms a sling around the anorectal junction (puborectal sling).

  – Is responsible for the angle formed between the rectum and the anal canal.
  – Functions as a sphincter to maintain anal continence during defecation.

Iliococcygeus part of the levator ani:
- Posterior component
  – inserted into anococcygeal ligament and tip of coccyx.
- Levator ani is attached to the pubic bones anteriorly, to the ischial spines posteriorly, and to a thickening in the obturator fascia (tendinous arch of levator ani) on each side.
- Ends in coccyx, anococcygeal ligament/ body and perineal body depending on the part of levator ani.

Coccygeus muscle extends from the ischial spines to the inferior sacrum and coccyx. Coccygeus is also known as ischiococcygeus

Functional significance of the levator ani muscle:
- Maintains the integrity of the pelvic floor.
- Is susceptible to damage during childbirth.
- Is important in maintaining the urinary continence.
- Preventing the prolapse of the rectum.
- Arises from a condensed fascia (tendinous arch) over the obturator muscle.

- Consists of:
  - Pubococcygeus.
  - Iliococcygeus.

  Nerve supply: Is innervated by ventral ramus of the S4 and perineal branch of the pudendal nerve.

Pelvic Fascia

- It includes parietal and visceral layer.
- Parietal layer lines the floor and walls of the pelvic cavity and is continuous with extraperitoneal tissue.
- Visceral layer covers the pelvic organs.
- Pelvic fascia is condensed to form puboprostatic or pubocervical ligaments, uterosacral and transverse cervical ligament.

URINARY BLADDER

- Hollow muscular organ.
- Empty bladder lies within the true pelvis.
- When full, it rises up into the abdominal cavity.
- In the fetus and newborn, even empty bladder is abdominal in position.
- Normal capacity is about 120–320 ml.
- *Shape:* Empty bladder is tetrahedral in shape. It has:
  - 4 angles—apex, neck and two lateral angles.
  - 4 surfaces—a superior, a posterior and two inferolateral surfaces.
  - 4 borders—a posterior, an anterior and two lateral borders.
- Distended bladder is ovoid in shape.

Relations

- Apex: Attached to the umbilicus by median umbilical ligament (urachus), represents obliterated allantoic diverticulum.
- Base (posterior surface) faces posteriorly:
  - *In male:* Rectovesical pouch, coils of intestine, seminal vesicles and vas deferens. Denonvillier's fascia (rectovesical septum) separates them and bladder from the rectum. Upper part of base covered by peritoneum (Figs 5.45 and 5.46).
  - *In female:* Not covered with peritoneum. Related to the anterior wall of the vagina and the uterus (cervix).
- Superolateral angles: Receive the ureters.

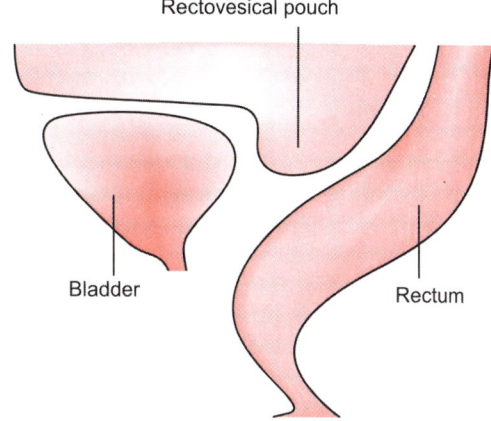

Fig. 5.45: Rectovesical pouch

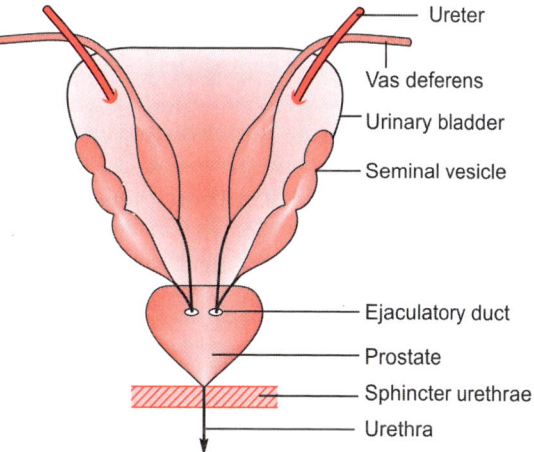

Fig. 5.46: Posterior aspect of bladder

- Neck or inferior angle: Opens into the urethra. Rests on the prostate in the male and the urogenital diaphragm in the female.
- *Superior surface:*
  - Is completely covered by peritoneum in the male and is related to the coils of the intestine.
  - In the female only the anterior 2/3rd is covered by peritoneum and is related to the uterovesical pouch. Posterior 1/3rd is not covered with peritoneum and is related to the cervix (supravaginal part) of the uterus.
- Inferolateral surfaces, related to obturator internus, pelvic diaphragm.

- Anterior aspect of bladder has no peritoneum, distended bladder may be punctured above pubic symphysis—suprapubic cystotomy.

Internal features of the urinary bladder:
- Thick muscle wall, Detrusor (stimulated by parasympathetic).
- Trigone, triangular region made up of smooth mucous membrane firmly attached to muscle coat. There are no folds in the mucosa of trigone but rest of bladder mucosa has folds called rugae.
- Ureteric orifices form lateral ends of triangle.
- Internal urethral orifice forms inferior angle of triangle.
- Interureteric fold extends between the ureteric orifices.
- Developed from absorbed mesonephric ducts.
- Detrusor muscle at the neck surrounds the urethra forming sphincter vesicae (internal urethral sphincter).
- Uvula is a projection in the trigone in males formed by median lobe of prostate. It projects into the interior and causes obstruction to flow of urine in benign prostatic hypertrophy.

Ligaments of the bladder: True and false ligaments.
- True ligaments are:
  - Lateral true ligament.
  - Posterior true ligament.
  - Medial puboprostatic ligament (in male).
  - Lateral puboprostatic ligament (in male).
  - Pubovesical ligaments (in female).
- False ligaments are:
  - Median umbilical fold.
  - Two medial umbilical folds.
  - Lateral and posterior false ligaments.

Blood Supply

- Superior and inferior vesical arteries (vaginal arteries in female instead of inferior vesical).
- Is drained by the vesical venous plexus to the internal iliac vein.

Nerve Supply

- Vesical plexus which is derived from inferior hypogastric plexus.
- Sympathetic from T11 to L2 segments. Inhibits contraction of detrusor and stimulates contraction of sphincter vesicae. (holds urine). (Sympathetic system is less important in control of bladder function relative to parasympathetic system).
- Parasympathetic from 2nd, 3rd, and 4th sacral segments of spinal cord, i.e. pelvic splanchnic nerves. Inhibits contraction of sphincter vesicae and stimulates contraction of detrusor (voids urine).
- *Higher centers in brain:* Distension of bladder by filling (urine) stimulates bladder contraction to void urine. This automatic reflex of bladder is suppressed by toilet training due to control by higher cortical centers on spinal neurons so that we can abstain from passing urine when we do not wish to.

- *Sensory (pain felt due to overstretching of bladder):* Fibers enter spinal cord:
  - via sympathetic, partly.
  - via parasympathetic, mainly.

- *Cystoscopy:* Visualization of interior of bladder using cystoscope (endoscope).
- *Cystogram:* Radiograph obtained with contrast media instilled into the bladder.
- *Ectopia vesicae:* Congenital anomaly due to defect in the anterior abdominal Wall and anterior wall of bladder so that bladder mucosa is exposed.

PROSTATE

- It is a fibromuscular gland present only in the male.
- Its secretion adds volume to semen.
- In the female, it is represented by the paraurethral glands (of Skene).
- It is situated in the pelvic cavity below the neck of the urinary bladder.
- It is about 8 gm.
- Resembles inverted cone.

Relations of the Prostate

It has:
- *Superior surface (base):* Related to the neck of the urinary bladder and pierced by the prostatic urethra (Fig. 5.47).
- *Apex:* Rests on the urogenital diaphragm.
- *Anterior surface* related to the body of pubis and retropubic space containing retropubic pad of fat. Upper part is attached to the pubis by puboprostatic ligaments. Prostatic urethra emerges out from its lower part.
- *Posterior surface:* Ejaculatory ducts pierce upper part of this surface. Rectovesical septum (Denonvillier's fascia) intervenes between this surface and the rectum.

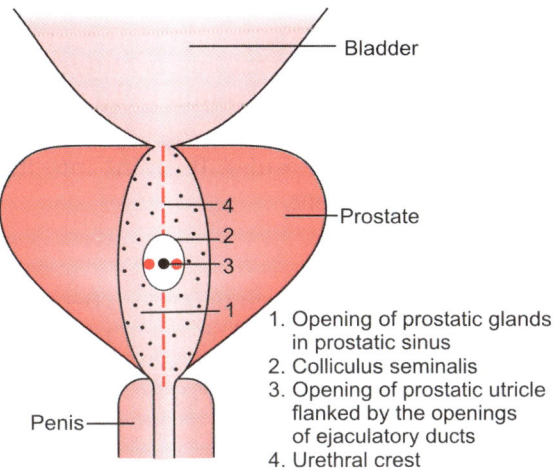

1. Opening of prostatic glands in prostatic sinus
2. Colliculus seminalis
3. Opening of prostatic utricle flanked by the openings of ejaculatory ducts
4. Urethral crest

Fig. 5.47: Prostatic urethra

- *Two inferolateral surfaces:* Related to the levator ani.

Capsule

- *It has 2 capsules:* True and false capsule.
- True capsule is the condensation of connective tissue of the gland.
- False capsule is formed by the pelvic fascia.
- Prostatic plexus of veins lie between the true and the false capsule.

Lobes of the Prostate

- The prostatic urethra passes vertically through the anterior part of the gland.
- The two ejaculatory ducts pierce the posterior surface of the gland and open into the posterior wall of the prostatic urethra. Thus the gland can be divided into 5 lobes:
- *Anterior lobe:* Fibrous, infront of the urethra.
- *Two lateral lobes:* On the sides of the urethra.
- *Posterior lobe:* Between the lateral lobes, but below the level of the ejaculatory ducts.
- *Median lobe:* Between the lateral lobes, but above the level of the ejaculatory ducts. It is commonly involved in benign enlargements of the prostate.

Blood Supply

- *Arteries:* Branches from internal pudendal, inferior vesical and the middle rectal arteries.
- *Venous drainage:* Prostatic venous plexus lies between the 2 capsules. It drains into the internal iliac veins.

There are valveless communications between prostatic and vertebral venous plexuses through which prostatic carcinoma can spread to the vertebral column and skull.

Lymphatic Drainage

Into the internal iliac, external iliac and sacral lymph nodes.

Nerve Supply

- Prostatic plexus of nerves from the hypogastric plexus.
- Parasympathetic fibres arise from S2, 3 and S4.

APPLIED ANATOMY

- Cancer can be palpated in per rectal (PR) examination.
- Benign enlargement due to hormonal imbalance after the age of 50 years. Usually affects the median lobe. The enlarged median lobe forms a projection into the bladder which may obstruct the internal urethral orifice by forming a sort of valve. More a person strains; more will be the obstruction.

URETHRA

It extends from the neck of the urinary bladder to the external urethral orifice.

Female Urethra

- 4 cm in length.
- Embedded in the anterior wall of the vagina.

- Passes through the deep perineal pouch.
- Paraurethral glands open into the wall of the urethra (homologous to the prostate in the male).

- Easy to pass catheters or cystoscope through it.

Male Urethra

- 20 cm in length. S-shaped in flaccid state of the penis.
- *Parts of the male urethra:* 3 parts—prostatic, membranous and spongy part.

Prostatic Part

- Passes through the prostate.
- It is the widest and the most dilatable part.
- It is spindle-shaped (middle part is dilated).
- Its posterior wall presents the following features (Fig. 5.47):
  - Urethral crest—vertical ridge in the midline.
  - Seminal colliculus: A spherical swelling in the middle of the urethral crest. Prostatic utricle opens on it in the middle.
  - Openings of the ejaculatory ducts are seen on each side of prostatic utricle on the seminal colliculus.
  - Prostatic sinuses—shallow depressions on each side of the urethral crest.
  - Ducts of the prostate gland open into the sinuses by minute openings.

Membranous Part

- Passes through the urogenital diaphragm to enter the bulb of the penis.
- It is the shortest, narrowest and the least dilatable part (after external urethral orifice).
- It is surrounded by the sphincter urethrae.
- Bulbourethral glands lie posterolateral to this part.

Spongy Part

- 15 cm in length.
- Passes through the bulb and corpus spongiosum of the penis to open at the external urethral orifice on the tip of the glans penis.
- There are two dilatations—intrabulbar fossa (at its beginning) and navicular fossa (in the glans penis).
- Ducts of the bulbourethral glands open into the spongy part at its beginning (intrabulbar fossa).

Sphincters of the urethra:
Two internal and external urethral sphincters:
- Internal urethral sphincter is made of smooth muscles and has sympathetic nerve supply.
- External urethral sphincter has skeletal muscle fibers and surrounds the membranous part. Supplied by the perineal branch of the pudendal nerve.
  Blood supply: Vessels of prostate and penis.

Lymphatic Drainage

- From the terminal (spongy) part to the deep inguinal lymph nodes.
- From the proximal (prostatic and membranous) part to the external and internal iliac nodes.

- *Hypospadias:* Urethra opens on the ventral surface of the penis.
- *Epispadias:* Urethral opening is seen on the dorsal surface of the penis.
- While performing urethral catheterization the curves of the urethra should be kept in mind.

DUCTUS DEFERENS

- It is also called vas deferens (Fig. 5.46).
- It is a tube 45 cm long.

- It begins at the tail of the epididymis and ends behind the prostate by uniting with the duct of seminal vesicle to form the ejaculatory duct.
- It begins from the tail of the epididymis.
- At the upper pole of the testis it enters the spermatic cord. It passes through the inguinal canal and reaches the deep inguinal ring.
- Here it curves round the lateral side of the inferior epigastric artery, crosses the external iliac vessels to enter the pelvis.
- Pelvic part crosses the obturator nerve and vessels and the ureter to reach the posterior surface of the urinary bladder medial to the seminal vesicle. Here it presents a dilatation called ampulla. It then descends to a point behind the prostate where it unites with the duct of seminal vesicle to form the ejaculatory duct. The ejaculatory duct pierces the prostate and ends by opening into the posterior wall of the prostatic urethra on the colliculus seminalis.
- *Blood supply:* Artery to the vas, a branch of the inferior/superior vesical artery.
- Lymphatic drainage is into the external iliac nodes.

Vasectomy (male steriliza-tion)—removal of a part of vas deferens and ligation of cut ends employed as a family planning (contraceptive) method.

SEMINAL VESICLE

- It is a long thin highly coiled tube situated behind the base of the urinary bladder (Fig. 5.46).
- Its duct joins with the vas deferens to form the ejaculatory duct.
- Its secretion forms bulk of the semen.

FEMALE REPRODUCTIVE ORGANS

Uterus

- Hollow muscular organ (Fig. 5.49).
- Lies in the pelvis between the bladder in front and the rectum behind.
- Flat anteroposteriorly.
- Pear-shaped.
- 7.5 cm length × 5 cm breadth × 2.5 cm thickness.
- During pregnancy it greatly increases in size.

Parts

- Fundus.
- Body.
- Cervix has two parts—vaginal and supravaginal part.
  - Fundus is the free rounded upper part of the uterus above the level of the opening of the uterine tubes.
  - Isthmus is a constriction that divides the uterus into larger upper part called the body and a smaller cylindrical lower part called the cervix.
  - The part of the cervix embedded in the anterior part of the upper end of the vagina is called vaginal part of the cervix and the part of the cervix above the vagina is called supravaginal part.

Normal anatomical position of the uterus:
- Anteverted, anteflexed.
- Long axis of the cervix is bent forwards over the long axis of vagina—anteversion (90°).
- The body of uterus is bent forwards over the cervix at the isthmus—anteflexion (125°).

Relations:
- *Anterior:* Anterior surface of the fundus and body are covered with peritoneum and are related to the uterovesical pouch and the superior surface of the urinary bladder. The supravaginal cervix is not covered by peritoneum and is related to the base of the urinary bladder.

- *Posterior:* Fundus, body and the supravaginal cervix are covered with peritoneum; related to the rectouterine pouch of Douglas and its contents, coils of small intestine and pelvic colon. The Douglas pouch separates the uterus from the rectum.

- *Lateral:*
  - Broad ligament extends from the uterus to the side walls of the pelvis.
  - Round ligament of the uterus.
  - Ligament of the ovary.
  - Uterine vessels.
  - Uterine tubes.
  - Ureters lie at the sides of the cervix on the lateral fornices of the vagina. They are crossed by the uterine arteries which ascend along the lateral borders of the uterus.
  - Transverse cervical ligaments or Mackenrodt's ligaments extend from the sides of the cervix and vagina to the lateral walls of the pelvis.

Interior of the Uterus

- The cavity of the uterus is a small cleft-like space. Triangular in outline.
- At the upper lateral angles are the openings of the uterine tubes.
- At the lower angle of uterine cavity is the internal os or opening of the cervical canal.

Cervical Canal

- Spindle-shaped.
- Above it opens into the uterine cavity at the internal os.
- Below it opens into the vagina through the external os.

- Median longitudinal ridges are seen in the mucosa of the anterior and posterior walls.
- Palmate folds extend laterally from the ridges like branches of a tree. This arrangement is called arbor vitae uteri.
- During pregnancy, upper 1/3rd of the cervical canal is taken up into the uterine cavity and is called the lower uterine segment.

Blood Supply of the Uterus

- *Arterial supply:*
  - Uterine arteries (mainly): Branches of the internal iliac arteries. They ascend between the layers of the broad ligament. Uterine artery crosses above the ureter near the supravaginal cervix to reach the sides of the uterus.
  - Ovarian arteries (partly): Branches of abdominal aorta
- *Venous drainage:*
  - Uterine, ovarian and vaginal veins which drain into the internal iliac veins.

Lymphatic Drainage

- From the cervix to the external and internal iliac lymph nodes, and sacral nodes.
- From the lower part of the body of the uterus to the external iliac lymph nodes.
- From the upper part of the body and fundus:
  - Mainly end in the aortic lymph nodes.
  - Few pass to the superficial inguinal lymph nodes.
- Lymph vessels near the openings of the fallopian tubes follow the round ligament to end in the superficial inguinal lymph nodes.

Nerve Supply

- Uterovaginal plexus.
- *Sympathetic:* T12, L1 segments cause uterine contraction and vasoconstriction.

- *Parasympathetic:* S2, S3, S4 cause uterine inhibition and vasodilatation.
  Uterus is also under hormonal influences.

Supports of the uterus (Fig. 5.50):
- Pelvic floor muscles.
- Perineal body.
- Urogenital diaphragm.
- Pubocervical ligaments.
- Transverse cervical ligaments.
- Uterosacral ligaments.
- Round ligaments of the uterus.

APPLIED ANATOMY

- IUCD (intrauterine contraceptive device) is a device which is placed in the uterus to prevent a pregnancy.
- Caesarian section is a delivery of the baby by making a surgical incision of the abdominal wall and uterus when normal delivery by vaginal route is not possible.
- Retroverted uterus is tilted backwards instead of being normally anteverted.
- Prolapse of the uterus is collapse or descent of uterus into vagina.
- Hysterosalpingography is radiological examination of uterine tubes and uterus after passing a radiopaque dye.
- Hysterectomy is surgical removal of uterus. The ureter is in danger of being inadvertently clamped or severed when the uterine artery is tied off.

Broad Ligament

- It is a peritoneal fold attaching the lateral borders of the uterus to the lateral pelvic wall (Fig. 5.48).
- It has two layers. Its upper free border encloses the fallopian tubes. The posterior layer is reflected backwards to the ovary as a fold called mesovarium.
- It assists in keeping the uterus in position.

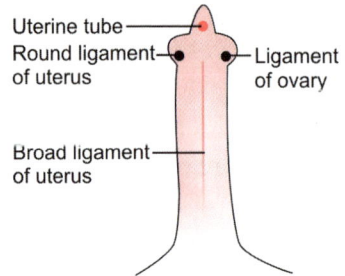

Fig. 5.48: Broad ligament

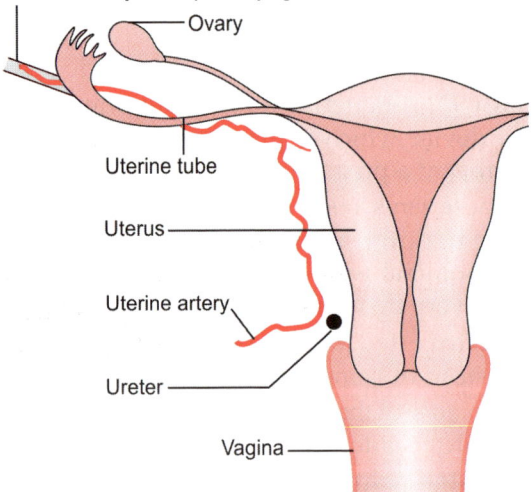

Fig. 5.49: Uterus, uterine tube and ovary

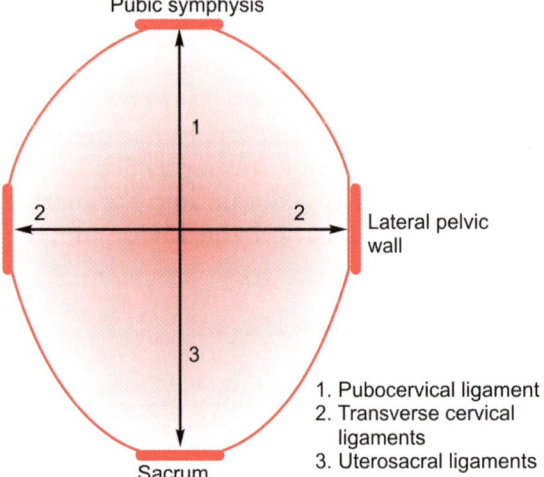

1. Pubocervical ligament
2. Transverse cervical ligaments
3. Uterosacral ligaments

Fig. 5.50: Supports of uterus

- Ovarian ligament.
- Uterine vessels.
- Lymphatics.
- Parametrial connective tissue.
- Nerves.
- Epoöphoron.
- Paroöphoron.

Round Ligament of the Uterus

- Extends from the lateral border of the uterus near the attachment of the fallopian tube, passes out through the inguinal canal, to be attached to the skin of the labium majus.
- It represents the embryonic gubernaculum.

FALLOPIAN TUBE

- Each tube is 10 cm long.
- Situated in the upper free margin of the broad ligament (Fig. 5.48).
- Extends from the upper end of the lateral border of the uterus to the ovary on the lateral pelvic wall (Fig. 5.49).

Parts of the Broad Ligament

- *Mesosalpinx:* Between the fallopian tube and the ligament of ovary.
- *Mesometrium:* Below the ligament of ovary.
- Infundibulopelvic ligament (suspensory ligament of ovary) is the part stretching between the infundibulum of the fallopian tube and ovary at one end and the lateral wall of the pelvis at the other end.

Contents of the broad ligament:
- Fallopian tube.
- Round ligament of the uterus.

- *It has two ends:*
  - Lateral ovarian end which has an opening into the abdominal cavity (more correctly peritoneal cavity) called abdominal ostium.
  - Medial uterine end opening to the uterine cavity.

Parts

1. Infundibulum which is expanded funnel-shaped lateral end. Has variable number of finger shaped fimbriae. One of the fimbria is long and attached to the ovary and called ovarian fimbria.
2. Ampulla which is the dilated part medial to the infundibulum.
3. Isthmus which is a narrow part medial to the ampulla.
4. Intrauterine or intramural part which pierces the muscular wall of the uterus to open to the uterine cavity by uterine ostium.
   - *Note:* Fertilization occurs in the ampulla.
   - *Blood supply:* Uterine and ovarian blood vessels.
   - *Lymphatic drainage* mainly follows ovarian vessels to aortic nodes. From intramural part it follows round ligament of uterus to superficial inguinal nodes.

CLINICAL POINTS

i. Tubal pregnancy (site of implantation is uterine tube instead of uterus).
ii. Tubectomy (a sterilization technique involving cutting and ligating cut ends of uterine tube as part of a family planning method).

OVARY

- Two in number, situated one on either side of the uterus in the ovarian fossa on the lateral pelvic wall (Fig. 5.49).
- Attached to the posterior layer of broad ligament by the mesovarium.

- Connected to the uterus by the ligament of the ovary.
- Almond-shaped.
- Its upper end is called tubal end. Lower end is called uterine end.
- A peritoneal fold, infundibulopelvic ligament stretches from the upper end to the lateral pelvic wall and transmits the ovarian vessels.
- Medial surface is overlapped by the uterine tube (fimbriated end).
- Lateral surface is related to the ovarian fossa, obturator nerve and vessels.
- *Ovarian fossa* seen on the lateral pelvic wall in which ovary is situated.
  - Boundaries of the ovarian fossa:
    - Posteriorly—ureter and internal iliac vessels.
    - Anteriorly—obliterated umbilical artery.
    - Floor—obturator nerve and vessels, peritoneum.
- *Blood supply:*
  - Ovarian artery: Direct branch from abdominal aorta.
  - Ovarian veins: Right ovarian vein ends in the inferior vena cava. Left ovarian vein ends in the left renal vein.
- Lymphatic drainage end in the aortic lymph nodes.
- *Nerve supply:* Sympathetic T10, T11. Parasympathetic from vagus nerve.

CLINICAL POINTS

Ovarian cysts are fluid-filled sacs seen in ovary which may or may not cause problems.

VAGINA

- Extends from the cervix of the uterus to the vaginal opening below in the cleft between the labia minora called the vestibule (Fig. 5.49).

- Lower end is the narrowest part.
- It is a fibromuscular canal.
- It is directed downwards and forwards. It makes an angle of 90° with the long axis of uterus.
- *Lumen:* Lower 1/3rd is H-shaped, middle 1/3rd is a transverse slit, upper 1/3rd is circular.
- Posterior wall is longer (9 cm) than the anterior (7.5 cm) wall.
- It has upper and lower ends, posterior and anterior wall, two lateral walls.
- Lower end opens into the vestibule and is guarded by the hymen in virgin.
- Upper end is pierced more anteriorly by the cervix. Thus a recess is formed between the cervix and the surrounding wall of the vagina. It is divided into 4 parts called vaginal fornices. They are—anterior, posterior, and 2 lateral fornices.
- *Relations:*
  - *Anterior wall:* Related to the urinary bladder, terminal parts of the ureters and urethra.
  - *Posterior wall:* Upper end is covered by peritoneum and is related to the rectovaginal pouch or pouch of Douglas. Below, to the rectum and perineal body.
  - *Lateral walls:* Upper end is related to the ureter crossed by the uterine artery, transverse cervical ligaments and levator ani.
- Interior of the vagina has an anterior and a posterior median longitudinal fold from which transverse ridges extend as rugae.
- *Blood supply:*
  - Uterine arteries, vaginal arteries, internal pudendal and middle rectal arteries. These arteries anastomose and form two longitudinal arterial chains, one on each of the anterior and posterior walls of the vagina in the midline. These are called vaginal azygos arteries.

- Venous drainage occurs into the internal iliac veins.
- *Lymphatic drainage:*
  - From the upper 1/3rd to the internal and external iliac nodes.
  - From the middle 1/3rd to internal iliac nodes.
  - From the lower 1/3rd to the superficial inguinal lymph nodes.
- *Nerve supply:*
  - Uterovaginal plexus.
  - Upper 4/5th is supplied by sympathetic and parasympathetic nerves (pain insensitive).
  - Lower 1/5th is supplied by the pudendal nerve branches (pain sensitive).

CLINICAL POINTS

- Abscess in the pouch of Douglas can be drained through the posterior fornix of vagina (culdocentesis).
- Vaginal prolapse may occur.
- PV (per vaginal examination): Urethra, bladder, rectum, rectovaginal pouch, cervix, ovary, fallopian tube, lateral pelvic wall, and ureters can be palpated. The size of the pelvis can also be assessed.

Female External Genitalia

- Also called vulva or pudendum (to feel ashamed).
- It includes mons pubis, labia majora, labia minora, clitoris, vestibule of vagina and greater vestibular glands.

INTERNAL ILIAC ARTERY

- It supplies almost all the pelvic viscera.
- *Origin:* It is the smaller of the two terminal branches of the common iliac artery.
- *Termination:* It ends by dividing into anterior and posterior divisions.

- *Extent:* It starts from in front of the sacroiliac joint and runs to the upper margin of the greater sciatic notch where it terminates by splitting into 2 divisions.
- *Relations:*
  - *Anteriorly:* Ureter, ovary and lateral end of the uterine tube in the female.
  - *Posteriorly:* Internal iliac vein, lumbo-sacral trunk.
  - *Laterally:* External iliac vein, psoas major and obturator nerve.
  - *Medially:* Covered with peritoneum and on the left side the sigmoid colon.
- *Branches:* Anterior and posterior divisions. Anterior division (branches).
  - Superior vesical.
  - Inferior vesical (in the male).
  - Middle rectal.
  - Uterine (in the female).
  - Vaginal (in the female).
  - Obturator.
  - Inferior gluteal.
  - Internal pudendal.
  Posterior division (branches)
  - Iliolumbar.
  - Lateral sacral.
  - Superior gluteal.
  Pelvic veins follow the arteries into the internal iliac vein.

The Sacral Plexus

- Formed by ventral rami of L4, L5, S1, S2, S3, S4.
- The sacral plexus is formed by the lumbosacral trunk, the anterior rami of the first, second, third and fourth sacral nerves.
- The lumbosacral trunk is formed by the union of the L4 and L5.
- The nerves arising are as follows:
  - Nerve to quadratus femoris.
  - Nerve to obturator internus.
  - Pudendal nerve S2, S3, S4.
  - Nerve to piriformis.
  - Superior gluteal L4, 5, S1.
  - Inferior gluteal L5, S1, 2.
  - Posterior cutaneous nerve of the thigh.
  - *Sciatic:*
    - Tibial......L4, 5, S1, 2, 3.
    - Common peroneal...... L4, 5, S1, 2.
  - Muscular branches to levator ani, coccygeus and external anal sphincter.
- The sacral plexus lies on the back of the pelvis between the piriformis and the parietal layer of pelvic fascia.
- The superior gluteal vessels run between the lumbosacral trunk and the first sacral nerve and the inferior gluteal vessels between the first and second sacral nerves.

Head and Neck

6

Osteology of Skull

- Cranium is the skull without the mandible.
- Skull includes the mandible.
- Calvaria is the part of the skull which encloses the brain (brain case).
- The remaining part forms facial skeleton.
- Bones of the top of the skull are ossified in membrane.
- There are membranous gaps in the new-born skull. These are called fontanelles.
  - There are 6 fontanelles: (Fig. 6.1)
    - ♦ 1 anterior.
    - ♦ 1 posterior.
    - ♦ 2 anterolateral (sphenoidal) fontanelles one on each side.
    - ♦ 2 posterolateral (mastoid) fontanelles one on each side.
  - The anterior fontanelle lies at the junction of frontal bone with the parietal bones (where coronal and sagittal sutures meet). It is fused at the end of second year.

Skull can be studied under the following headings:
- Norma verticalis (as viewed from above).
- Norma frontalis (as viewed from the front).

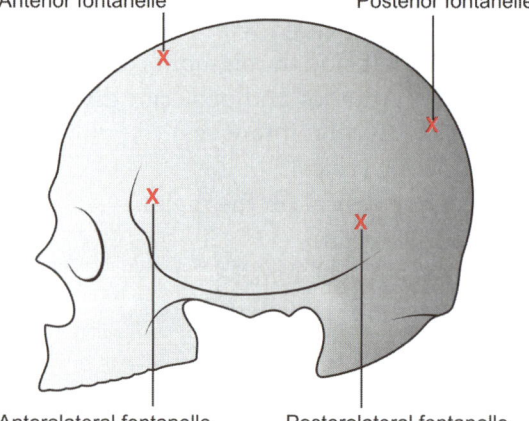

Anterior fontanelle   Posterior fontanelle

Anterolateral fontanelle   Posterolateral fontanelle

Fig. 6.1: Fontanelles

- Normal occipitalis (as viewed from behind).
- Norma lateralis (as viewed from the sides, there are two views here, right and left).
- Norma basalis (as viewed from below).
- Interior of base of the skull.

Norma Verticalis

- In this view, there is a transversely running coronal suture and anteroposteriorly extending sagittal suture (Fig. 6.2).
- Bregma is the junction of coronal suture with the sagittal suture.
- Anterior fontanelle is located at the bregma in the infant skull.
- Frontal bone is normally one bone (formed by fusion of 2 halves) but sometimes there

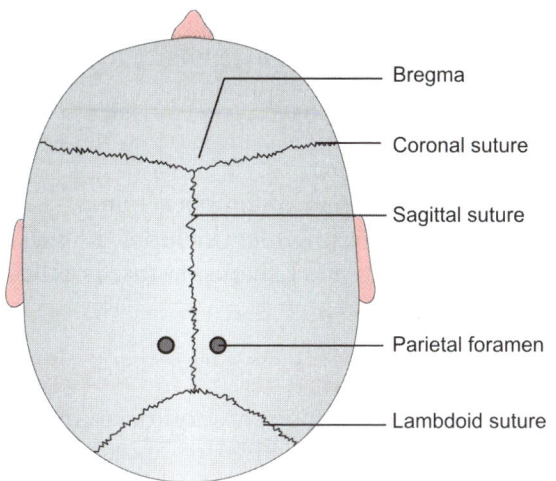

Fig. 6.2: Norma verticalis

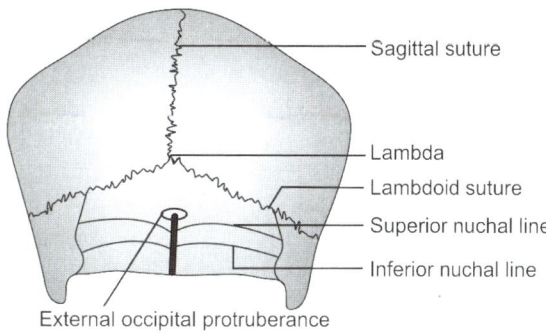

Fig. 6.3: Norma occipitalis

may be a suture between the two halves of the frontal bone (not fused completely) called "metopic suture".

- On either side of the sagittal suture near its posterior end there are parietal foramen.
- Parietal emissary vein traverses this foramen. Emissary veins are the valveless veins which connect the extracranial veins with the intracranial venous sinuses. They help to maintain the intracranial venous pressure. If there were to be increased pressure intracranially, the blood is shunted out through the emissary veins.

They are sometimes vehicles of transmission of infection from extracranial source intracranially.

- There are tuberosities over the parietal bones called the parietal tuberosities.
- Similarly there are frontal tuberosities over the front of frontal bone.

Norma Occipitalis

- This is the posterior view of the skull (Fig. 6.3).

- There are parieto-occipital sutures in this view. The two parieto-occipital sutures together are named "the lambdoid suture" because of its resemblance to letter lambda. The point of junction of lambdoid suture with the sagittal suture is called "lambda".
- There is a prominent protruberance midway between foramen magnum and lambda called the external occipital protruberance.
- External occipital crest is a median crest which descends from the external occipital protruberance to the posterior margin of the foramen magnum.
- Superior nuchal line is a convex arch which extends laterally from the external occipital protruberance.
- Inferior nuchal line is a convex line which extends laterally from the middle of the external occipital crest.
- Identify the occipitomastoid and parietomastoid sutures.
- Masotid process is a nipple like projection at the inferolateral angle of the norma occipitalis.

Norma Lateralis

- This is the lateral view of the skull (Fig. 6.4).
- The prominent structure in this view is zygomatic arch.

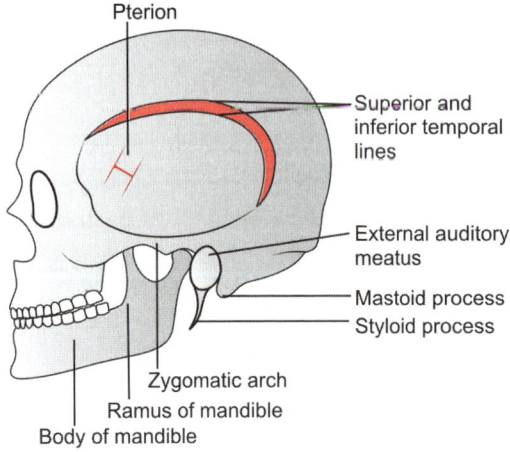

Pterion

Superior and
inferior temporal
lines

External auditory
meatus

Mastoid process
Styloid process

Zygomatic arch
Ramus of mandible
Body of mandible

Fig. 6.4: Norma lateralis

- The zygomatic arch is formed by the union of two processes:
  1. Temporal process of the zygomatic bone.
  2. Zygomatic process of temporal bone.
- Opening of external acoustic meatus is seen.
- *Note:* Place your little finger into your external acoustic (auditory) meatus and move the jaw. You can appreciate the movements of the temporomandibular joint. The temporomandibular joint is placed just anterior to the external acoustic meatus in front of the tragus of the external ear.
- There are two temporal lines on the norma lateralis. The temporal lines arch over the parietal bones. The two lines are:
  1. The superior temporal line.
  2. The inferior temporal line.
- Temporal fascia is attached to the superior temporal line while temporalis muscle is attached to the inferior temporal line.
- *Note:* You can feel the contractions of the temporalis muscle when you move your mandible up.
- Temporal fossa is made up of four bones and lies superior to the zygomatic arch.

- The four bones which meet in the anterior part of the floor of the temporal fossa are:
  1. Greater wing of sphenoid.
  2. Parietal bone.
  3. Frontal bone.
  4. Squamous part of temporal bone.
- The small circle which includes all these four bones in an H-shaped suture is called the "pterion".

CLINICAL POINTS

The pterion is an important surgical landmark. It corresponds to the anterior branch of the middle meningeal artery in the interior of the cranium. In the injuries to the side of the head, this artery may be involved resulting in bleeding. "Burr hole" is the operation of choice to remove the intracranial blood clot.

- Similarly the following bones meet at the posterior end of the norma lateralis of the skull.
  1. Parietal bone.
  2. Occipital bone.
  3. Temporal bone.

The point where all these bones meet is called "asterion".
- There is a fossa inferior to the level of the zygomatic arch. This is called "infra-temporal fossa".
- The boundaries of the infratemporal fossa are:
  - Laterally, the ramus of the mandible.
  - Medially, the lateral pterygoid plate.
  - Anteriorly, the posterior surface of the body of the maxilla.
  - Posteriorly, it is open.
  - Superiorly, roof which is formed medially by greater wing of sphenoid and opens laterally into temporal fossa.
  - Inferiorly, floor is open.
  - Medially, it leads into a small fissure called pterygomaxillary fissure.

- The pterygomaxillary fissure lies between the lateral pterygoid plate and the maxilla.
- The pterygomaxillary fissure leads into a small fossa called "pterygopalatine fossa".

Norma Basalis

The anterior part of the norma basalis has alveolar process of maxilla bearing teeth. The adult dental formula is (Fig. 6.5):

$$\frac{M3 \quad PM2 \quad C1 \quad I2 \quad || \quad I2 \quad C1 \quad PM2 \quad M3}{M3 \quad PM2 \quad C1 \quad I2 \quad || \quad I2 \quad C1 \quad PM2 \quad M3}$$

Total: 32 teeth

The dental formula of deciduous teeth is:

M2 C1 I2 | | I2 C1 M2
M2 C1 I2 | | I2 C1 M2

Total : 20 teeth

I—Incisor, C—Canine
PM—Premolar, M—Molar

There is an incisive fossa behind the incisor teeth.

The hard palate is formed by the paired:
1. Palatine processes of maxilla.
2. Horizontal processes of palatine bone.

- The suture between the palatine processes of maxilla (intermaxillary suture), between the horizontal plates of palatine bones (interpalatine suture) and the suture between the palatine process of maxilla and horizontal process of palatine bone together appears like a cross, therefore, it is called "cruciform suture".
- Palatine glands cause small impressions on the hard palate.
- There is a groove extending from the greater palatine foramen to the incisive fossa. This groove is for the greater palatine artery.
- The posterior end of the hard palate is a free margin which gives attachment to the soft palate.
- Palatine crest is a small crest just anterior to the posterior margin of the hard palate.
- Greater palatine foramen transmits the greater palatine nerve and vessels.
- Lesser palatine foramina are two or more in number and transmit the lesser palatine nerves and vessels and they lie posterior to the greater palatine foramen.
- The projection of the middle of the posterior border of the hard palate is called the posterior nasal spine.

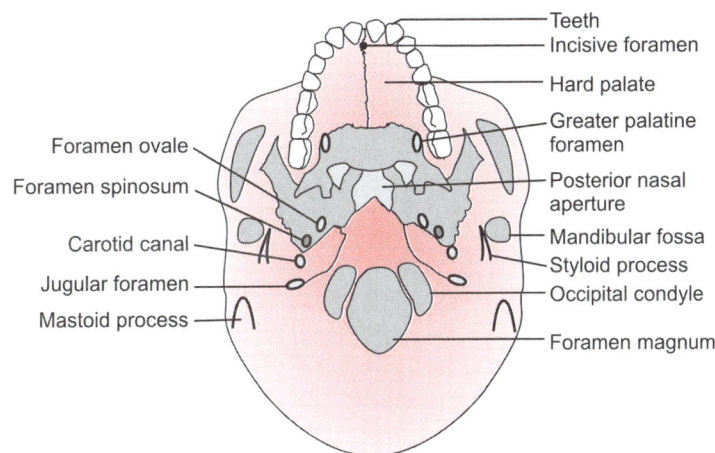

Fig. 6.5: Norma basalis

- Posterior nasal apertures are the two openings superior to the posterior border of the hard palate.
- The posterior nasal apertures are also called choanae and vomer bone separates the two choanae.
- The lateral boundary of the posterior nasal aperture is formed by the pterygoid process.
- The pterygoid process is divided into the lateral and medial pterygoid plates.
- The lower end of the medial pterygoid plate has a hook-shaped process called pterygoid hamulus.
- The tensor palati muscle hooks around the pterygoid hamulus and stretches the soft palate.
- The lateral pterygoid plate is wider than medial as it gives origin to the pterygoid muscles.
- The medial pterygoid plate does not give attachment to the pterygoid muscles.
- The pterygoid fossa is the depression between the lateral and medial pterygoid plates.
- Scaphoid fossa lies just behind the upper aspect of medial pterygoid plate.

Foramen ovale is a large oval foramen which lies in the greater wing of sphenoid bone.

Four structures pass through the foramen ovale:

1. Mandibular nerve
2. Accessory meningeal artery
3. Lesser petrosal nerve
4. Emissary vein
   (Remember mnemonic **MALE**)

- Foramen spinosum lies posterolateral to the foramen ovale. Middle meningeal artery passes through it. It is called foramen spinosum as it lies by the side of the spine of the sphenoid bone.

- In the posterolateral part of the greater wing of the sphenoid is the spine of the sphenoid bone.
- Auditory tube (eustachian tube) lies between the greater wing of the sphenoid bone and the petrous part of the temporal bone.
  - Foramen lacerum is an irregular opening between the apex of the petrous part of the temporal bone and the body of the sphenoid. In living it is covered by cartilage and no important structure traverses it except an emissary vein.
  - Petrous part of the temporal bone: It is stone hard. There is a circular opening in it. This is called carotid canal and internal carotid artery passes through it.
  - An irregular foramen between the petrous part of the temporal bone and the occipital bone is called the "jugular foramen".
  - Following structures pass through the jugular foramen:
    - Glossopharyngeal nerve.
    - Vagus nerve.
    - Accessory nerve.
    - Inferior petrosal sinus.
    - Sigmoid sinus continues as the internal jugular vein.

  - Occipital condyles:

    These are the convex articular surfaces of the occipital bone. They form the atlantooccipital joints with the corresponding articular surfaces of the atlas.

  - Anterior condylar canal: It lies in front of the occipital condyle. This is also called the hypoglossal canal. The hypoglossal nerve (XII) passes through it.

  - The posterior condylar canal is often absent. When present an emissary vein passes through it.

– The styloid process: There is a prominent styloid process anteromedial to the mastoid process in the norma basalis.

– Stylomastoid foramen: It lies between the styloid and mastoid processes. Facial nerve emerges from it.

Identify the following structures in the midline in the base of the skull (anterior to posterior):

- Incisor teeth
- Incisive fossa
- Intermaxillary suture
- Interpalatine suture
- Posterior nasal spine
- Vomer
- Body of the sphenoid
- Basiocciput
- Foramen magnum.

Norma Frontalis

- Orbits are the prominent sockets seen in this view (Fig. 6.6).
- Eyeballs are located in the orbits.
- There is a prominent anterior nasal aperture which is piriform in shape. The inferior part of the piriform opening has a spine called anterior nasal spine.

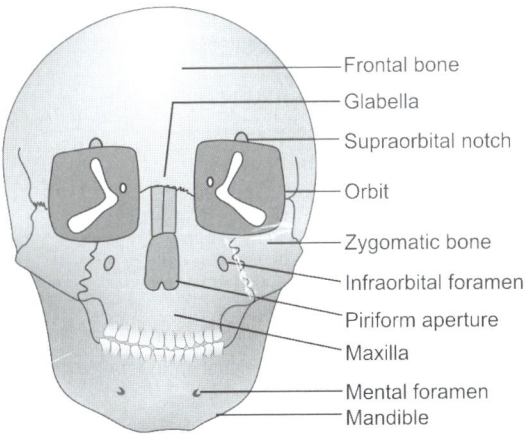

Fig. 6.6: Norma frontalis

- There is an elevation just above the root of the canine tooth. It is called "canine eminence". There are two depressions on either side of it:
  - Medial to the canine eminence there is incisive fossa and lateral to it canine fossa.
- There is a foramen or notch at the junction of medial one-third with the lateral two-thirds of the superior border of the orbit. This is called supraorbital foramen or notch. Supraorbital nerve and vessels pass through it.
- There is infraorbital foramen inferior to the orbit in line with the supraorbital foramen. Infraorbital nerve and vessels pass through it.
- In the same line, there is another foramen in the mandible called the mental foramen through which mental nerve and vessels pass.
- Nasal bones are the two short bones at the root of the nose. They are very delicate and are often fractured.
- Medial wall of the orbit is formed by the frontal process of maxilla, lacrimal bone and the orbital plate of the ethmoid bone.
- Superior orbital fissure, inferior orbital fissure and optic canal open into the orbit. Optic canal and superior orbital fissure are connected to the middle cranial fossa while the inferior orbital fissure is connected to the infratemporal fossa and pterygopalatine fossa.

Interior of the Cranium

It is divided into three fossae:
1. Anterior cranial fossa
2. Middle cranial fossa
3. Posterior cranial fossa

Anterior Cranial Fossa

- Its floor is mainly formed by the orbital plate of the frontal bone. This forms the roof of the orbit. Orbital plates are bilateral though the frontal bone is single (Fig. 6.7).

- The ethmoid bone is sandwiched between the two orbital plates.
- The cribriform plate is present on either side of the crista galli. The olfactory nerves (first cranial nerve) pass through the openings in the cribriform plate.
- Jugum sphenoidale is the smooth part of the sphenoid bone which lies behind the cribriform plate of ethmoid bone.
- The most posterior part of the anterior cranial fossa is the lesser wing of the sphenoid bone.
- There is an optic canal between the two roots joining the lesser wing of the sphenoid bone with its body. Optic nerve (the second cranial nerve) passes through it. Ophthalmic artery passes through the optic canal along with the optic nerve.

Middle Cranial Fossa

- The anterior boundary of the middle cranial fossa is the lesser wing of the sphenoid bone (Fig. 6.7).

- The posterior boundary of the middle cranial fossa is formed by the petrous part of the temporal bone.
- The following structures are in the midline of the middle cranial fossa:
  1. Sulcus chiasmaticus
  2. Tuberculum sellae
  3. Hypophyseal fossa or pituitary fossa
  4. Dorsum sellae
     - 2, 3, 4 together constitute the sella turcica.
- The medial end of the lesser wing of the sphenoid bone is called "the anterior clinoid process".
- The lateral end of the dorsum sellae is called the posterior clinoid process.
- Pituitary fossa is the depression in the body of the sphenoid which lodges the pituitary gland.

Superior Orbital Fissure

- It is a fissure which connects the middle cranial fossa with the orbit. It lies between the lesser wing and greater wing of the sphenoid.

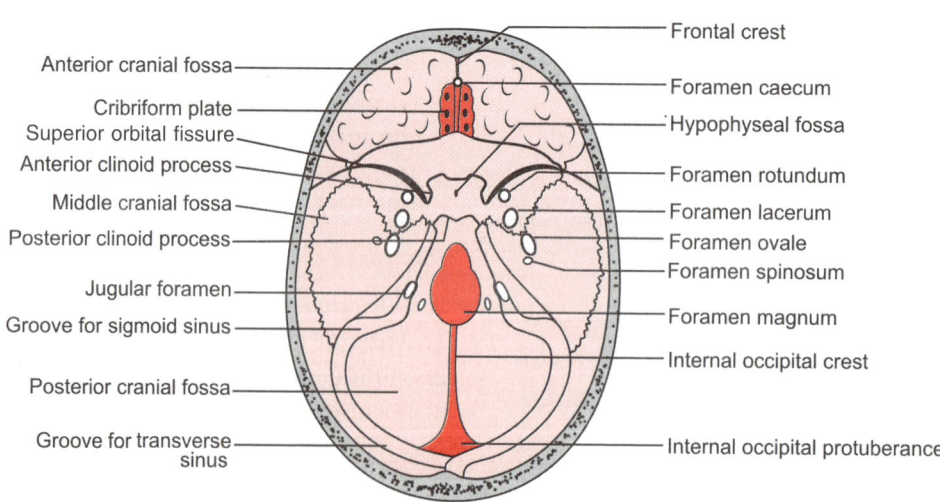

Anterior cranial fossa
Cribriform plate
Superior orbital fissure
Anterior clinoid process
Middle cranial fossa
Posterior clinoid process
Jugular foramen
Groove for sigmoid sinus
Posterior cranial fossa
Groove for transverse sinus

Frontal crest
Foramen caecum
Hypophyseal fossa
Foramen rotundum
Foramen lacerum
Foramen ovale
Foramen spinosum
Foramen magnum
Internal occipital crest
Internal occipital protuberance

Fig. 6.7: Middle cranial fossa

- It is wide medially and narrows laterally.
- Following structures pass through the superior orbital fissure:
  1. Oculomotor (III) nerve.
  2. Trochlear (IV) nerve.
  3. Three branches of ophthalmic division of trigeminal nerve (V).
  4. Abducens nerve (VI).
  5. Ophthalmic veins.
- *Foramen rotundum* is a round foramen in the greater wing of the sphenoid bone posterior to the medial end of the superior orbital fissure. Maxillary nerve passes through it.
- Posterolateral to the foramen rotundum, there is foramen ovale in the greater wing of the sphenoid bone which transmits the mandibular nerve.
- *Foramen spinosum* lies posterolateral to the foramen ovale in the middle cranial fossa and middle meningeal artery passes through it. The groove for the middle meningeal artery can be seen leading away from the foramen spinosum.

Posterior Cranial Fossa

- It lies behind the petrous part of the temporal bone (Fig. 6.7).
- There is a large foramen magnum in this fossa.
- Between the dorsum sellae and the foramen magnum there is a sloping surface called "clivus".
- Internal acoustic meatus lies on the anterolateral wall of the posterior cranial fossa.
- Two cranial nerves pass through the internal acoustic meatus:
  1. Facial nerve (VII)
  2. Vestibulocochlear (statoacoustic) nerve (VIII).

Jugular foramen: It lies between the petrous part of the temporal bone and the occipital bone.

The following structures pass through the jugular foramen:
1. Glossopharyngeal nerve (IX)
2. Vagus nerve (X)
3. Accessory nerve (XI)
4. Inferior petrosal sinus
5. Sigmoid sinus continues as the internal jugular vein.

Hypoglossal canal transmits the hypoglossal nerve (XII).

Interior of Cranial Vault

It shows:
- Groove for superior sagittal sinus. Lips of the groove provide attachment to falx cerebri (Fig. 6.8).
- Frontal crest provides attachment to apex of falx cerebri.
- Arachnoid (granular) foveolae are pits on either side of sagittal groove formed by arachnoid granulations.
- Grooves for middle meningeal vessels.

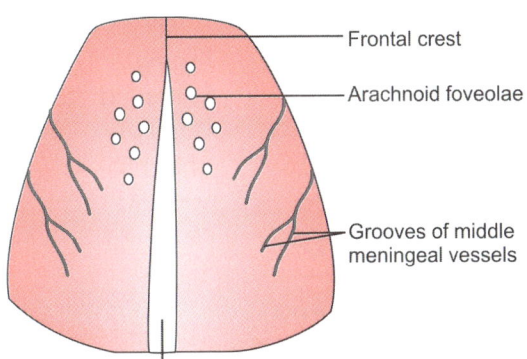

Fig. 6.8: Interior of cranial vault

Following is the list of the cranial nerves and the foramen through which they pass:

Olfactory	Cribriform plate of the ethmoid
Optic	Optic canal
Oculomotor	Superior orbital fissure
Trochlear	Superior orbital fissure
	Branches of ophthalmic (superior orbital fissure)
Trigeminal	Maxillary (foramen rotundum)
	Mandibular (foramen ovale)
Abducent	Superior orbital fissure
Facial	Leaves the posterior cranial fossa through internal acoustic meatus. Exits the skull through the stylomastoid foramen
Vestibulocochlear	Internal acoustic meatus
Glossopharyngeal	Jugular foramen
Vagus	Jugular foramen
Accessory	Jugular foramen
Hypoglossal	Anterior condylar canal (hypoglossal canal)

Following are the paired and unpaired bones of the skull:

Paired	Unpaired
Parietal	Frontal
Temporal	Sphenoid
Maxillae	Ethmoid
Lacrimal	Mandible
Inferior nasal concha	Vomer
Zygomatic	Occipital
Palatine	Nasal

Cervical Vertebrae

- Total 7 in number.
- All are characterized by presence of foramen transversarium in the transverse process (Fig. 6.9).
- C1 (atlas), C2 (axis) and C7 (vertebra prominens) are atypical.
- Typical cervical vertebrae (C3–C6) are characterized by:
  - Bifid spine
  - Small body
  - Foramen transversarium in transverse process
- *Atlas: (unique features) (Fig. 6.10)*
  - No body
  - No spine
  - Anterior and posterior arches
  - Anterior and posterior tubercles
  - 2 lateral masses

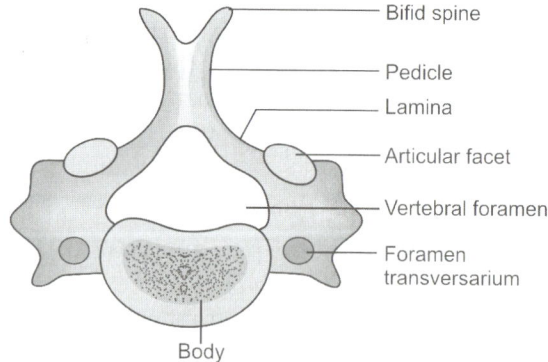

Fig. 6.9: Typical cervical vertebra

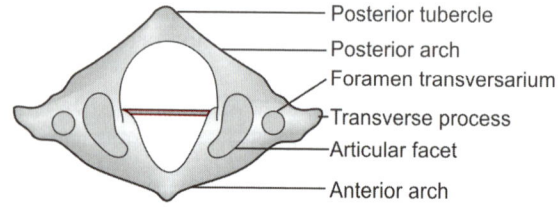

Fig. 6.10: Atlas

- *Axis: (unique features)*
  - Dens or odontoid process (Fig. 6.11)
- *Vertebra prominens: (unique features)*
  - Long prominent spine.

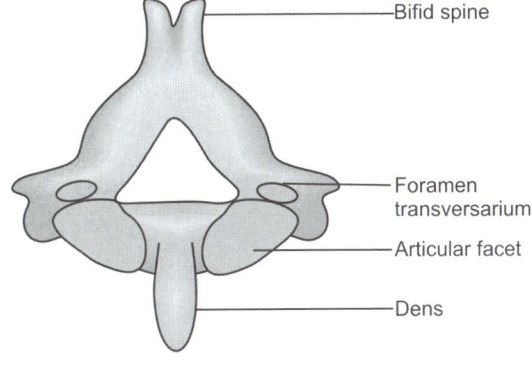

Fig. 6.11: Axis

Mandible

- Is lower jaw bone.
- Has a body and 2 rami (Figs 6.12 and 6.13).
- At birth it is 2 separate halves which fuse to form one bone in 1st year.
- Body is horse shoe-shaped; having outer and inner surfaces and upper and lower borders.

- Upper border or alveolar margin bears sockets for teeth.
- Ramus is quadrilateral.
  - It has outer and inner surfaces, upper and lower borders and anterior and posterior borders.
  - Upper border has 2 processes namely: coronoid process and condylar process.
    - ♦ Condylar process includes head and neck.

Nerves related to Mandible

Nerve	Area of mandible to which they are related
Masseteric	Mandibular notch
Auriculotemporal	Medial aspect of neck
Inferior alveolar	Enters mandibular foramen and runs in mandibular canal
Mental	Emerges from mental foramen
Lingual	Below lower 3rd molar tooth
Mylohyoid	Mylohyoid groove
Mandibular branch of facial	Along body

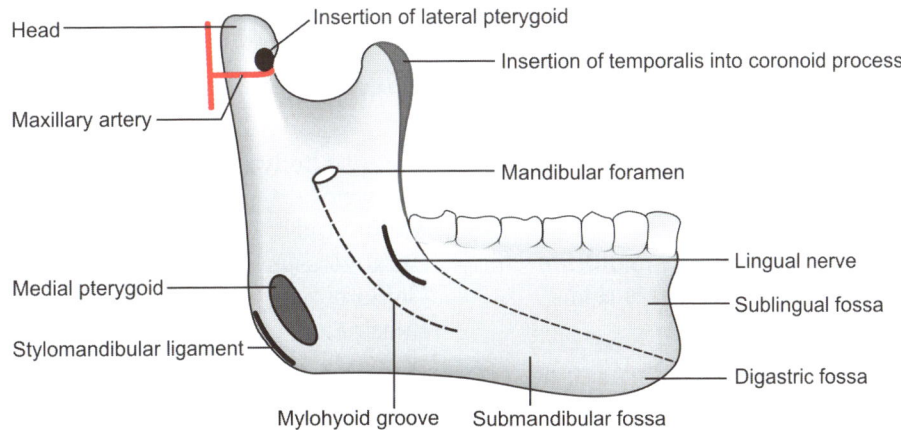

Fig. 6.12: Mandible (medial aspect)

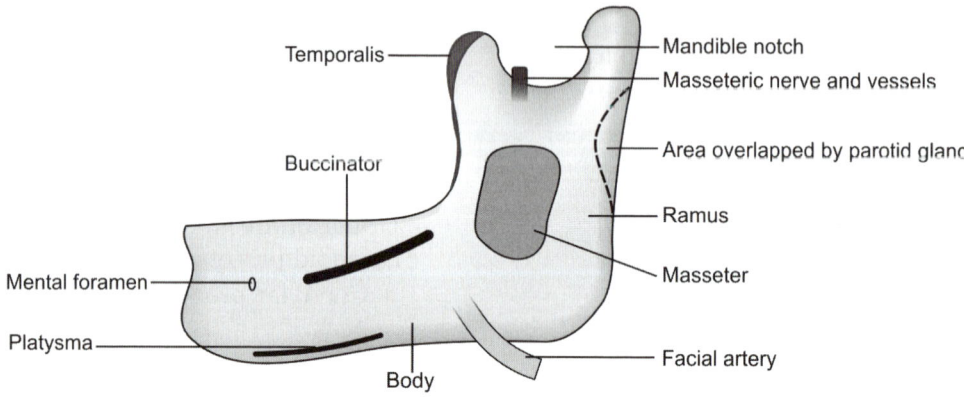

Fig. 6.13: Mandible (lateral aspect)

Arteries related to Mandible

Artery	Area of mandible to which they are related
External carotid	Behind the neck of mandible where it terminates into 2 terminal branches—maxillary and superficial temporal
Maxillary	Medial to the neck
Superficial temporal	Behind the neck
Inferior alveolar	Enters mandibular foramen and runs in mandibular canal
Mental	Emerges from mental foramen
Facial	Lower border (base) of mandible at anteroinferior angle of masseter

Glands related to Mandible

Gland	Area of mandible to which they are related
Sublingual	Sublingual fossa
Submandibular	Submandibular fossa
Parotid	Posterior border of ramus

Ligaments attached to Mandible

Ligament	Area of mandible to which they are attached
Lateral temporomandibular (from root of zygoma)	Lateral aspect of neck
Sphenomandibular (from spine of sphenoid)	Lingula
Pterygomandibular (from pterygoid hamulus)	Posterior limit of mylohyoid line
Stylomandibular (from styloid process)	Angle

Muscles taking Origin from Mandible

Muscle	Area of mandible from which they take origin
Anterior belly of digastric	Digastric fossa
Mylohyoid	Mylohyoid line
Genioglossus	Upper genial tubercles
Geniohyoid	Lower genial tubercles
Buccinator	Oblique line below molar teeth
Superior constrictor	Posterior limit of mylohyoid line

Muscles inserting into Mandible

Muscle	Area of mandible into which they are inserted
Temporalis	Coronoid process
Masseter	Lateral surface of ramus
Lateral pterygoid	Front of neck of mandible
Medial pterygoid	Inner surface of angle
Platysma	Lower border

Age Changes in Mandible (Fig. 6.14)

Age	Angle	Mental foramen
Children	140° or more	Near to lower border (base)
Adults	120°	Midway between upper and lower borders
Old	140°	Near to alveolar margin (upper border)

Hyoid Bone

- U-shaped.
- Situated in front of neck at C3 vertebral level.
- Has a body, 2 lesser horns and 2 greater horns (cornua).
- Lesser cornu provides attachment to stylohyoid ligament.
- Tip of greater cornu provides attachment to lateral thyrohyoid ligament.

- The thyrohyoid membrane is separated from body of hyoid bone by a bursa.
- Lesser cornu and superior part of body are derived from 2nd pharyngeal arch.
- Greater cornu and inferior part of body are derived from 3rd pharyngeal arch.

SCALP

- This is the soft tissue that covers the top of the skull. It has long hairs arising from its skin.
- *Extent:*
  - It extends from the eyebrows in front to the superior nuchal lines behind.
  - On either side it is bounded by the superior temporal lines.
- It is made up of five layers. Each letter of the word scalp acts as mnemonic and denotes a layer of scalp (Fig. 6.15):
  - S: Skin
  - C: Connective tissue
  - A: Aponeurotic layer
  - L: Loose areolar tissue layer
  - P: Pericranium
- *Skin of the scalp:* It is thicker than the skin of many other parts. It has long hairs.There are many sebaceous glands. These glands secrete oily sebum which lubricates hair and skin.

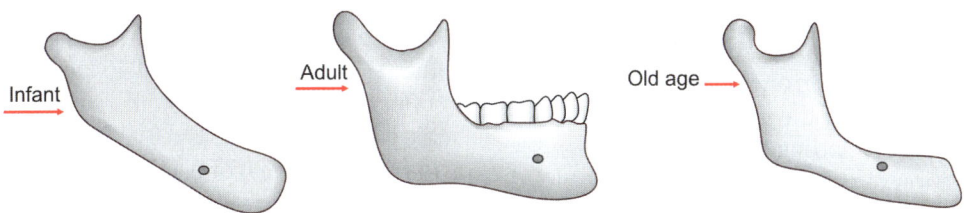

Fig. 6.14: Age changes in mandible

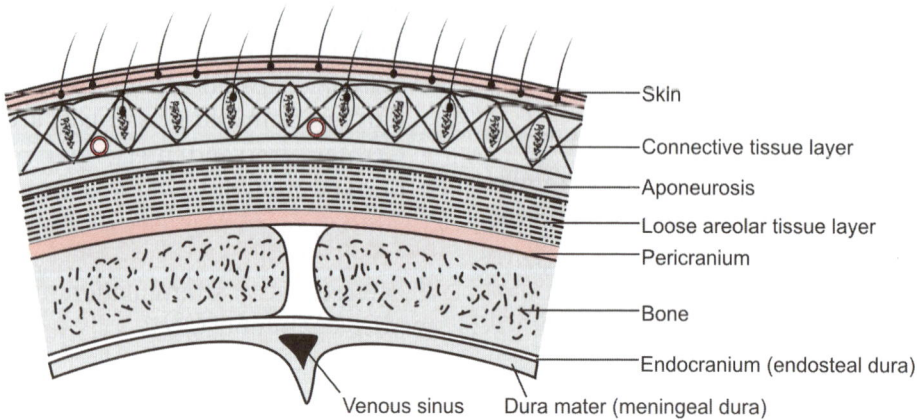

Fig. 6.15: Layers of scalp

Often they form cysts (a fluid- filled cavity following the blockage of its duct). Therefore, sebaceous cysts are very common in the skin of the scalp. The skin is connected to the underlying connective tissue layer and it is not easy to separate the two layers.

- *Connective tissue layer:*
  - This layer is made up of tough connective tissue. It contains the blood vessels and nerves. The connective tissue is unyielding.

That is the reason why the anesthetic medication injected into this layer is not easily dispersed. It may not possible to anesthetize a given area of skin by one injection. That is the reason why a physician prefers to give more than one prick around the area to be anesthetized.

  - The blood vessels traverse the connective tissue layer. The outer coats of the vessels are connected to the surrounding connective tissue. When one of these vessels is cut, the cut end of the vessel is not collapsed as the surrounding connective tissue exerts traction over the margin of the cut blood vessel. Therefore, the wounds of the scalp bleed profusely. They also heal quickly as

rich blood supply brings the products necessary for healing.

Remember: Wounds of the scalp bleed profusely but heal quickly.

  - The connective tissue layer is connected to the overlying skin and underlying aponeurotic layer.
- *Aponeurotic layer:*
  - This is the aponeurosis of the occipito-frontalis muscle. Occipital belly of occipitofrontalis muscle lies in the posterior part of the scalp while its frontal part lies in its anterior part (Fig. 6.17).
  - Therefore, this layer can be more appropriately called a musculoaponeurotic layer. This layer is fused with the overlying connective tissue.

CLINICAL POINT

Any small cut wound of skin and connective tissue does not require a suture as the cut ends remain opposed and heal well. However, if the aponeurotic layer is also cut (transversely), a suture is necessary as the two bellies (occipital and frontal bellies) of occipitofrontalis muscle pull the aponeurosis in opposite directions and tend to enlarge (gape) the wound.

Surgeon's scalp: The first three layers of the scalp, (the skin, connective tissue and aponeurotic layers) remain fused with each other. Whenever long hairs are caught in a winding machine, all these three layers are torn as one layer. As this is a surgical emergency which requires the involvement of a surgeon, it is termed "surgeons scalp". (In olden days the prisoners were used to be punished by scalping). Even when a scalp flap is made the three layers remain together.

Loose areolar tissue space:

– This is a potential space which lies between the musculoaponeurotic and pericranial layers. The veins which traverse this space are connected with the intracranial dural venous sinuses by the valveless emissary veins.

Hence, infection from extracranial source can spread intracranially leading to meningi-tis. The blood or pus can spread easily in it due to its somewhat spongelike nature. Therefore, the loose areolar tissue space is often termed the "dangerous space of the scalp".

– Any collection of blood or other fluid in this space usually gravitates down to the upper eyelid. That is the reason why boxers after a bad punch to the scalp, end up with black eye.

– Safety valve mechanism of loose areolar tissue space: If intracranial hemorrhage is accompanied by the fracture of a cranial bone and tearing of duramater and pericranium, the blood collected intracranially can pass through the fracture of the bone and settle in the potential loose areolar tissue space till it is filled with blood. This delays the onset of pressure symptoms inside the cranial cavity. This is called safety valve mechanism.

• *Pericranium:*

– This is the outer periosteum of the skull. It is firmly attached to the sutures. It is not attached to the bones of the vault of the skull.

Should there be any collection of blood between the bone and the pericranium, it is usually restricted to the outline of the bone. This is called the "cephalhema-toma". For example, hemotoma over the left parietal bone results in a swelling over the area of left parietal bone and it does not spread beyond it because of firm attachment of pericranium to the sur-rounding sutures along the margins of this bone.

– *Caput succedaneum:* In difficult deliveries, the skull of the newborn may be pressurized resulting in the venous congestion of the head. The swelling following the venous congestion of the scalp is called caput succedaneum.

Nerve Supply of the Scalp

There are five nerves in front of the auricle. Out of them four are sensory and one motor. The four sensory and one motor nerves are (Fig. 6.16):

1. Supratrochlear.
2. Supraorbital.
3. Zygomaticotemporal.
4. Auriculotemporal.
5. The motor nerve is the temporal branch of the facial nerve.

There are five nerves behind the auricle. Out of them four are sensory and one motor. The four sensory and one motor nerves are (Fig. 6.16):

1. Great auricular nerve (ventral rami of C2 and C3 from the cervical plexus).
2. Lesser occipital nerve (ventral ramus of C2 from the cervical plexus).
3. Greater occipital nerve (dorsal ramus of C2).

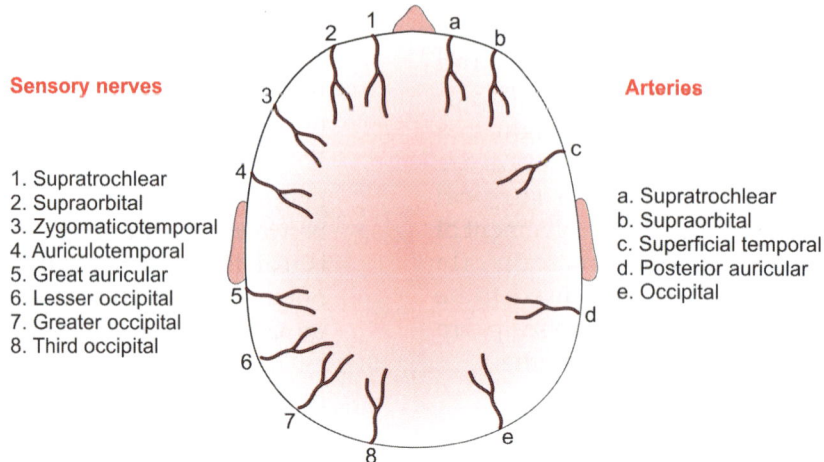

Sensory nerves

1. Supratrochlear
2. Supraorbital
3. Zygomaticotemporal
4. Auriculotemporal
5. Great auricular
6. Lesser occipital
7. Greater occipital
8. Third occipital

Arteries

a. Supratrochlear
b. Supraorbital
c. Superficial temporal
d. Posterior auricular
e. Occipital

Fig. 6.16: Arteries and sensory nerves supplying scalp

4. Third occipital nerve (dorsal ramus of C3).
5. The motor nerve is the posterior auricular branch of the facial nerve.

The arteries supplying the scalp are five in number on each side (Fig. 6.16):

1. Supratrochlear.
2. Supraorbital.
3. Superficial temporal.
4. Posterior auricular.
5. Occipital.

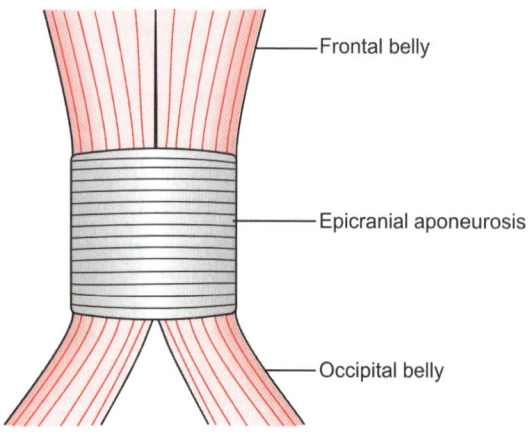

Frontal belly

Epicranial aponeurosis

Occipital belly

Fig. 6.17: Occipitofrontalis

The veins accompany the corresponding arteries. Therefore, the five veins are:

1. Supratrochlear.
2. Supraorbital.
3. Superficial temporal.
4. Posterior auricular.
5. Occipital.

Lymphatic Drainage of the Scalp

Lymph vessels do originate in the scalp but there are no lymph nodes in the scalp. That is the reason why an enlarged mass of the scalp can never be an enlarged lymph node. Lymph vessels of the scalp drain into the pericervical collar of lymph nodes around the junction of head with the neck.

- It drains into the following four lymph nodes:
  - Submandibular
  - Parotid
  - Posterior auricular (retroauricular)
  - Occipital

All these lymph nodes drain into the deep cervical lymph nodes that lie along the internal jugular vein.

FACE

It extends from the free margin of hair line superiorly to the lower border of the mandible inferiorly. On either side it is bounded by the auricles.

The skin of the face is mainly supplied by the branches of the trigeminal nerve (Fig. 6.21). The trigeminal nerve has three branches:
1. Ophthalmic (V1)
2. Maxillary (V2)
3. Mandibular (V3)

The three branches of ophthalmic nerve which supply the face are:
1. Nasociliary
2. Frontal
3. Lacrimal
  - Frontal nerve divides into supraorbital and supratrochlear branches.
  - External nasal and infratrochlear come from the nasociliary.

The three branches of maxillary nerve which supply the face are:
1. Infraorbital
2. Zygomaticofacial
3. Zygomaticotemporal

The three branches of mandibular nerve are:
1. Mental
2. Buccal
3. Auriculotemporal

The skin over the angle of the mandible is supplied by the great auricular nerve.

The motor nerves of face: All motor branches supplying the muscles of face come from the facial nerve. It is the 7th cranial nerve. It passes through the parotid gland. Facial nerve gives five branches to the face. They are (Fig. 6.20):
1. Temporal
2. Zygomatic
3. Buccal
4. Marginal mandibular
5. Cervical

Fascia in the Face

- There is no deep fascia in the face.
- The muscles of the face are directly inserted into the skin of the face.
- If deep fascia were to be there, it would have come in the way of expression.
- However, the deep fascia forms the parotid sheath on the side of the face and also covers the buccinator muscle.
- Edema of the face is very common.
- Fluid tends to get collected in the superficial tissues just deep to the skin. This is common in the eyelids.

Muscles of Facial Expression (Fig. 6.18)

- They are developed from the second pharyngeal arch (branchial arch).
- They are supplied by the facial nerve.
- They are directly inserted into the skin of the face.

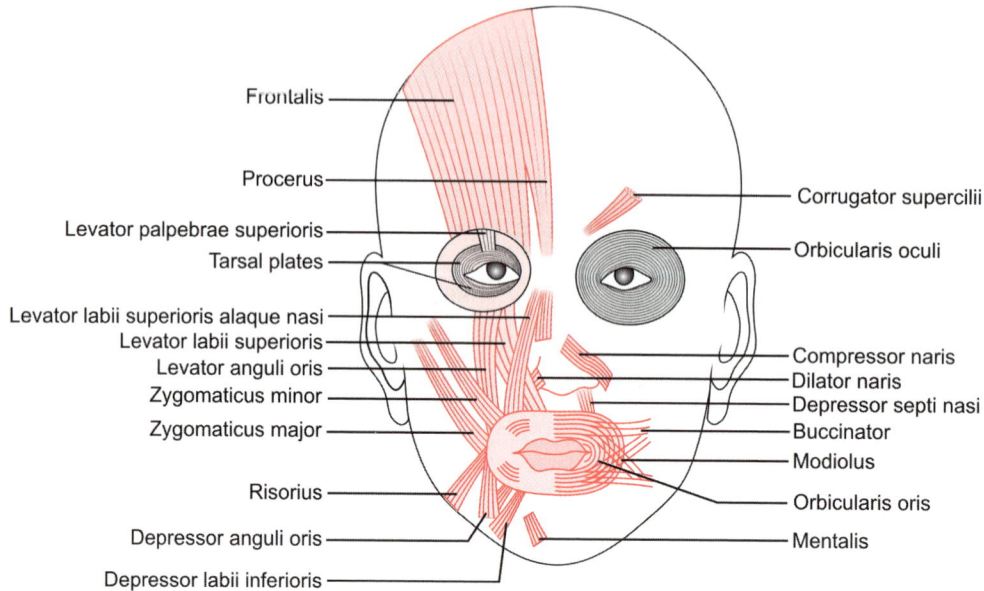

Fig. 6.18: Muscles of face

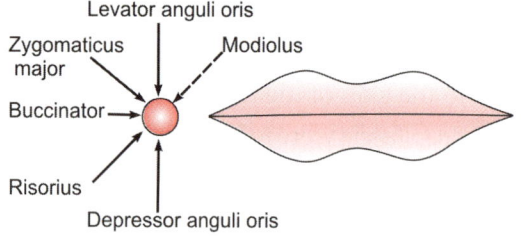

Fig. 6.19: Modiolus

- They are arranged as sphincters around the orifices. They also help as dilators of the orifices.
- The important muscles are:
  1. *Frontalis:* It is the part of occipitofrontalis muscle and it produces transverse wrinkles over the forehead.
  2. *Orbicularis oris:* It is the sphincter of the mouth. Its fibers encircle the mouth and blend with the other facial muscles. It helps in whistling and sucking. It is very important in speech and mastication. It can keep the mouth closed (lips approximated) very strongly against resistance.
  3. *Buccinator:* It is the muscle of the cheek. It bridges the gap between the maxilla and mandible. It forms the lateral wall of the vestibule of the mouth. It feeds the food to the grinding teeth. It is well developed in trumpeters. When it is paralyzed, as in the facial nerve palsy, the food gets accumulated in the vestibule of the mouth. This muscle is pierced by the parotid duct.
  4. *Orbicularis oculi:* It surrounds the orbit and acts like the sphincter muscle of the eye. It is divided into three parts:
     a. The orbital part which forcefully closes the eyelids.
     b. The palpebral part which closes lightly as in sleeping.

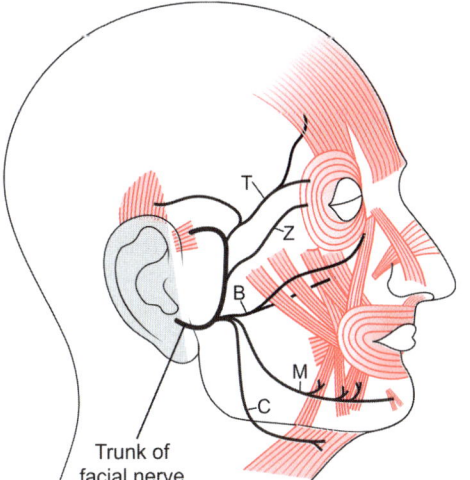

Trunk of
facial nerve

T. Temporal branch, Z. Zygomatic branch,
B. Buccal branch, M. Mandibular branch,
C. Cervical branch

Fig. 6.20: Motor nerve supply of face

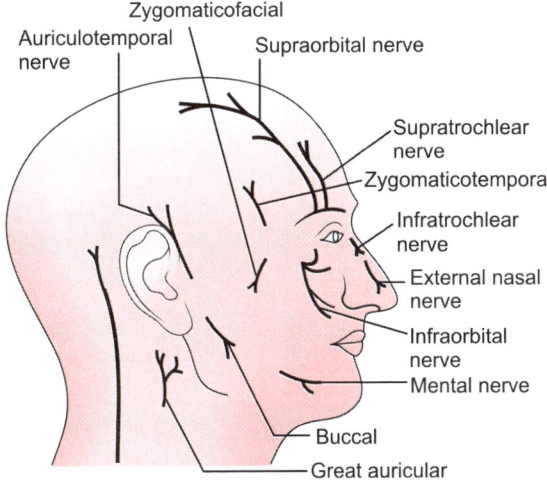

Zygomaticofacial
Auriculotemporal
nerve
Supraorbital nerve
Supratrochlear
nerve
Zygomaticotemporal
Infratrochlear
nerve
External nasal
nerve
Infraorbital
nerve
Mental nerve
Buccal
Great auricular

Fig. 6.21: Sensory nerve supply of face

c. Lacrimal part which helps in the drainage of lacrimal fluid by dilating lacrimal sac.

5. *Procerus:* It produces transverse wrinkles over the bridge of the nose.

6. *Zygomaticus major:* It is often called the smiling muscle as it widens the face (as in expressing the word "cheese").

Following muscles alter the shape of the mouth:
- Depressor anguli oris
- Levator anguli oris
- Levator labii superioris
- Depressor labii inferioris
- Orbicularis oris.

Arteries of the Face

- The main artery of the face is the facial artery.
- The transverse facial artery also supplies the face.
- The branches of facial artery anastomose richly with the branches of the opposite artery.
- The forehead is supplied by the supra-orbital and supratrochlear branches of the ophthalmic artery branch of the internal carotid artery.

Facial Artery

- It is the main artery of the face.
- It arises from the external carotid artery.
- It winds round the lower border of the mandible at the anteroinferior angle of the masseter muscle.
- Its course is tortuous in the face.
- It goes towards the angle of the mouth and later runs on the side of the nose and continues as the angular artery at the medial angle of the eye.
- Its branches in the face are:
  - Inferior labial
  - Superior labial
  - Lateral nasal
- It gives muscular branches and anastomosis with the branches of the opposite facial artery.

- The wounds of the face bleed profusely and heal quickly (similar to the rule of blood vessels in the scalp). That is the reason why plastic surgery operations of the face are successful.
- Facial pulse is felt where facial artery winds round the inferior border of mandible.
- When a blood vessel of the lip is injured, it bleeds from both the cut ends and, therefore, pressure has to be applied on both sides.
- Facial artery lies anterior to the facial vein.

Facial Vein

- It begins at the medial angle of the eye as angular vein. The angular vein is formed by the union of supratrochlear and supra-orbital veins.
- It receives tributaries corresponding to the branches of the facial artery.
- It is straight and lies posterior to the facial artery.
- It has no valves.
- It comes close to the facial artery near the anteroinferior angle of the masseter muscle and crosses the lower border of the mandible.
- In the neck it is joined by the anterior division of the retromandibular vein. It opens in the internal jugular vein.
- Connections:
  - At the medial angle of the eye near its commencement it is connected to the superior ophthalmic vein. Superior ophthalmic vein opens into the cavernous sinus. Through this route infection is spread to the cavernous sinus from the face. Angular vein → superior ophthalmic vein → cavernous sinus.
  - Following is another route of spread of infection from the facial vein to the cavernous sinus: Facial vein → deep facial vein → pterygoid venous plexus → emissary vein → cavernous sinus.

Therefore, triangular area covering the upper lip and nose is called the dangerous area of the face (Fig. 6.22) as any infection in this area can be spread to the cavernous sinus leading to cavernous sinus thrombosis.

Lymphatic drainage of face: It is shown in Fig. 6.23.

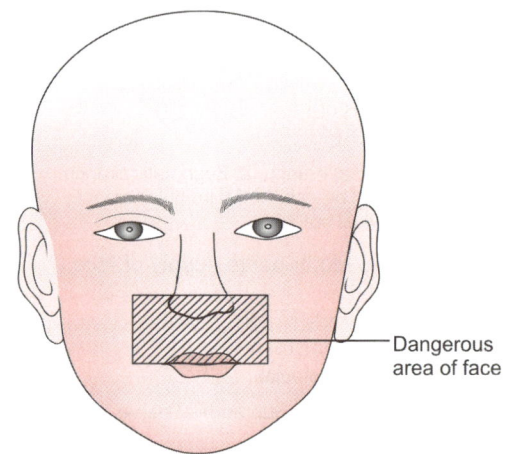

Fig. 6.22: Dangerous area of face

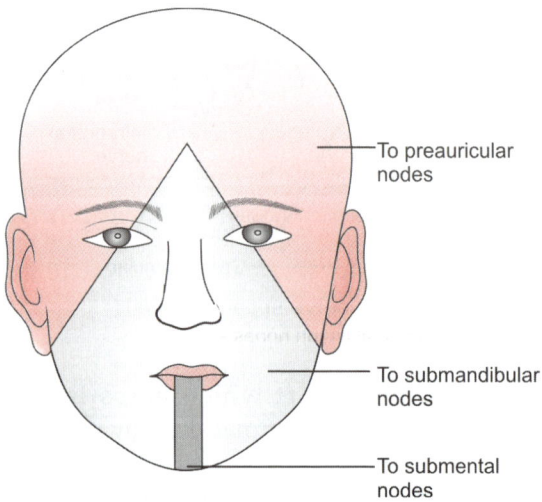

Fig. 6.23: Lymphatic drainage of face

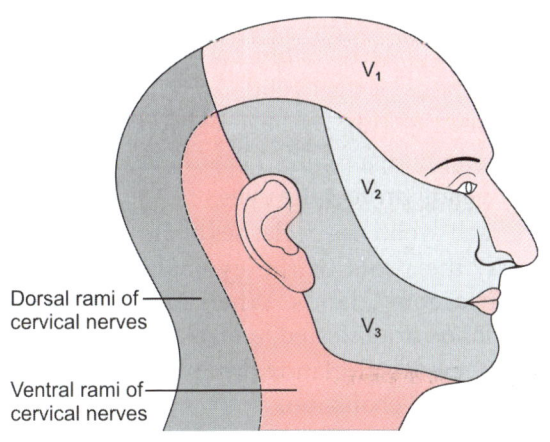

V1. Ophthalmic nerve V2. Maxillary nerve
V3. Mandibular nerve

Fig. 6.24: Sensory innervation of head and neck

Lymphatic Drainage of Head and Neck

- Superficial drainage of lymph occurs into superficial cervical lymph nodes. They are arranged as a collar at the junction of head and neck. They include submental, submandibular, parotid, mastoid and occipital nodes (Fig. 6.25).

- Deep drainage of all lymph from head and neck occurs into deep cervical lymph nodes either directly or indirectly after passing through superficial lymph nodes. They include:
  - *Anterior deep cervical:* It consists of pretracheal, paratracheal, prelaryngeal and thyroid nodes.
  - *Lateral deep cervical:* It consists of superior deep cervical, inferior deep cervical and retropharyngeal nodes. Jugulodigastric node is a member of the superior group and juguloomohyoid is a member of the inferior group (Fig. 6.25).

CLINICAL ANATOMY

- *Neck dissection* involves surgical removal of structures of the neck affected by spread of cancer. It may be of the following types:

Surgical procedure	Structures removed
Radical neck dissection	Removal of all ipsilateral cervical lymph nodes below the body of mandible +

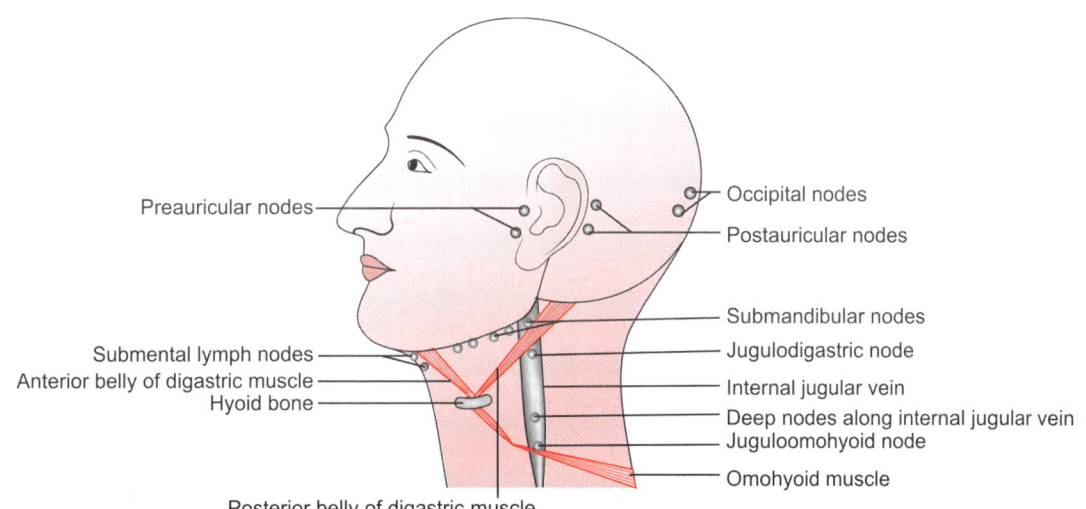

Fig. 6.25: Cervical lymph nodes

	11th cranial nerve, IJV and SCM
Modified radical neck dissection	Same as above but preserves one or more of either the 11th cranial nerve, IJV or SCM
Extended radical neck dissection	Radical neck dissection + additional lymph node groups or other non-lymphatic structures (neural, muscular or vascular) that are not removed in radical neck dissection
Selective neck dissection	Selective lymph node groups instead of all the lymph node groups of radical neck dissection

Eyelid

Eyelid is made up of the following layers (Fig. 6.26):

- Skin
- Thin layer of superficial fascia
- Orbicularis oculi
- Tarsal plate: It is a fibrous plate which forms the basis of the eyelid.
- Tarsal glands
- Conjunctiva
- Eyelids protect the eyes.
- Each eyelid has eyelashes at the free margin.
- At the roots of the eyelashes there are sebaceous glands. When these sebaceous glands are infected, a stye results.
- When tarsal glands are infected it results in tarsal chalazion.
- Levator palpebrae superioris elevates the upper eyelid.
- There is a smooth muscle in the upper eyelid called the superior tarsal muscle. It is supplied by the sympathetic nerves from the cervical sympathetic chain.

Therefore, in Horner's syndrome there is ptosis, constriction of pupil and loss of sweating on the same side of the face.

Lacrimal Apparatus

It includes the lacrimal gland, lacrimal ducts, conjunctival sac, lacrimal puncta, lacrimal canaliculi, lacrimal sac and nasolacrimal duct.

1. Lacrimal gland
   - Secretes the tears (fluid) (Fig. 6.27).

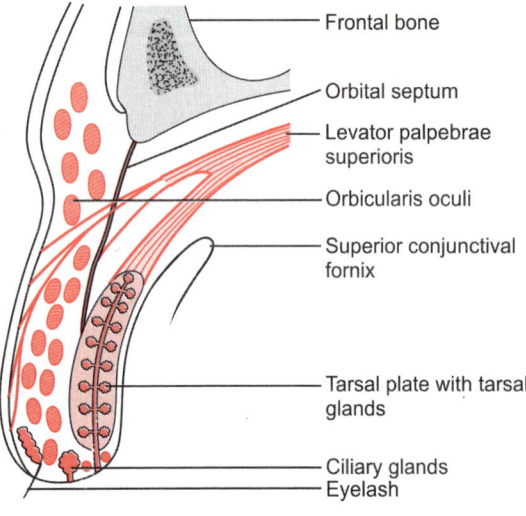

Fig. 6.26: Eyelid

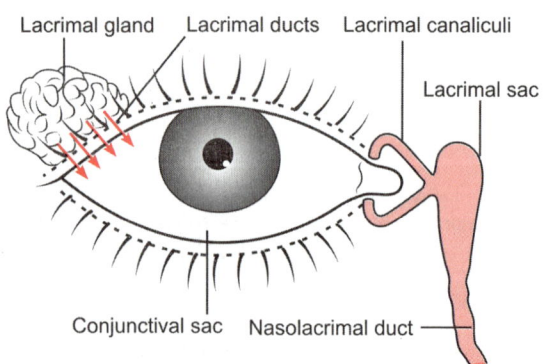

Fig. 6.27: Lacrimal apparatus

– Is supplied by the secretomotor fibers from the pterygopalatine ganglion. These fibers reach the gland as follows (in that order):

Lacrimatory nucleus (superior salivatory nucleus), nervus intermedius of 7th cranial nerve, geniculate ganglion, greater petrosal nerve, nerve of pterygoid canal, pterygopalatine ganglion, zygomatic nerve, zygomaticotemporal nerve, its communication to lacrimal nerve and then reaches the gland through lacrimal nerve.

- Sensory innervation of the gland comes from the lacrimal nerve, a branch of the ophthalmic nerve.
- The gland has two parts: The superficial (palpebral) and deep (orbital) parts.
- The ducts of the deep part traverse the superficial part. Therefore, the removal of the superficial (palpebral) part is akin to the removal of the whole gland.

2. Conjunctival sac is the space between the palpebral conjunctiva and ocular (bulbar) conjunctiva. The point of continuation of palpebral conjunctiva with the ocular conjunctiva is called the conjunctival fornix. The superior conjunctival fornix lies deep to the upper eyelid while the inferior conjunctival fornix lies deep to the lower eyelid.

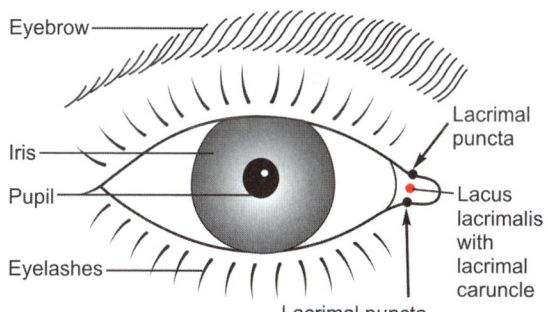

Eyebrow

Iris

Pupil

Eyelashes

Lacrimal puncta

Lacrimal puncta

Lacus lacrimalis with lacrimal caruncle

Fig. 6.28: Surface features of eye (right)

- Lacrimal secretion is poured into the lateral part of the superior conjunctival fornix through the lacrimal ducts. It is swept medially by the blinking of eyelids. This keeps the front of the eyeball moist and the cornea is nourished.

> If lacrimal fluid is not there, it results in blindness because of damage due to drying.

- The lacrimal fluid is collected in the lacus lacrimalis at the medial angle of the eye.

3. Lacrimal part of the orbicularis oculi contracts, which makes the puncta to be dipped into the lacus lacrimalis and the negative pressure in the lacrimal sac helps the fluid to be sucked into them.

4. The fluid passes through the lacrimal canaliculi into the lacrimal sac. Nasolacrimal duct carries the fluid from the lacrimal sac into the inferior meatus of the nose. Here the fluid passes backwards into nasopharynx to be swallowed.

Parotid Gland

- It is the largest serous salivary gland.
- It is present on the side of the face.
- The parotid duct opens into the vestibule of the mouth.

It has the following surfaces and borders:
- Superficial surface
- Superior surface
- Apex
- Anteromedial surface
- Posteromedial surface
- Anterior border
- Posterior border
- Medial border

Superficial Surface

It is related to the following structures:
- Skin
- Superficial fascia
- Superficial group of parotid lymph nodes

- Parotid fascia which is the deep fascia of the neck extending upwards to enclose the parotid gland.

Superior Surface

It is related to the following structures:
- External acoustic meatus
- Auriculotemporal nerve
- Superficial temporal vessels

Anterior border is related to the following structures:
- Zygomatic branch of the facial nerve
- Transverse facial artery
- Parotid duct
- Buccal branch of the facial nerve
- Marginal mandibular branch of the facial nerve.

Apex

Following structures exit at the apex of the parotid gland:

- Cervical branch of the facial nerve
- Retromandibular vein (2 divisions)

Anteromedial Surface

It is concave and winds around the posterior border of the ramus of the mandible. It is related to the following structures (Fig. 6.29):
- Masseter muscle
- Ramus of the mandible
- Medial pterygoid muscle.

Posteromedial Surface

It is related to the following structures:
- Posterior belly of digastric
- Sternocleidomastoid muscle
- Styloid process and three muscles attached to it
  1. Styloglossus
  2. Stylopharyngeus
  3. Stylohyoid

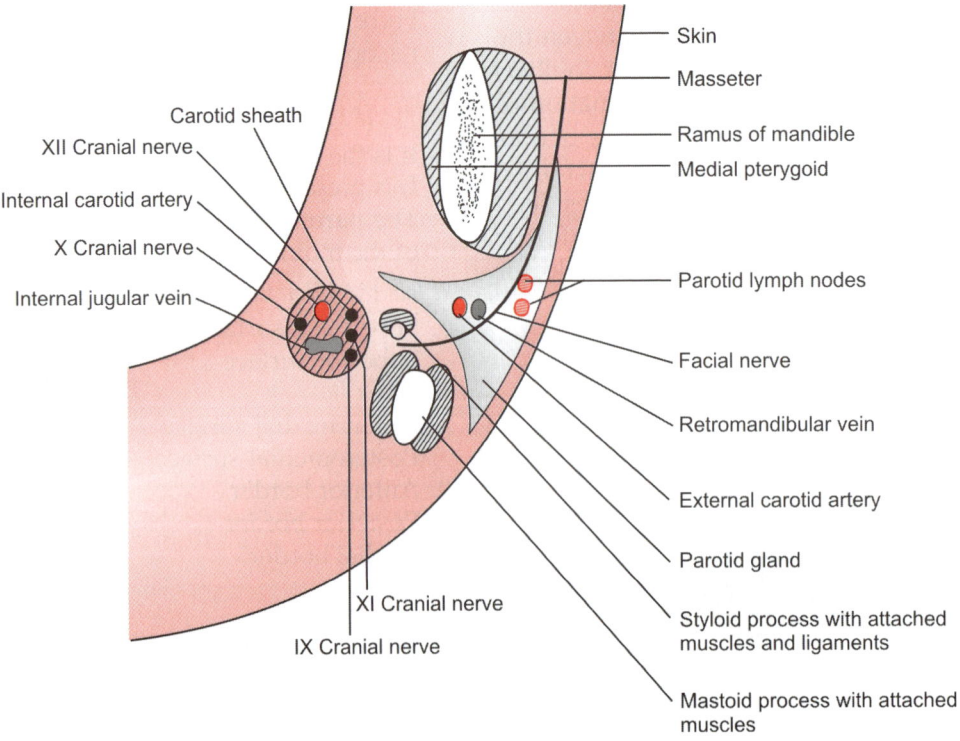

Fig. 6.29: Relations of parotid gland (horizontal section)

Facial nerve enters the parotid gland by piercing the posteromedial surface (Fig. 6.29).

The styloid process and group of structures associated with it separate the parotid gland from the internal carotid artery and internal jugular vein.

Structures present inside the parotid gland (Fig. 6.29)

- Facial nerve and its five branches
- Retromandibular vein and its two tributaries, superficial temporal vein and maxillary vein.
- External carotid artery and the proximal parts of its two terminal branches, superficial temporal artery and the maxillary artery lie in it. The transverse facial artery, a branch of superficial temporal artery arises inside the gland.
- External carotid artery is accompanied by sympathetic plexus of nerves.

Parotid Duct

- It is about 2 to 2.5 inches long.
- It lies over the masseter muscle and then bends medially to pierce the buccal pad of fat, buccopharyngeal fascia, buccinator muscle and then opens into the vestibule of the mouth at the level of the crown of the upper second molar tooth.
- Accessory parotid gland lies anterior to it.
- The duct lies between the transverse facial artery (and upper buccal branch of 7th nerve) above and the (lower) buccal branch of facial nerve below.

Sialogram is the radiography of the salivary gland duct system after injecting contrast medium into the duct of the salivary gland. Any blockage (due to sialolith or calculus) can be identified.

Parasympathetic secretomotor fibers to the gland:

Inferior salivatory nucleus in the brainstem
↓
Glossopharyngeal nerve
(its tympanic branch to tympanic plexus)
↓
Tympanic plexus
↓
Lesser petrosal nerve
↓
Otic ganglion (relay in this ganglion)
↓
Postganglionic fibers pass through → Auriculotemporal nerve → Parotid gland

Blood supply: Branches of the external carotid artery.

Sensory supply: Branches of great auricular nerve and auriculotemporal nerve.

CLINICAL ANATOMY

Frey's syndrome:

Auriculotemporal nerve carries fibers (sympathetic) to sweat glands and also (parasympathetic) to parotid gland. During regeneration following injury to the auriculotemporal nerve, the wrong ends may get connected (of sympathetic and parasympathetic). In that case, whenever there is taste stimulation or thought of food, it results in the sweating of the skin over the area of the distribu-tion of auriculotemporal nerve (which should normally have caused salivation). This is called Frey's syndrome.

Parotitis associated with swelling of parotid gland is painful because the parotid fascia is tough and unyielding. Masticatory movements become painful because of the relation of the gland to the temporo-mandibular joint and mandible.

Styloid Apparatus

It includes (fig. 6.30):
1. Styloglossus muscle
2. Stylopharyngeus muscle
3. Stylohyoid muscle
4. Stylohyoid ligament

Deep Fascia of the Neck

It is divided into three layers:
1. The superficial layer of this deep fascia is called the investing layer of cervical fascia (Fig. 6.31).
2. The middle layer is called the pretracheal fascia.
3. The innermost layer is called the prevertebral fascia.

The investing layer of the cervical fascia:
- This is shaped like a cylinder and it is attached superiorly to the following structures:
  1. Lower border of the mandible.
  2. Angle of the mandible.
  3. Styloid process (it forms the stylomandibular ligament between the styloid process and the angle of the mandible).

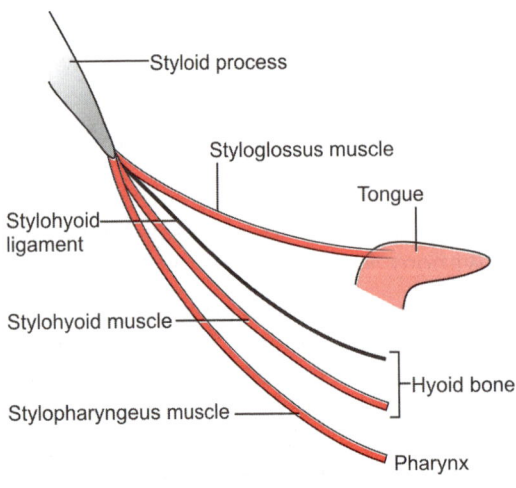

Styloid process

Styloglossus muscle

Tongue

Stylohyoid ligament

Stylohyoid muscle

Hyoid bone

Stylopharyngeus muscle

Pharynx

Fig. 6.30: Styloid apparatus

4. Mastoid process (between angle of mandible and mastoid process it splits and encloses the parotid gland).
5. Superior nuchal line.
6. External occipital protuberance.
- Along its upper attachment it splits twice to enclose two glands, the submandibular and parotid on each side.
- In the middle it encloses two muscles; on each side it encloses the trapezius and sternocleidomastoid muscles. In between these two muscles, the investing layer of cervical fascia forms the roof of the posterior triangle.
- Along its lower attachment, it splits twice to enclose two spaces:
  i. Suprasternal space (Burns)
  ii. Supraclavicular space
- Inferiorly the investing layer attaches to:
  i. Manubrium
  ii. Clavicles
  iii. Spines and acromion of scapulae
- *Anteriorly:* Continuous with opposite side.
- *Posteriorly:* Attaches to C7 spine and ligamentum nuchae.

Pretracheal Fascia

- This is the fascia of the visceral compartment of the neck (Fig. 6.31).
- It encloses the thyroid gland and the trachea and oesophagus.
- It is prominent in front of the trachea and, therefore, it is called the pretracheal fascia.
- Extends superiorly from hyoid bone; inferiorly into thorax blending with fibrous pericardium.
- Laterally it fuses with carotid sheath.

Prevertebral Fascia

- It covers the prevertebral muscles and forms the floor of the posterior triangle (Fig. 6.31).

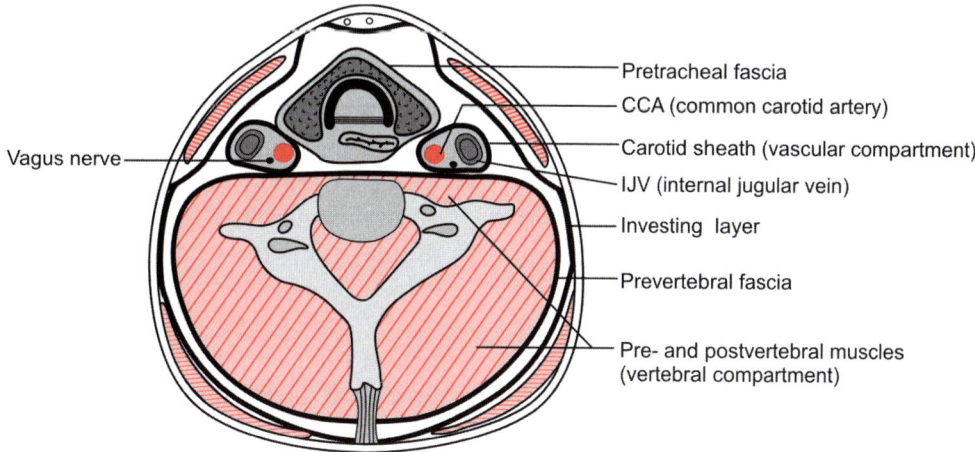

Fig. 6.31: Deep cervical fascia (horizontal section)

- It forms the posterior boundary of the retropharyngeal space in the median region.
- It extends from base of skull to anterior longitudianl ligament of T3 vertebra.
- Laterally it is lost deep to trapezius.

Carotid Sheath

It is a tubular condensation of the deep cervical fascia extending from skull base to root of neck containing common and internal carotid arteries and internal jugular vein and vagus nerve (Fig. 6.31).

Sternocleidomastoid Muscle (SCM)

- *Origin:* It arises from the manubrium sterni and the medial 1/3rd of the clavicle.
- *Insertion:* It is inserted into the mastoid process and the lateral half of the superior nuchal line.
- Between its sternal and clavicular heads there is a depression called the lesser supraclavicular fossa. This fossa contains the internal jugular vein. This relation is important while performing central cannulation.
- It is a very important muscle as it is related to many structures and it separates the anterior and the posterior triangles.
- Triangle anterior to the muscle is called the anterior triangle while the triangle posterior to it is called the posterior triangle.
- *Action:*
  - When both muscles contract, it pulls the head forwards. It also helps to lift the head from the horizontal position as getting up from bed.

– It turns the face to the opposite side and bends the head to the same side.

– It helps in the deep inspiration as it can elevate the sternum and indirectly the first rib.

- *Nerve supply:* It is supplied by the spinal part of accessory nerve. Branches of 2nd and 3rd cervical nerves carry proprio-ceptive fibers of the sternomastoid muscle.

- *Torticollis (wry neck):*
  – Congenital torticollis is most common variety.
- Head is tilted to the same side and face turned to the opposite side.
- Fibrosis and shortening of SCM is the cause.
- Treatment is by surgery.
  – Other causes of torticollis are also recognized.

The following structures (nerves) are related to the middle of posterior border of the sternomastoid muscle (nerve point of neck):

- Lesser occipital nerve
- Great auricular nerve
- Accessory nerve
- Transverse cutaneous nerve of neck
- Supraclavicular nerves

Posterior Triangle

- It lies posterior to the sternocleidomastoid muscle (SCM) (Fig. 6.33).

- It lies on the side of the neck.

Boundaries

- *Anterior boundary:* It is formed by the posterior border of the SCM.
- *Posterior boundary:* It is formed by the anterior border of trapezius muscle.
- *Apex:* Directed superiorly where SCM and trapezius meet.

- *Base* is formed by the intermediate third of the clavicle.
- *Roof:* It is formed by the skin, superficial fascia, platysma and investing layer of cervical fascia. The investing layer of cervical fascia has the spinal part of accessory nerve in its thickness. External jugular vein crosses the SCM obliquely.

Nerve Point of the Neck

- It is at the level of middle of the posterior border of the SCM (Fig. 6.32).
- Following nerves emerge at this point:
  1. Accessory nerve
  2. Lesser occipital nerve
  3. Great auricular nerve
  4. Transverse cutaneous nerve of neck
  5. Supraclavicular nerves.

Floor of the Posterior Triangle

- It is formed by the following muscles (from above downwards they are):
- Splenius capitis
- Levator scapulae

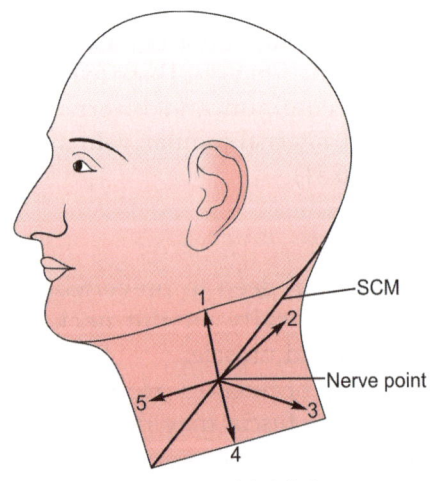

1. Great auricular, 2. Lesser occipital, 3. Accessory, 4. Supraclavicular, 5. Transverse cutaneous nerve of neck

Fig. 6.32: Nerves emerging at nerve point

- Scalenus medius
- All these muscles are covered by the prevertebral fascia.
- At the anteroinferior angle scalenus anterior may appear (but largely it lies deep to the SCM).
- At the apex, sometimes part of the semispinalis capitis may appear.
- At the posteroinferior angle scalenus posterior appears.

In the lower part of the triangle, the trunks of the brachial plexus lie between the scalenus medius and scalenus anterior deep to prevertebral fascia.

Nerves Present in the Posterior Triangle

1. Spinal part of accessory nerve.
2. Cutaneous and muscular branches of cervical plexus.
   Following branches of cervical plexus cross the triangle:
   - Lesser occipital nerve
   - Great auricular nerve
   - Transverse cutaneous nerve of neck
   - Supraclavicular nerves.
3. Following nerves of brachial plexus are seen:
   - Trunks of the brachial plexus
   - Nerve to serratus anterior
   - Dorsal scapular nerve
   - Suprascapular nerve
   - Nerve to subclavius

Arteries Present in the Posterior Triangle

1. Third part of the subclavian artery.
2. Suprascapular artery.
3. Transverse cervical artery (divides into superficial and deep branch at the anterior border of levator scapulae).
4. Occipital artery.
   - The deep branch of the transverse cervical artery may arise independently from the third part of the subclavian artery in the triangle and it is called the dorsal scapular artery.
   - *Note:* The transverse cervical artery and suprascapular arteries are the branches of the thyrocervical trunk which arises from the first part of the subclavian artery.
   - *Note:* The deep branch of the transverse cervical artery lies deep to the levator scapulae and the superficial branch of the transverse cervical artery lies deep to the trapezius muscle.

Veins of the Posterior Triangle

1. The external jugular vein and its tributaries: anterior jugular vein, transverse cervical vein and suprascapular vein.
2. The subclavian vein (usually not in triangle; but behind clavicle).

Lymph Nodes of the Posterior Triangle

Lymph nodes are situated along the external jugular vein. These are called the superficial cervical lymph nodes. These nodes might get matted or enlarged in tuberculosis or in cancer. In such case when these nodes are removed, a great care has to be exercised to retain the accessory nerve which is in close relation to these lymph nodes.

Divisions

- The posterior triangle is divided into two triangles by the inferior belly of the omohyoid muscle.
- The triangle superior to the inferior belly of the omohyoid is called the occipital triangle (Fig. 6.33).
- The triangle inferior to the inferior belly of the omohyoid is called the supraclavicular triangle (Fig. 6.33). The depression over the supraclavicular triangle is called the greater supraclavicular fossa.

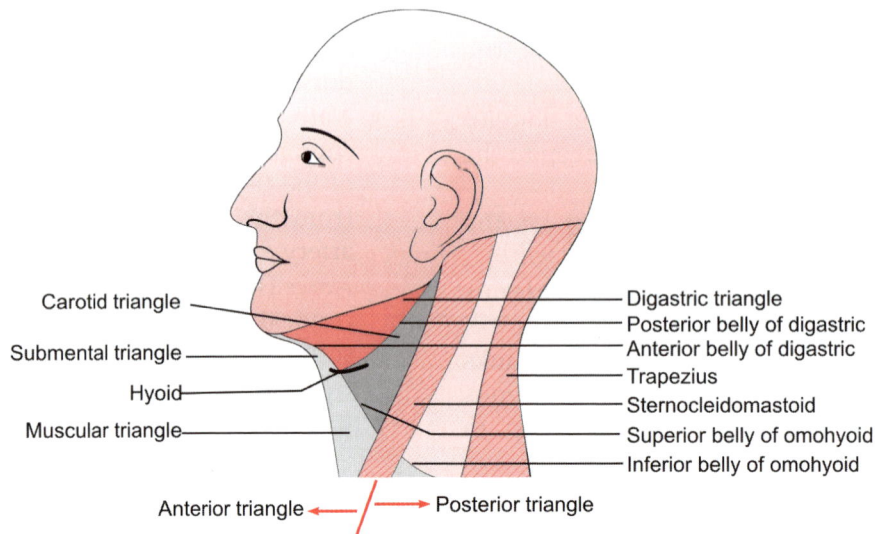

Carotid triangle — Digastric triangle
Submental triangle — Posterior belly of digastric
Hyoid — Anterior belly of digastric
Muscular triangle — Trapezius
— Sternocleidomastoid
— Superior belly of omohyoid
— Inferior belly of omohyoid
Anterior triangle ←— / —→ Posterior triangle

Fig. 6.33: Triangles of the neck

The third part of the subclavian artery can be compressed against the first rib in the greater supraclavicular fossa. This is the way to control the bleeding from a major vessel of the upper limb.

External Jugular Vein

- It is formed by the union of the posterior division of the retromandibular vein with the posterior auricular vein.
- It crosses the sternocleidomastoid muscle.
- It is accompanied by the great auricular nerve.
- It lies superficial to the investing layer of the cervical fascia in the roof of the posterior triangle.
- In the lower part it pierces the roof of the posterior triangle.
- The external jugular vein opens into the subclavian vein.
- It receives the following three veins (tributaries):
  1. Transverse cervical
  2. Suprascapular
  3. Anterior jugular

When the external jugular vein is accidentally injured in the posterior triangle by a sharp knife, where it pierces the investing layer of the cervical fascia; its lumen remains open and does not get collapsed. This may turn out to be dangerous. Through this air may be sucked into the vein and subsequently into the right atrium. This air embolism may prove fatal.

Injury to the cervical branch of facial nerve during surgical dissections of the neck causes paralysis of platysma resulting in skin folds.
- Subclavian vein or internal jugular vein puncture is done for right cardiac catheterization or placement of central venous line in these veins.
- *Subclavian vein puncture:* In the infra-clavicular approach the needle is passed

along the inferior aspect of the middle of the clavicle; the needle being aimed in the direction of the jugular notch.

- *Internal jugular vein puncture:*
  - Right IJV is preferred as it is larger.
  - The needle is passed into the area between sternal and clavicular heads of SCM in a downward direction.
- Jugular venous pressure:
  - IJV is used as no valves exist between IJV and right atrium.
  - For the same reason it correlates well with the right atrial pressure.
  - EJV is not reliable because of valves in it.

Muscles of the Back

- Arranged in layers (Fig. 6.34).
- Divided into extrinsic and intrinsic muscles.
- Intrinsic muscles are the true muscles of the back (deep group).
- Extrinsic muscles include the superficial and intermediate group.
- Superficial group includes trapezius, latissimus dorsi, levator scapulae and rhomboid muscles.
- Intermediate group includes serratus poste-rior group; namely superior and inferior.
- Deep or intrinsic group consists of erector spinae and many other muscles like multifidus, rotatores, suboccipital, inter-spinal and intertransverse muscles (Fig. 6.35).

Erector Spinae

- Or sacrospinalis extends from the sacrum to the skull.
- It is a muscle complex that is made of 3 columns.
- From medial to lateral the 3 columns are spinalis, longissimus and iliocostalis (Figs 6.34 and 6.36).
- It extends the trunk.

Suboccipital Triangle

- This is a triangle that is placed very deeply in the back of neck below the occipital bone.
- The following structures have to be identified and reflected before the suboccipital triangle is approached:
  - Skin
  - Superficial fascia
  - Deep fascia
  - Trapezius muscle

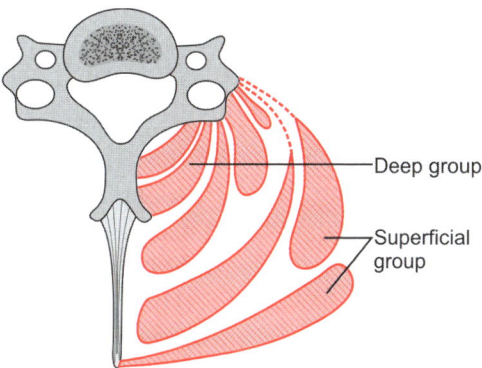

Deep group

Superficial group

Fig. 6.34: Muscles of the back

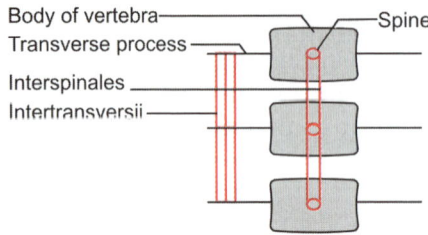

Fig. 6.35: Intertransverse and interspinal muscles

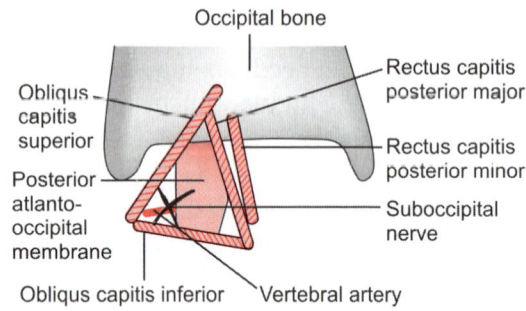

Fig. 6.37: Suboccipital triangle

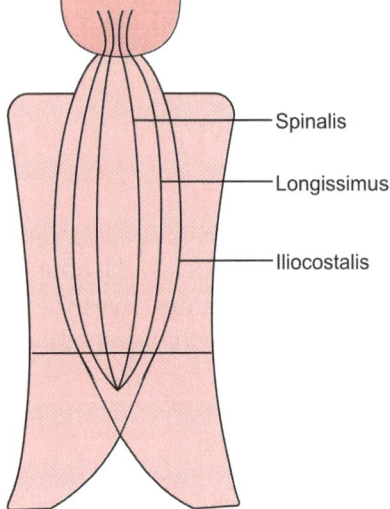

Fig. 6.36: Erector spinae

- Splenius capitis (directed upwards and laterally and is inserted into the mastoid process and lateral 1/3rd of superior nuchal line).
- Semispinalis capitis (directed upwards and medially and is inserted into the medial part of the area between the superior and inferior nuchal lines).

The suboccipital triangle lies deep to the semispinalis capitis muscle (roof).

Following muscles form the boundaries of the suboccipital triangle (Fig. 6.37):

- *Superomedially:* Rectus capitis posterior major arises from the spine of C2 and is inserted into the lateral part of the area between the inferior nuchal line and the posterior margin of foramen magnum.
- *Inferiorly:* Obliqus capitis inferior arises from the spine of second cervical vertebra and is inserted into the transverse process of atlas.
- *Superolaterally:* Obliqus capitis superior arises from the transverse process of the atlas and is inserted into the lateral part of the area between into the superior and inferior nuchal lines.

The following structures are found in the floor of the triangle:
- Posterior atlantooccipital membrane, posterior arch of atlas.

Contents of the Triangle

1. Third part of the vertebral artery.
2. Dorsal ramus of first cervical nerve (suboccipital nerve). This nerve supplies all the small muscles of the suboccipital triangle.
3. Connective tissue.
4. Suboccipital plexus of veins.

The roof is formed by the semispinalis capitis muscle.

Greater occipital nerve (medial branch of dorsal ramus of C2) is the thickest cutaneous nerve of the body. It winds round the obliqus capitis inferior muscle and pierces the semispinalis capitis and trapezius to supply the skin of the back of the scalp.

APPLIED ANATOMY

- Should there be vertebral insufficiency then vertigo results when the head is turned backwards as in taking reverse in a vehicle. This is due to the winding course of the vertebral artery in the suboccipital triangle.
- The suboccipital triangle is used to approach the posterior cranial fossa in operations dealing with the posterior fossa and cerebellum.
- This is also used in cisternal puncture of cisternal magna to withdraw CSF. Cisternal puncture may be preferred when lumbar puncture is contraindicated.

Note: Rectus capitis posterior minor arises from the atlas and is inserted into the medial part of the area between the inferior nuchal line and the posterior margin of the foramen magnum.

Curvatures of the Vertebral Column

- The adult vertebral column has 4 curvatures. They are:
  1. Cervical convexity
  2. Thoracic concavity
  3. Lumbar convexity
  4. Sacral concavity
- Thoracic and sacral curvatures are primary curvatures present in the fetus (Fig. 6.38).
- Later secondary curvatures are added as follows:
  - With head holding or raising head (at 3–4 months) anterior cervical convexity is formed.
  - With standing (end of 1st year) anterior lumbar convexity develops.

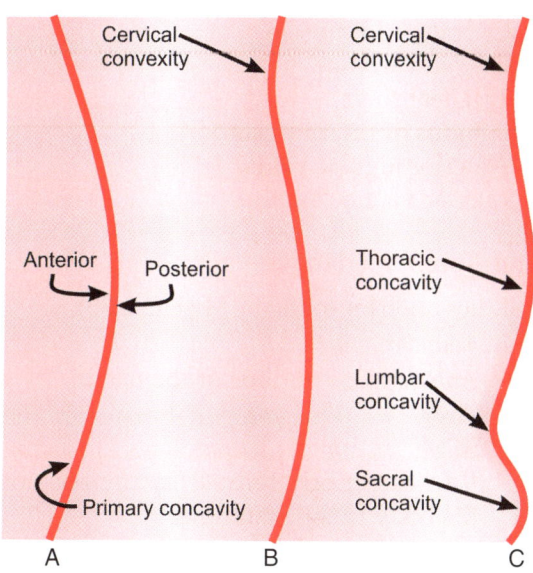

Fig. 6.38: Vertebral column curvatures

- Movements of vertebral column
  - Flexion
  - Extension
  - Lateral flexion
  - Rotation

- Abnormal curvatures of vertebral column.
  - Kyphosis—increased convexity backwards
  - Lordosis—increased convexity forwards
  - Scoliosis—increased convexity to the side.

Anterior Part of the Neck

The following structures lie in the median region of the neck:
- Symphysis menti.
- Mylohyoid raphe.
- Anterior bellies of digastric muscle meet.
- Submental lymph nodes.
- Hyoid bone (body).
- Thyrohyoid ligament.
- Thyroid cartilage.
- Cricothyroid ligament.

- Cricothyroid muscle.
- Cricoid cartilage.
- Tracheal rings.
- Isthmus of thyroid gland.
- Anterior jugular veins.
- Jugular venous arch.

The Anterior Triangle

- It lies anterior to the SCM (Fig. 6.33).
- *Its boundaries are:*
  - *Anterior:* The midline of the neck.
  - *Posterior:* The anterior border of the SCM.
  - *Base:* Superiorly formed by the base of the body of the mandible.
  - *Apex* is directed downwards towards the manubrium sterni.
- *It is divided into the following triangles:*
  - *The submental triangle:* Only half of this triangle is included in the corresponding anterior triangle.
  - *The digastric triangle:* This is also called "the submandibular triangle".
  - *The carotid triangle:* Where carotid arteries and internal jugular vein lie.
  - *The muscular triangle:* Mainly formed by the muscles and contains thyroid gland.

The Submental Triangle

The boundaries are (Fig. 6.33):
- Base is formed by the hyoid bone.
- Apex is formed by the symphysis menti.
- On either side it is bounded by the anterior bellies of digastric muscle.

The roof is formed by the following:
- The skin
- Superficial fascia
- Investing layer of cervical fascia
  The floor is formed by the mylohyoid muscle.

  Contents: Commencement of the anterior jugular veins and submental lymph nodes.

The Digastric Triangle

It is also called "submandibular triangle".

The boundaries are (Fig. 6.33):
- Superiorly the base is formed by the lower border of the body of the mandible.
- Anteroinferiorly it is bounded by the anterior belly of digastric.
- Posteroinferiorly it is bounded by the posterior belly of digastric and stylohyoid muscles.
- Apex is formed by the intermediate tendon of digastric muscle at the hyoid bone.

The roof is formed by the following:
- Skin
- Superficial fascia
- Platysma
- Cervical branch of facial nerve
- Investing layer of cervical fascia

Contents:
- Facial vein
- Submandibular gland and submandibular lymph nodes
- Facial artery.

Note: The facial artery runs deep to the gland and later it lies between the gland and mandible before it winds around the lower border of the body of the mandible. Facial vein lies superficial to the submandibular gland.

The floor is formed by:
- Mylohyoid muscle
- Hyoglossus muscle

The Carotid Triangle

The boundaries are (Fig. 6.33):
- *Superior:* The posterior belly of digastric and stylohyoid muscles.
- *Anteroinferior:* Superior belly of omohyoid.
- *Posteroinferior:* The anterior border of the SCM.

The roof is formed by the following:
- The skin.

- Superficial fascia.
- Platysma.
- Transverse cutaneous nerve of neck.
- Investing layer of cervical fascia.

The floor is formed by the following:
- *Anteriorly:* Thyrohyoid muscle and hyoglossus.
- *Posteriorly:* Middle and inferior constrictor of pharynx.

Contents:
The contents of the anterior triangle are:
- The common carotid artery
- The internal carotid artery
- The external carotid artery and its branches
- The internal jugular vein and its tributaries

The common carotid artery divides at the level of the upper border of the thyroid cartilage into external and internal carotid arteries.

Note: The common carotid artery does not give any branch and the internal carotid artery does not supply any structure outside the skull).

Branches of the external carotid artery in the carotid triangle (Fig. 6.45):

1. The ascending pharyngeal artery (arises on the medial side).
2. The superior thyroid artery.
3. The lingual artery.
4. The facial artery.
5. The occipital artery arises from the posterior aspect of the artery and runs along the lower border of the posterior belly of digastric muscle.
   - 2, 3 and 4 arise from the front of the artery.

The internal jugular vein and its tributaries:
Tributaries of the internal jugular vein in the carotid triangle are:
- Facial vein (as common facial vein)
- Lingual vein

- Occipital vein
- Superior and middle thyroid veins
- Ascending pharyngeal vein

Carotid sheath: This is the thickening of the deep fascia around the major vessels of the neck. It contains the following structures:
- The common carotid artery up to the level of the upper border of thyroid cartilage and internal carotid artery superior to that level.
- The internal jugular vein lies lateral to the arteries.
- The vagus nerve lies within the carotid sheath between the artery and vein on a deeper plane.

The Muscular Triangle

The boundaries are (Fig. 6.33):
- *Posterosuperior:* Superior belly of omohyoid
- *Posteroinferior:* Anterior border of SCM
- *Medial:* Midline of the neck.

Contents:
- Sternohyoid
- Sternothyroid
- Thyroid and parathyroid glands.

The Submandibular Gland

It lies in the submandibular triangle. The superficial relations of the submandibular gland are:

1. Skin
2. Superficial fascia
3. Platysma
4. Cervical branch of facial nerve
5. Submandibular lymph nodes
6. Submandibular fossa of mandible
7. Facial vein
8. Investing layer of cervical fascia forming the capsule of the gland.

Medial relations of Submandibular Gland

- It is related to mylohyoid and hyoglossus muscles and the structures that lie superficial to them (Fig. 6.39).
- a. Structures lying superficial to the mylohyoid muscle:
  1. Anterior belly of digastric
  2. Submental artery and accompanying vein
  3. Nerve to mylohyoid
  4. Submandibular gland
- b. Structures lying superficial to hyoglossus muscle (from above downwards):
  1. Styloglossus muscle
  2. Lingual nerve
  3. Submandibular ganglion
  4. Submandibular duct
  5. Hypoglossal nerve
  6. Veins accompanying hypoglossal nerve.
  7. Structures 1, 2, 4, 5 and 6 pass between mylohyoid and hyoglossus muscles.

  [Submandibular gland lies superficial to all these structures (a) and (b)].

  Other medial relations include stylohyoid ligament, glossopharyngeal nerve, stylohyoid muscle and posterior belly of digastric.

  The submandibular gland has two parts: The superficial and deep.

- The superficial part lies superficial to mylohyoid muscle.
- The small deep part lies between the mylohyoid and hyoglossus muscle. It lies in the intermuscular interval between these two muscles.

Note:
- The facial artery grooves the submandibular gland, makes an S-bend and traverses the space between the gland and the medial surface of the mandible before it winds round the anteroinferior part of the masseter muscle (Fig. 6.40).
- The facial vein crosses superficial to the gland (Fig. 6.40).

Secretomotor Pathway

The fibers reach the gland in the following order: Superior salivatory nucleus, nervus intermedius of facial nerve, geniculate ganglion of facial nerve, chorda tympani, lingual nerve, submandibular ganglion, postganglionic fibers to submandibular and sublingual glands.

Hyoglossus Muscle

- It is a quadrilateral muscle which arises from the hyoid bone and is inserted into the side of the tongue.

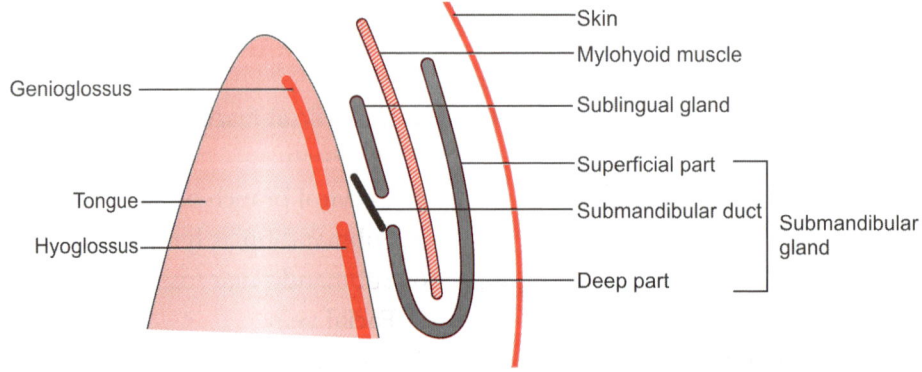

Fig. 6.39: Relations of submandibular gland (horizontal section)

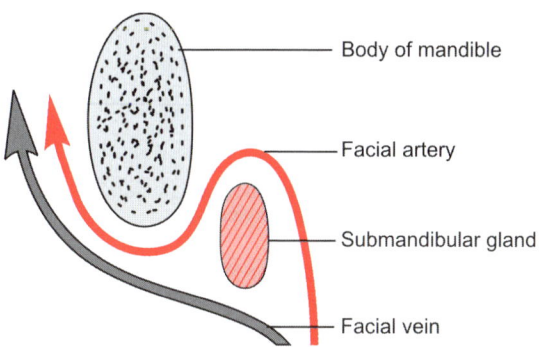

Body of mandible

Facial artery

Submandibular gland

Facial vein

Fig. 6.40: Relation of facial vessels to submandibular gland

- Its anterior part is partly overlapped by the mylohyoid muscle. The deep part of the submandibular gland lies in the interval between the two muscles.
- Structures lying superficial to the hyoglossus are already described under submandibular gland.
- The following structures lie deep to the hyoglossus muscle:
  1. The glossopharyngeal nerve
  2. Stylohyoid ligament
  3. Lingual artery and accompanying veins
  4. Stylopharyngeus
- *Action:* It depresses the side of the tongue.
- *Nerve supply:* Hypoglossal nerve.

The nerve supply and attachments of the following muscles are important:
- *Stylohyoid:* Arises from the styloid process and is inserted into the hyoid bone. It usually splits at its insertion. It is supplied by the facial nerve.
- *Posterior belly of the digastric muscle:* It arises from mastoid notch on the medial side of the mastoid process. It is inserted by its intermediate tendon to the hyoid bone; which is common to it and its anterior belly. Nerve supply of the posterior belly of digastric is facial nerve.

- Remember that facial nerve exits through the stylomastoid foramen which lies between the styloid process and mastoid process and, therefore, the facial nerve supplies these two muscles, stylohyoid and posterior belly of digastric. These muscles are derived from the second branchial arch.
- *Nerve supply of the anterior belly of digastric:* It is supplied by the nerve to mylohyoid which supplies the mylohyoid and anterior belly of digastric muscles.

The muscles attached to mandible and supplied by the mandibular nerve are:
- Lateral pterygoid
- Medial pterygoid
- Temporalis
- Masseter
- Mylohyoid
- Anterior belly of digastric

Hypoglossal nerve in the anterior triangle:
- It passes forwards between the internal jugular vein and the internal carotid artery and crosses the internal carotid and external carotid below the level of the posterior belly of digastric muscle.
- It crosses superficial to the loop of lingual artery, hyoglossus muscle and later supplies all the extrinsic and intrinsic muscles of the tongue except palatoglossus muscle.
- It carries C1 fibers and part of these fibers leave the hypoglossal nerve as the superior root of ansa cervicalis and the remaining fibers supply thyrohyoid and geniohyoid muscles.

Ansa Cervicalis
- This is a loop of C1, C2 and C3 fibers (Fig. 6.41).
- C1 fibers reach the ansa as its superior root from the hypoglossal nerve.

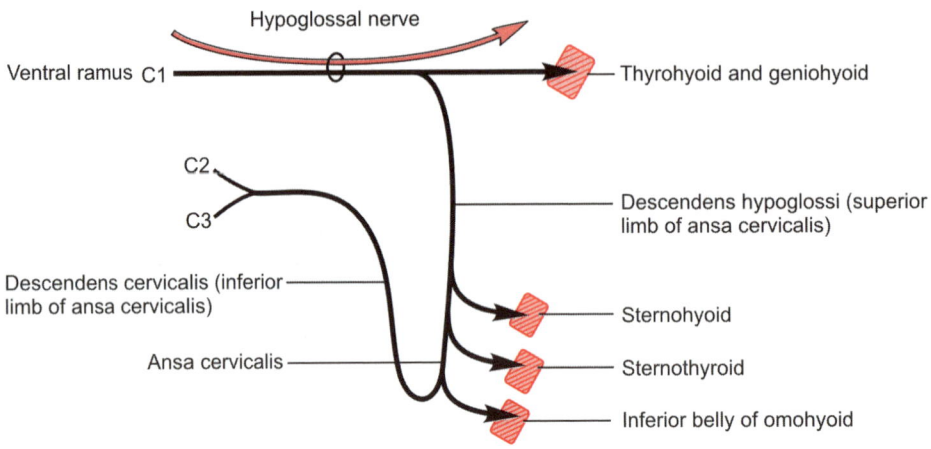

Hypoglossal nerve

Ventral ramus C1 ——————→ Thyrohyoid and geniohyoid

C2

C3 —————————— Descendens hypoglossi (superior limb of ansa cervicalis)

Descendens cervicalis (inferior limb of ansa cervicalis)

Ansa cervicalis ———————— Sternohyoid

———————— Sternothyroid

———————— Inferior belly of omohyoid

Fig. 6.41: Ansa cervicalis

- C2 and C3 fibers form the inferior root of the ansa cervicalis. These fibers come from the cervical plexus.
- The ansa cervicalis lies anterior to carotid sheath. It supplies three muscles:
  1. Omohyoid (inferior belly)
  2. Sternohyoid
  3. Sternothyroid
  Ansa cervicalis and its superior root supply all the infrahyoid muscles except the thyrohyoid. The superior root of ansa cervicalis supplies superior belly of omohyoid.
  1. The thyrohyoid is supplied by C1 fibers through the hypoglossal nerve.
  2. The geniohyoid muscle is also supplied by C1 fibers through the hypoglossal nerve but you should know that geniohyoid is a suprahyoid muscle (above the level of hyoid bone).

Cervical Plexus

- It is formed by the ventral rami of C1, C2, C3 and C4 roots. Part of the C4 may contribute to the brachial plexus (Fig. 6.42).
- C2, C3 and C4 divide into upper and lower branches to form loops.

- C1 does not divide into upper and lower branch.
  The loop between the C2 and C3 gives the following branches:
- The lesser occipital (C2).
- The great auricular (C2 and C3).
- The transverse cervical (C2 and C3).
  The loop between the C3 and C4 gives the supraclavicular nerves (C3 and C4).
  Apart from this, the cervical plexus supplies the prevertebral muscles, rectus capitis anterior, rectus capitis lateralis, longus colli and longus capitis.
- Phrenic nerve (C3, 4 and 5) arises from the cervical plexus.

- *Cervical plexus block:* Anesthetic agents can be injected at the nerve point along the posterior border of the sternomastoid muscle.

Thyroid Gland

- It is a ductless endocrine gland present in the anterior median region of the neck
- It is covered by the pretracheal fascia which forms its false capsule.

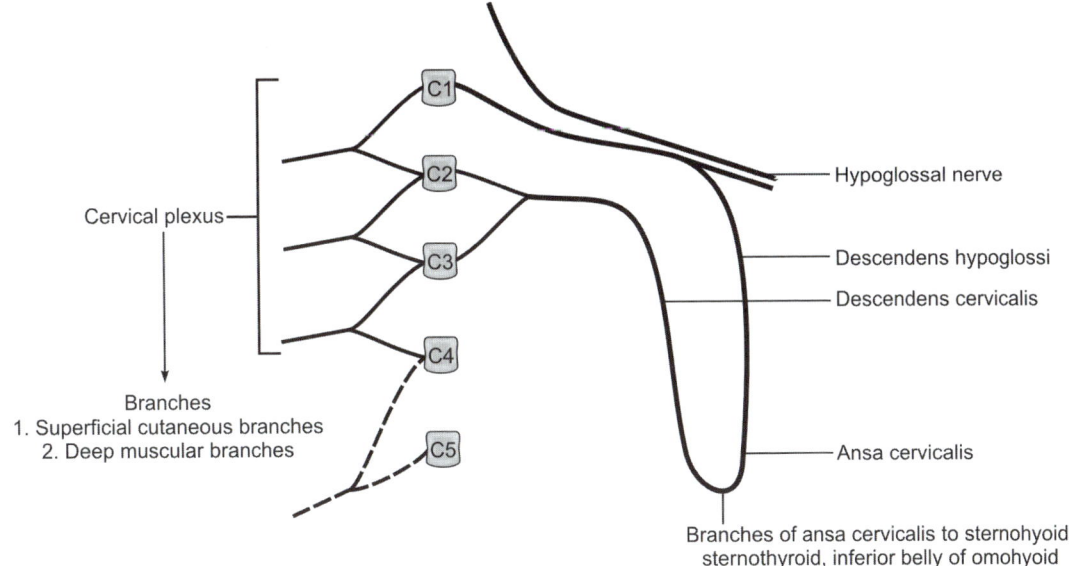

Fig. 6.42: Cervical plexus

- The true capsule is the condensed connective tissue of the gland.
- The gland has right and left lobes and an isthmus.
- Isthmus lies in front of the second, third and fourth tracheal rings.
- Each lobe has a superior pole which is limited by the attachment of sternothyroid to the oblique line of thyroid cartilage.
  Note: That is the reason why any enlargement of gland is never directed upwards.
- Inferior pole usually lies at the level of fifth tracheal ring.
- Each lobe has a superficial, medial and posterolateral surfaces:

Superficial surface is related to the following muscles: Sternohyoid, sternothyroid and lower part of sternomastoid muscles.

Medial surface is related to the following structures:
- *2 tubes:* Trachea and oesophagus.
- *2 nerves:* External and recurrent laryngeal nerve.

- *2 muscles:* Cricothyroid and inferior constrictor muscle of pharynx.

Posterolateral surface is related to the carotid sheath and its contents:
- The common carotid artery
- The internal jugular vein
- The vagus nerve

Arterial supply of the thyroid gland:
1. Superior thyroid artery
2. Inferior thyroid artery
3. Thyroidea ima
1. Superior thyroid artery, a branch of the external carotid artery and the inferior thyroid artery, a branch of the thyrocervical trunk. The superior thyroid artery is accompanied by the external laryngeal nerve which supplies the cricothyroid muscle. The external laryngeal nerve lies closely related to the artery.

That is the reason why the superior thyroid artery is ligated with care to avoid injury to the external laryngeal nerve (Fig. 6.44).

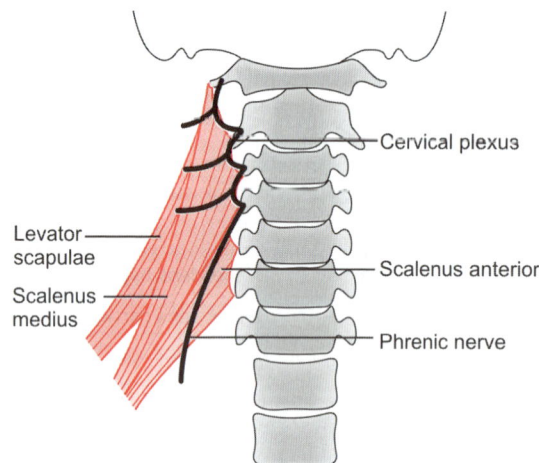

Fig. 6.43: Scalene muscles and phrenic nerve

2. The inferior thyroid artery is a branch of the thyrocervical trunk and it turns medially at the level of 6th cervical vertebra and goes behind the carotid sheath and in front of vertebral vessels. As it approaches the gland, it is closely related to the corresponding recurrent laryngeal nerve.

That is the reason why the inferior thyroid artery is ligated with care to avoid injury to the recurrent laryngeal nerve (Fig. 6.44).

If recurrent laryngeal nerve is injured, it results in the hoarseness of the voice as all the muscles of the larynx are supplied by the recurrent laryngeal nerve except cricothyroid.

3. The other artery which often supplies the thyroid gland is the thyroidea ima. It arises either from the arch of aorta or the brachiocephalic artery and ascends in front of trachea to reach the lower end of the isthmus of thyroid gland.

It is inadvertently cut during tracheostomy operations. Should the thyroidea ima be cut, it may retract into the thorax behind manubrium and this may pose a difficulty for the surgeon to get the bleeding stopped.

Venous drainage of thyroid gland:
Three paired veins usually drain the thyroid gland:
1. The superior thyroid vein
2. The middle thyroid vein
3. The inferior thyroid vein.

1. Out of these three, only the superior thyroid vein accompanies the corresponding artery and opens into the internal jugular vein.
2. The middle thyroid vein does not accompany any artery and it directly opens into the internal jugular vein.
3. The inferior thyroid veins, the right and left, emerge at the lower border of the isthmus and cross the front of the trachea. It is here that they are prone to be injured. They might get cut and start bleeding during tracheostomy operation. They open into the corresponding brachiocephalic vein. Often the right and left inferior thyroid veins join together to form a single inferior thyroid vein which usually opens into the left brachiocephalic vein. It does not accompany the corresponding artery.

Lymphatic Drainage

Lymph vessels of thyroid are drained into the following lymph nodes:
1. Prelaryngeal
2. Pretracheal
3. Paratracheal
4. Deep cervical lymph nodes
5. Some lymph vessels may open into thoracic duct or into the right lymphatic duct.

Parathyroid Glands

- They are two in number on each side (Fig. 6.44).
- There are superior and inferior pairs of parathyroid glands.
- They lie between the true and false capsules.

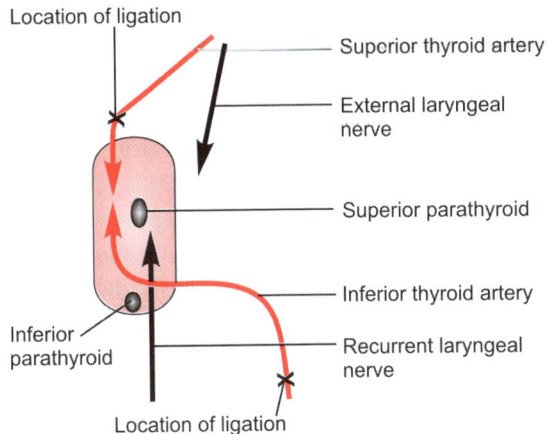

Location of ligation

— Superior thyroid artery

— External laryngeal nerve

— Superior parathyroid

Inferior parathyroid

— Inferior thyroid artery

— Recurrent laryngeal nerve

Location of ligation

Fig. 6.44: Posterior aspect of lobe of thyroid gland

- They are essential for life and that is the reason why all care should be taken to retain them during the thyroidectomy operations. Partial or subtotal thyroidectomy is preferred.
- The superior parathyroid lies little more than 1 cm above the level of inferior thyroid artery entry into the gland along the posterior border of thyroid gland. This border is indicated by the vertical anastomosis between the superior and inferior thyroid arteries.
- The inferior parathyroid gland lies little more than 1 cm below the level of inferior thyroid artery entry into the thyroid gland on the posterior border.
- The superior parathyroid gland is developed from the fourth pouch and the inferior parathyroid gland is developed from the third pouch along with thymus. That is the reason why the inferior parathyroid gland may descend into the thorax along with the thymus.
- Superior parathyroid is also called parathyroid IV.
- Inferior parathyroid is also called parathyroid III.

- *Blood supply of parathyroid glands:*
  i. Mainly by the inferior thyroid artery but the anastomosis between the superior and inferior thyroid artery also supplies.
  ii. Veins drain with those of the thyroid.
- Lymph vessels drain with those of the thyroid into the deep cervical lymph nodes.
- *Nerve supply:* Sympathetic branches coming from the cervical sympathetic ganglia supply parathyroid glands.

- *Tetany:* If parathyroids are removed, there is generalized convulsion caused by lowered calcium level. This is termed tetany.

Subclavian Artery

- The right subclavian artery is a branch of the brachiocephalic artery.
- The left subclavian artery is a branch of the arch of aorta.
- The left subclavian has both thoracic and cervical courses.
- The right subclavian has only the cervical course.
- The right subclavian and the cervical course of the left subclavian arteries:
  – They begin at the level of the corresponding sternoclavicular joints.
  – They terminate at the outer border of the first rib and continue as the corresponding axillary artery.
- Subclavain artery is divided into three parts by the scalenus anterior muscle.
  – The first part lies medial to the scalenus anterior muscle.
  – The second part lies behind the scalenus anterior muscle.
  – The third part lies lateral to the scalenus anterior.
- *First part of the subclavian artery:*
  – *Anterior relations:* Skin, superficial fascia, investing layer of cervical fascia, SCM,

internal jugular vein, ansa subclavia and vagus nerve.

– Anteroinferiorly there is subclavian vein which is joined by the internal jugular vein to form the corresponding brachiocephalic vein at medial border of scalenus anterior.

– *Posterior:* It is related to the apex of the lung, cervical pleura, suprapleural membrane and ansa subclavia.

Branches of the first part:

• The internal thoracic artery which runs inferiorly.

• The vertebral artery which runs superiorly.

• The thyrocervical trunk.

Thyrocervical trunk arises along the medial border of the scalenus anterior and gives three branches:

• Suprascapular

• Transverse cervical

• Inferior thyroid

Inferior thyroid turns medially behind the internal jugular vein and the common carotid artery at the level of the 6th cervical vertebra. It gives glandular branches to thyroid and the ascending cervical artery. It also gives the inferior laryngeal artery.

• The first part of the subclavian artery is hooked around on the right side by the right recurrent laryngeal nerve. However the left recurrent laryngeal nerve does not hook around the left subclavian artery.

• *Ansa subclavia:* It is a loop of sympathetic fibers which connect the middle cervical with the inferior cervical sympathetic ganglia. This loop goes around the first part of right and left subclavian arteries.

• *Second part of the subclavian artery:*
  – It lies behind the scalenus anterior.

– *Anterior relations:* Skin, superficial fascia, investing layer of cervical fascia, subclavian vein, transverse cervical artery, suprascapular artery, sternomastoid and scalenus anterior muscle

– *Posterior relations:* Suprapleural membrane, cervical pleura and apex of lung.

Scalenus anterior syndrome: The lower trunk of brachial plexus and the second part of the subclavian artery are compressed by the spasm of scalenus anterior muscle as seen with the cervical rib. Then the patient feels pain or numbness on the medial side of the hand and forearm and there is weak radial pulse on the corresponding side of the limb.

Adson's test: In scalenus anterior syndrome the radial pulse becomes weak when the head is hyperextended and turned to the affected side.

Branches:

• Costocervical trunk is the only branch of the second part. The costocervical trunk arches over the cervical pleura and reaches the neck of the first rib where it divides into the deep cervical and superior intercostal arteries.

• *Third part of the subclavian artery:*

  – Lies lateral to the scalenus anterior in the lower part of the posterior triangle (supraclavicular triangle).

  – This artery is usually pressed against the first rib in the greater supraclavicular fossa to stop the bleeding from a ruptured upper limb artery.

  – Often deep branch of the transverse cervical artery arises from it and when present, this branch is called dorsal scapular artery.

The Vertebral Artery

- It arises from the first part of the subclavian artery.
- It is divided into four parts:
  - The first part lies in a triangle bounded medially by the longus colli muscle and laterally by the scalenus anterior muscle. The base is formed by the first part of the subclavian artery. The first part extends from its origin to the foramen transversarium of the 6th cervical vertebra.
  - The second part lies in the foramen transversaria of upper six cervical vertebrae. It gives spinal branches.
  - The third part lies in the suboccipital triangle superior to the posterior arch of the atlas. It gives muscular branches to the muscles of the region (Fig. 6.37).
  - The fourth part of the vertebral artery is present inside the cranium. It passes through the foramen magnum. It pierces the duramater and arachnoidmater.

The two vertebral arteries unite at the lower border of the pons to form a basilar artery.

The fourth part of the vertebral artery gives five branches:

1. Anterior spinal artery
2. Posterior spinal artery
3. Posterior inferior cerebellar artery
4. Medullary branches
5. Meningeal branches

The Common Carotid Artery

- The right common carotid artery is a branch of the brachiocephalic trunk at the level of right sternoclavicular joint.
- The left common carotid artery is a branch of the arch of aorta. It enters the neck behind the left sternoclavicular joint.
- The common carotid artery lies inside the carotid sheath medial to the internal jugular vein. The vagus nerve lies inside the carotid sheath posterolateral to the artery (Fig. 6.31).
- It divides at the level of the upper border of the thyroid cartilage which corresponds to the level of the disc between the C3 and C4 vertebrae.
- Its two terminal branches are (Fig. 6.45):
  i. The external carotid
  ii. The internal carotid
- Common carotid artery does not give any branch.
- Anteriorly it is related to the following:
  i. SCM
  ii. Sternohyoid
  iii. Sternothyroid
  iv. Ansa cervicalis
- Superior belly of omohyoid crosses the artery at the level of C6 vertebra. At this point of crossing juguloomohyoid lymph node is situated. This is the lymph node of the tongue.

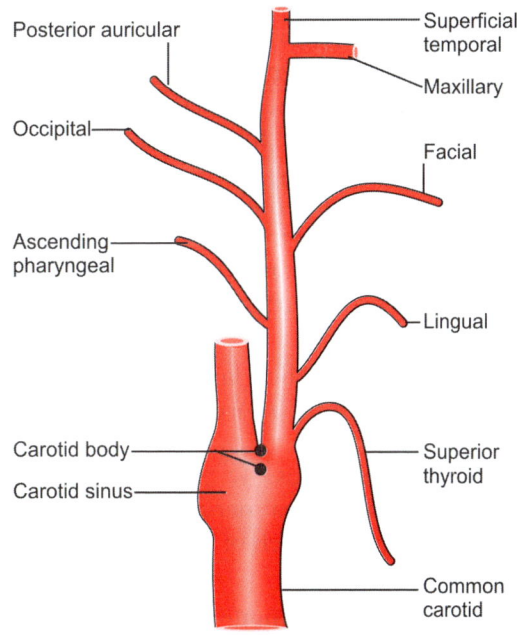

Fig. 6.45: External carotid artery branches

- Posteriorly it is related to the following:
  i. Inferior thyroid artery
  ii. Cervical sympathetic chain
  iii. Transverse processes of lower cervical vertebrae

The pulsations of common carotid artery are easily felt against the anterior tubercle of the transverse process of 6th cervical vertebra (carotid tubercle). The artery can be compressed against this tubercle.

Internal Carotid Artery

- This is the continuation of the common carotid artery (Fig. 6.45) and is one of its terminal branches. It begins at the level of the upper border of the thyroid cartilage which corresponds to the disc between C3 and C4.
- It lies inside the carotid sheath.
- Both internal and external carotid arteries lie deep to posterior belly of digastric and stylohyoid muscles. These muscles act like strap to these arteries and serve to keep them fastened to their place.
- Below the level of the posterior belly of digastric muscle, hypoglossal nerve crosses anterior to the internal carotid artery.
- Above the level of the digastric muscle, the internal carotid artery is separated from the external carotid artery by the following structures:
  1. Part of the parotid gland posterior to the external carotid artery.
  2. Styloid process.
  3. Stylopharyngeus.
  4. Glossopharyngeal nerve.
  5. Pharyngeal branch of vagus.

  Posterior relation:
  – Superior sympathetic ganglion
  – Prevertebral muscles

- Internal carotid artery does not give any branch in the neck. All its distribution is inside the cranial cavity.

- Thick plaques may block the internal carotid arteries partially or completely. In such cases endarterectomy operation is performed. During these operations one has to be careful of various nerves met in the region (9th, 10th, 11th and 12th cranial nerves).

Carotid Sinus and Body

- *Carotid sinus:* It is the dilatation of the proximal part of the beginning of the internal carotid artery and sometimes the distal part of the common carotid artery (Fig. 6.45). There are baroreceptors in it which are stimulated by pressure changes in the artery. This is supplied by the carotid sinus nerve, a branch of the glossopharyngeal nerve.

- *Hypersensitive carotid sinus:* In some individuals the carotid sinus is hypersensitive and any pressure on the artery leads to bradycardia and fall in blood pressure. In such cases the common carotid pulse should not be taken.

- *Carotid body:* It is the chemoreceptor present at the bifurcation of the common carotid artery (Fig. 6.45). It monitors oxygen saturation in blood.

Temporal Region

It includes temporal and infratemporal fossae (Fig. 6.46).

Temporal Fossa

- It forms floor of the temporal region.
- It is present on the side of the head.

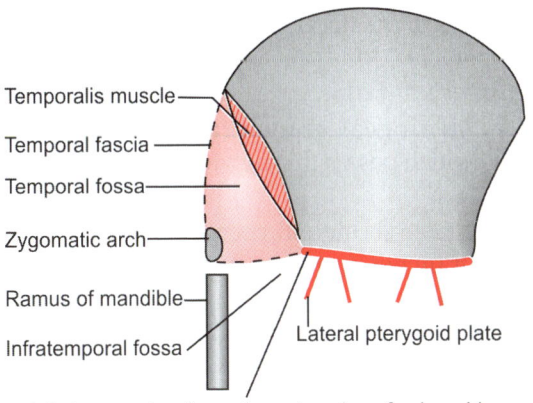

Temporalis muscle
Temporal fascia
Temporal fossa
Zygomatic arch
Ramus of mandible
Infratemporal fossa
Lateral pterygoid plate
Infratemporal surface of greater wing of sphenoid

Fig. 6.46: Temporal and infratemporal fossae

Boundaries:
- *Superior:* Superior temporal line.
- *Inferior:* Zygomatic arch; deep to which it is continuous with infratemporal fossa.
- *Anterior:* Frontal process of zygomatic bone.
- Roof is formed by the skin, superficial fascia and temporal fascia.
- Floor of the fossa has four bones:
  1. Parietal
  2. Greater wing of sphenoid
  3. Squamous part of temporal
  4. Frontal

Contents:
1. Temporalis muscle
2. Deep temporal nerves
3. Deep temporal arteries
4. Accompanying veins

Pterion: It is an important landmark in the floor of the temporal fossa. It is a small area which includes all the four bones of the floor of the temporal fossa in an H-shaped suture. It corresponds to the anterior branch of the middle meningeal artery.

Infratemporal Fossa

- *Boundaries:*
  - *Anterior:* Posterior surface of the body of the maxilla.
  - *Posterior:* Open but bounded by the styloid and mastoid process of temporal bone.
  - *Lateral:* Ramus of the mandible.
  - *Medial:* Lateral pterygoid plate and pterygomaxillary fissure.
- Pterygomaxillary fissure connects the infratemporal fossa with the pterygo-palatine fossa.

Contents:
1. Lateral pterygoid.
2. Medial pterygoid.
3. Mandibular nerve, its branches and otic ganglion (Figs 6.47 and 6.48).
4. Maxillary artery and its branches.
5. Pterygoid venous plexus.

Lateral pterygoid:
- It has two heads.
- The upper head arises from the roof of the infratemporal fossa formed by the greater wing of the sphenoid bone.
- The lower head arises from the lateral surface of the lateral pterygoid plate.
- It is inserted into the front of the neck of the mandible and articular disc of TMJ.
- *Action:* Opens the mouth by drawing the mandible forwards along with the disc.
- *Nerve supply:* The anterior division of the mandibular nerve.

Medial Pterygoid Muscle

- It has two heads. The superficial and deep.

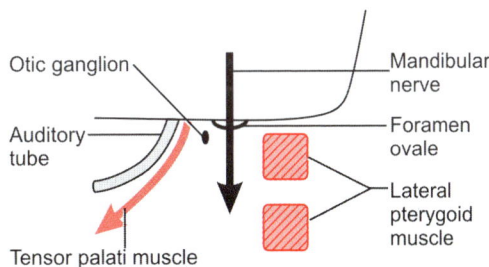

Otic ganglion
Auditory tube
Tensor palati muscle
Mandibular nerve
Foramen ovale
Lateral pterygoid muscle

Fig. 6.47: Infratemporal fossa

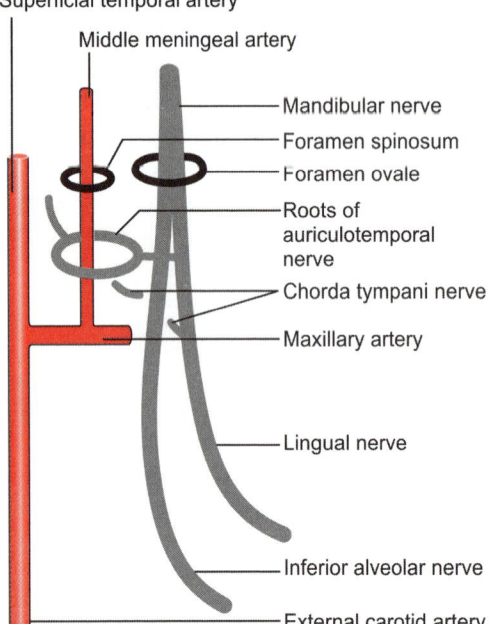

Fig. 6.48: Mandibular nerve

- Superficial head arises from the maxillary tuberosity, an elevation behind the last molar tooth.
- Deep head arises from the medial surface of the lateral pterygoid plate.
- It is inserted into the medial side of the angle of the mandible.
- *Action:* It elevates the mandible.
- *Nerve supply:* Supplied by the nerve to medial pterygoid from main trunk of mandibular nerve.

Mandibular Nerve

- It is one of the 3 divisions of the trigeminal nerve.
- It is both sensory and motor. It is the nerve of the first branchial arch and supplies the muscles of mastication.
- It passes through the foramen ovale.
- Otic ganglion lies medial to the trunk of the mandibular nerve.

- Trunk of the nerve divides into anterior and posterior divisions.
- *Branches:* Trunk gives two branches:
  - Meningeal branch (nervous spinosus which passes through foramen spinosum) and
  - Nerve to medial pterygoid which gives branches to tensor tympani and tensor palati.

The anterior division of the mandibular nerve is mainly motor but contains some sensory fibers. The branches are:

1. The deep temporal branches
2. Nerve to lateral pterygoid
3. Nerve to masseter
4. Its sensory fibers pass through the buccal nerve which supplies the skin over the buccinator and the mucous membrane deep to the buccinator muscle.

The posterior division of mandibular nerve is mainly sensory but contains some motor fibers. The branches are:

1. Auriculotemporal nerve
2. Inferior alveolar nerve
3. Lingual nerve
4. Motor fibers pass through the nerve to mylohyoid, a branch of the inferior alveolar nerve, before it enters the mandibular foramen.

Auriculotemporal Nerve

- It is a branch of the posterior division of the mandibular nerve.
- It has two roots (Fig. 6.48).
- Both the roots join to form a loop. Within this loop, the middle meningeal artery ascends.
- This nerve supplies
  1. A joint (TMJ)
  2. Gland (parotid) [It carries postganglionic parasympathetic fibers to the parotid gland].
  3. Skin of the temporal fossa.

Inferior Alveolar Nerve

- It enters the mandibular foramen.
- It gives the nerve to mylohyoid which supplies mylohyoid and anterior belly of digastric muscles before it enters the mandibular foramen.
- It supplies the teeth of the lower jaw and gives the mental nerve which emerges at mental foramen and supplies the skin over the chin and lower lip.

Lingual Nerve

- It descends as follows:
  - First between lateral pterygoid and tensor palati.
  - Next between lateral and medial pterygoid.
  - It then lies between ramus of mandible and medial pterygoid.
  - It is then related inferior to lower 3rd molar tooth.
  - It extends forwards over the hyoglossus muscle; reaches between genioglossus and mylohyoid where it winds round the submandibular duct.
- Chorda tympani joins the lingual nerve at an acute angle in the infratemporal fossa.
- The chorda tympani is a branch of the facial nerve and it carries the taste fibers from the anterior two-thirds of the tongue.

Therefore, lingual nerve distal to the joining of chorda tympani nerve carries three types of sensations:

1. General sensation from the anterior two-thirds of the tongue.
2. Taste sensation from the anterior two-third of the tongue except the mucous membrane over circumvallate papillae.
3. Secretomotor fibers to the submandibular and sublingual salivary glands.

Submandibular ganglion is connected to the lingual nerve by 2 roots.

Maxillary Artery

- It arises from the external carotid artery in the substance of the parotid gland.
- It passes anteriorly deep to the neck of the mandible.
- It crosses the lower head of the lateral pterygoid muscle and runs medially between the two heads of the lateral pterygoid and enters the pterygopalatine fossa through the pterygomaxillary fissure (Fig. 6.49).
- It is divided into three parts by the lower head of the lateral pterygoid muscle.
- Sometimes it may go deep to the lower head of the lateral pterygoid muscle.

First part: It extends from its origin to the lower border of the lower head of the lateral pterygoid muscle. It gives the following branches:

1. Deep auricular
2. Anterior tympanic
3. Middle meningeal
4. Accessory meningeal
5. Inferior alveolar (runs downwards).

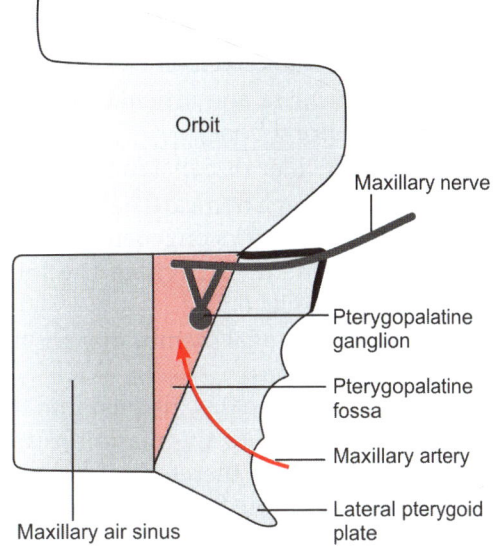

Fig. 6.49: Pterygopalatine fossa

Second part: It crosses either superficial or deep to the lower head of the lateral pterygoid muscle. It gives the following branches (remember all are muscular):

1. Deep temporal arteries (to temporalis).
2. Masseteric artery (to masseter).
3. Artery to medial pterygoid (to medial pterygoid).
4. Artery to lateral pterygoid (to lateral pterygoid).
5. Buccal artery (to buccinator).

Third part: It runs between the two heads of the lateral pterygoid and then enters the pterygopalatine fossa through the pterygomaxillary fissure. It gives the following branches:

1. Posterior superior alveolar artery
2. Infraorbital artery
3. Sphenopalatine artery
4. Pharyngeal artery
5. Greater palatine artery
6. Artery of pterygoid canal.

Temporomandibular Joint

- It is a condylar variety of synovial joint.
- Articular surfaces (Fig. 6.51):
  - Head of the mandible below.
  - Mandibular fossa and articular tubercle above (temporal bone).
  - It has an articular disc inside the joint.
- The articular disc is a fibrocartilaginous disc which makes the two incongruent articular surfaces congruent. It divides the joint cavity into two (Fig. 6.51).
  - There are 2 synovial membranes for the 2 separate cavities.
  - The lateral pterygoid is inserted into the front of the neck of the mandible and articular disc and, therefore, it helps in opening the mouth by drawing the mandible forwards.
- *Fibrous capsule:* It is attached to the margins of the mandibular fossa superiorly and to

the margins of the neck of the mandible inferiorly.

- *Ligaments:*
  - Lateral ligament is a strong ligament of this joint (Fig. 6.50).
  - Accessory ligaments are:
    - ♦ Stylomandibular ligament (thickened part of the investing layer of cervical fascia)
    - ♦ Sphenomandibular ligament (extends from the spine of the sphenoid to the

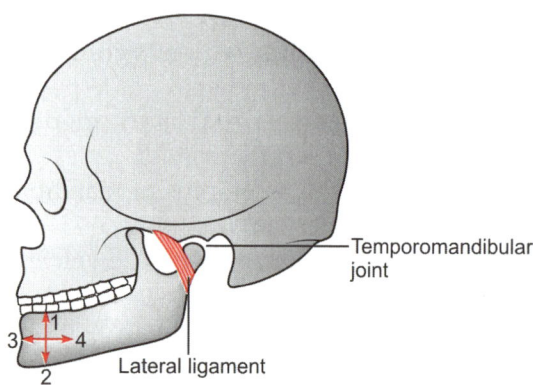

Fig. 6.50: Movements of mandible at temporomandibular joint

1. Elevation 2. Depression 3. Protraction 4. Retraction

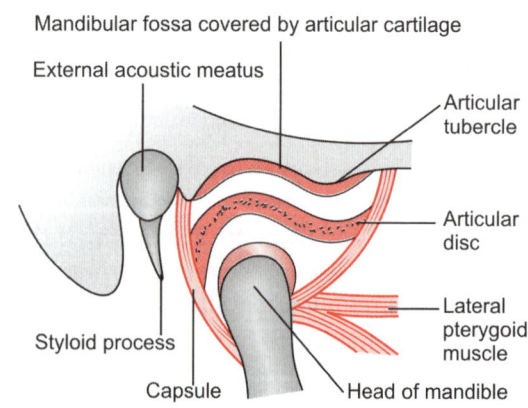

Fig. 6.51: Temporomandibular joint

lingula of the mandible. It represents the dorsal part of the first arch cartilage).

- *Movements:*
  - Upper compartment lies above the disc and lower compartment lies below the disc.
  - Gliding movements of protraction (forwards) and retraction (backwards) take place in upper compartment while hinge (rotatory) movements of elevation and depression occur in the lower compartment.
- Movements of the temporomandibular joint and the muscles associated with such movements (Fig. 6.50):
  - *Depression* (Opening of the mouth): Lateral pterygoid and gravity. Also assisted by the anterior belly of digastric, geniohyoid.
  - *Chewing* (Side to side movement): Alternative contraction of protractors of one side and retractors of opposite side.
  - *Elevation:* Temporalis, masseter and medial pterygoid.
  - *Protraction:* Lateral and medial pterygoid.
  - *Retraction:* Posterior fibers of the temporalis.
- *Nerve supply of the joint:*
  - Auriculotemporal nerve.
  - Nerve to masseter.

Dislocation of the TMJ
- It is dislocated anteriorly when the head slips forwards over the articular tubercle. The patient cannot close the mouth after this dislocation. While reducing this dislocation, the attending physician pads his fingers to prevent his fingers being crushed by the sudden reduction of the head of the mandible into its socket.
- When a dental surgeon exerts too much downward pressure on the mandible, it might result in the anterior dislocation of the TMJ.

Muscles of Mastication

1. Temporalis
2. Lateral pterygoid
3. Medial pterygoid
4. Masseter
   - All of them are derived from the first branchial arch and are supplied by the mandibular division of the trigeminal nerve.
- *Temporalis:*
  - Arises from the temporal fossa and temporal fascia and is inserted into the coronoid process and anterior border of ramus of the mandible.
  - It helps in elevation of mandible and posterior fibers helps in retraction of mandible.
- *Masseter:*
  - It arises from the zygomatic arch and is inserted into the lateral side of the ramus of the mandible.
  - It helps in protraction and elevation of mandible.

TONGUE

- It is a skeletal muscle mass covered by mucosa.
- Helps in chewing, swallowing, taste and speech.
- Attached by muscles to hyoid, styloid process, palate and mandible.
- It has following parts: root, tip and body.
- Dorsum is divided into oral and pharyngeal parts by V-shaped sulcus terminalis. Foramen cecum is a median pit in sulcus terminalis (Fig. 6.52).
- Dorsum of tongue (oral part) shows:
  - Papillae of filiform, fungiform and circumvallate type. Circumvallate papillae are arranged anterior and parallel to sulcus terminalis.
- Dorsum of tongue (pharyngeal part) shows:
  - Lingual tonsil.

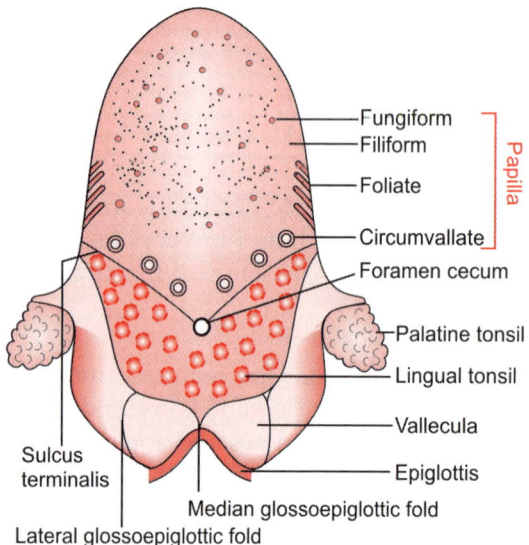

Fig. 6.52: Tongue

- Inferior surface shows:
  - From medial to lateral - frenulum linguae in midline, on each side deep lingual vein and a fold called plica fimbriata.

Muscles of Tongue

- Median fibrous septum divides tongue into right and left halves; each half comprising 4 intrinsic and 4 extrinsic muscles.

- All are supplied by hypoglossal nerve except palatoglossus by pharyngeal plexus.
- *Action:* Intrinsic muscles alter shape of tongue while the extrinsic muscles alter the position of tongue.

Extrinsic (Fig. 6.53)	*Intrinsic*
Genioglossus	Superior longitudinal
Hyoglossus	Inferior longitudinal
Styloglossus	Transverse
Palatoglossus	Vertical

APPLIED ANATOMY

Hypoglossal nerve palsy: When patient is asked to protrude his tongue; tip of tongue deviates to paralyzed side because of unopposed action of the genioglossus of the normal side. (To understand this correlate the action of genioglossus while seeing a picture of origin and insertion of this muscle.)

Nerve Supply of Tongue

- Anterior 2/3rd—general sensation is by lingual nerve; taste is by chorda tympani branch of facial nerve.
- Posterior 1/3rd and circumvallate papillae—general sensation and taste by glossopharyngeal nerve.

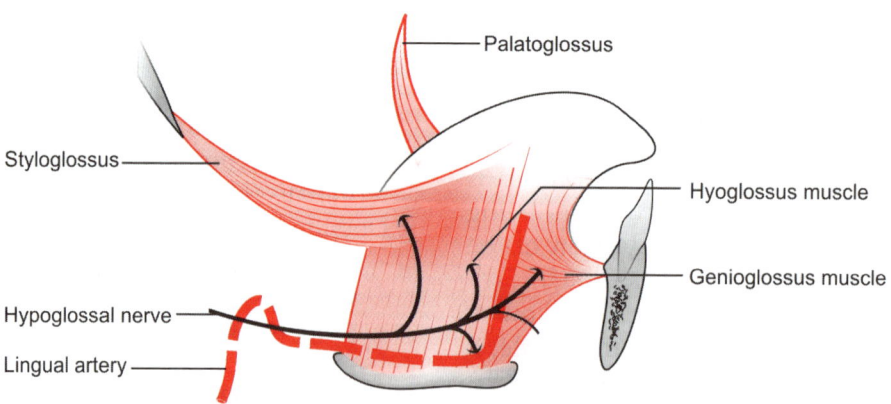

Fig. 6.53: Muscles of tongue (extrinsic)

- Posterior most part of tongue is by internal laryngeal branch of vagus.

Arterial supply: Lingual artery.

Lingual artery is divided into 3 parts by hyoglossus muscle.

1. I part before hyoglossus
2. II part deep to hyoglossus
3. III part along anterior border of hyoglossus (deep lingual artery).

Veins

- Dorsal lingual along lingual artery.
- Deep lingual veins.

Lymphatic Drainage

- Tip drains bilaterally to submental nodes.
- Margins drain unilaterally to submandibular nodes.
- Posterior 1/3rd and area near midline drains bilaterally to upper deep cervical lymph nodes.
- Lymph node of tongue is juguloomohyoid since most of the lymph of tongue drains into them ultimately.

PALATE

Palate consists of 2 parts: hard palate and soft palate.

Hard Palate

- The hard palate (bony) is formed anteriorly by the palatine processes of the maxillae and posteriorly by the horizontal plates of the palatine bones (Fig. 6.56).

Soft Palate

- It is a movable fibromuscular fold attached to posterior border of hard palate (Fig. 6.56).

Muscles of Soft Palate

1. Levator palati (elevates soft palate) (Fig. 6.55).

2. Tensor palati (tenses soft palate).
3. Musculus uvulae.
4. Palatoglossus.
5. Palatopharyngeus.

Arterial supply: Branches of maxillary, facial and ascending pharyngeal artery.

Nerve supply: All muscles by pharyngeal plexus (cranial accessory through vagus) except tensor palati by mandibular nerve. Soft palate also receives general sensory fibers, secretomotor fibers to glands and taste fibers. Taste fibers come from facial nerve.

PALATINE TONSIL

- Along with tubal tonsils, pharyngeal tonsils and lingual tonsils it forms Waldeyer's ring in relation to the oropharyngeal isthmus guarding the entry of respiratory and gastrointestinal tract.
- Lies between the palatoglossal and palatopharyngeal arches (Fig. 6.56).
- Its bed is formed by the pharyngobasilar fascia, superior constrictor, buccopharyngeal fascia and glossopharyngeal nerve.
- *Arterial supply:* Mainly by tonsillar branch of facial artery.
- *Lymphatic drainage:* Jugulodigastric node.
- *Nerve supply:* Tonsillar branch of glossopharyngeal nerve.

APPLIED ANATOMY

Frequent infection (tonsillitis) predisposes to its surgical removal (tonsillectomy) when the knowledge of its relations becomes important.

Adenoiditis

- Adenoids or nasopharyngeal tonsils are present at the junction of roof and posterior wall of nasopharynx.
- In children its inflammation (adenoiditis) and swelling causes airway obstruction leading to mouth breathing.

- Facial appearance is termed adenoid facies characterized by:
  - Expressionless face.
  - Pinched nose due to absence of air flow.
  - Open mouth due to mouth breathing.

PHARYNX

- It is a fibromuscular tube.
- Attached above to base of skull.
- Below it is continuous with oesophagus at the level of C6 vertebra.
- It is divided into nasopharynx, oropharynx and laryngopharynx (Fig. 6.57).
- Pharyngeal musculature consists primarily of superior, middle and inferior constrictors externally (Figs 6.54 and 6.58) and longitudinal muscles namely stylopharyngeus (from styloid process), palatopharyngeus (from soft palate) and salpingopharyngeus (from auditory tube) internally.
- Pharyngobasilar fascia lines the inner aspect and buccopharyngeal fascia lines the external aspect of pharyngeal constrictors.
- Inferior constrictor has two parts: thyropharyngeus and cricopharyngeus.

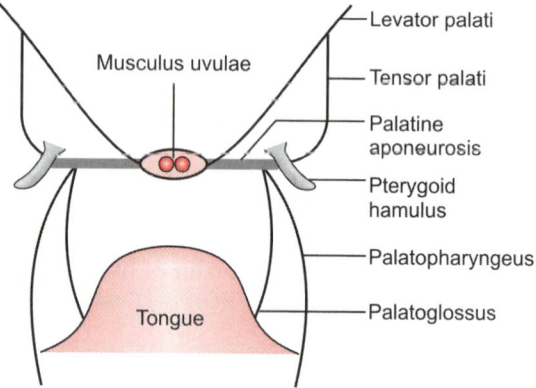

Fig. 6.55: Muscles of soft palate

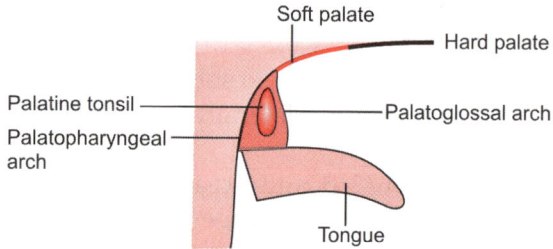

Fig. 6.56: Palatine tonsil

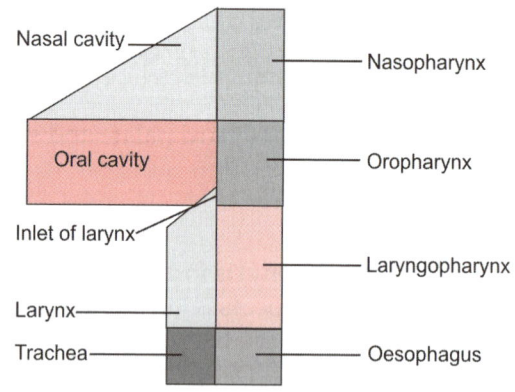

Fig. 6.57: Subdivisions of pharynx

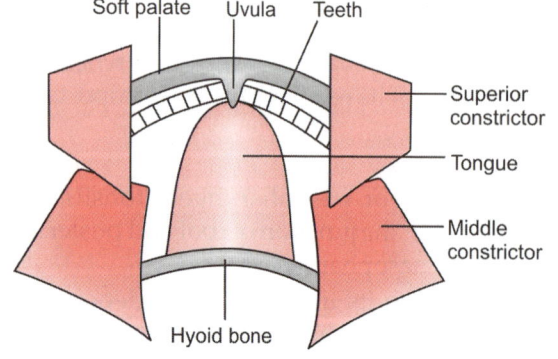

Fig. 6.54: Tongue (as seen from pharynx)

In the gap between the base of skull and upper border of superior constrictor 2 structures pass:
1. Auditory tube
2. Levator palati muscle

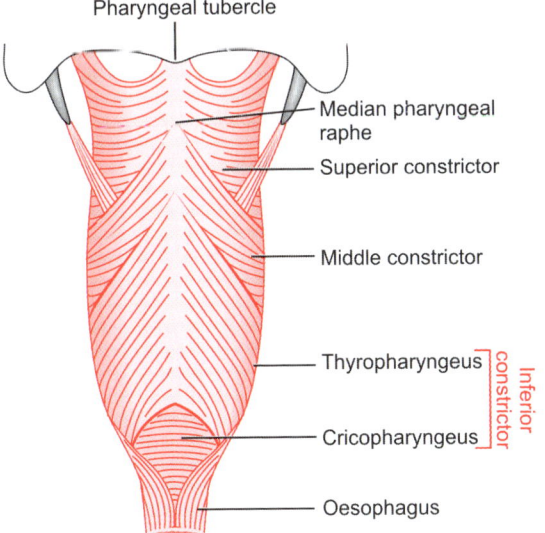

Fig. 6.58: Pharyngeal constrictors

In the gap between the superior constrictor and middle constrictor 2 structures pass:
1. Stylopharyngeus.
2. Glossopharyngeal nerve.

In the gap between middle constrictor and inferior constrictor 2 structures pass:
1. Internal laryngeal nerve.
2. Superior laryngeal vessels.

In the gap between lower border of inferior constrictor and oesophagus 2 structures pass:
1. Recurrent laryngeal nerve.
2. Inferior laryngeal vessels.

Nerve supply: Pharyngeal plexus mainly on middle constrictor formed by pharyngeal branch of vagus (containing fibers of cranial accessory nerve), pharyngeal branch of glosso-pharyngeal nerve, and pharyngeal branch of superior cervical sympathetic ganglion.

NOSE

Nasal Septum

It is made of septal cartilages, perpendicular plate of ethmoid and vomer.

Blood supply of nasal septum:
Little's area or Kisselbach's area in antero-inferior part of nasal septum is a site of rich anastomoses between branches of spheno-palatine, anterior ethmoidal, greater palatine and superior labial branches of facial artery. Nose picking results in bleeding (epistaxis).

Deviated nasal septum (DNS) is a condition in which nasal septum does not lie in the middle and is deviated to one side. It may be asymptomatic.

However, at times the nasal septum may be grossly deviated and impinge on the lateral wall of the nose thereby causing obstruction to the passage of air. This may require surgery.

Lateral Wall of Nose

- Formed by upper and lower nasal cartilages, nasal, frontal process of maxilla, superior and middle nasal concha of ethmoid, palatine, medial pterygoid plate of sphenoid, lacrimal and inferior nasal concha.
- There are 3 shelves on lateral wall namely superior, middle and inferior nasal concha
- Above superior nasal concha is spheno-ethmoidal recess, sphenoidal sinus opens into it (Figs 6.59 and 6.60).
- Between superior and middle concha is superior meatus, posterior ethmoidal sinus opens into it.
- Between middle and inferior concha is middle meatus, frontal, maxillary, anterior and middle ethmoidal sinuses open into it.
- Below inferior concha is inferior meatus, nasolacrimal duct opens into it.

Paranasal Sinuses

- There are air-filled spaces present in some bones surrounding the nasal cavity.
- Lined by mucous membrane continuous with that of nasal cavity.

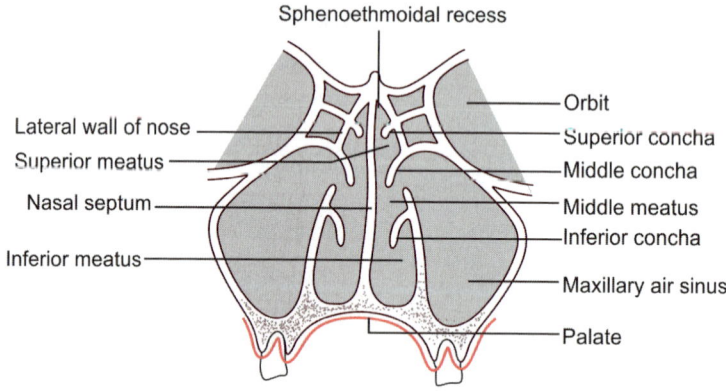

Fig. 6.59: Coronal section showing nasal cavity

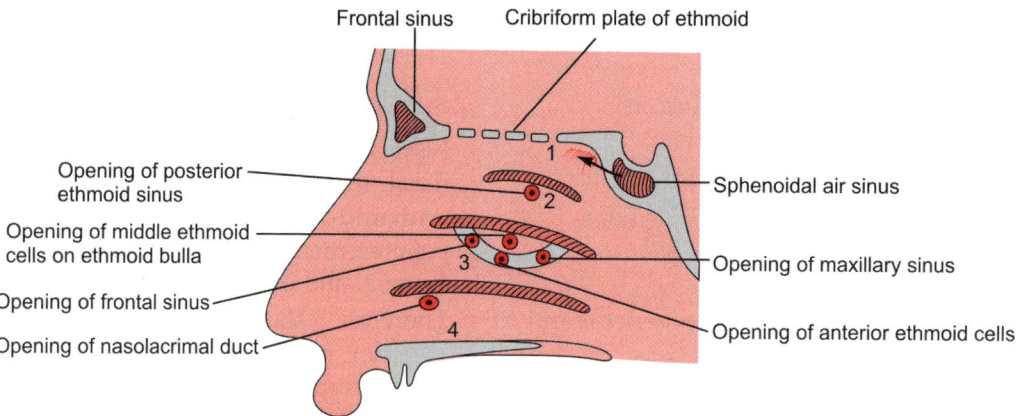

1. Sphenoethmoidal recess, 2. Superior meatus, 3. Middle meatus, 4. Inferior meatus

Fig. 6.60: Lateral wall of nose (concha cut)

- They include frontal, maxillary, sphenoid and ethmoidal sinuses.
- Ethmoidal sinuses include anterior, middle and posterior.

Functions

- Makes skull lighter.
- Add resonance to voice.

Maxillary Sinus

- Largest sinus.
- Lies in body of maxilla (Fig. 6.61).
- Drains into middle meatus.
- It is pyramidal in shape.

- Its opening is at a disadvantageous position on its medial wall nearer the roof. Therefore, secretions can accumulate before being drained and hence, increase risk of infection.
- Floor is related to upper teeth and hence, maxillary sinusitis is associated with toothache.

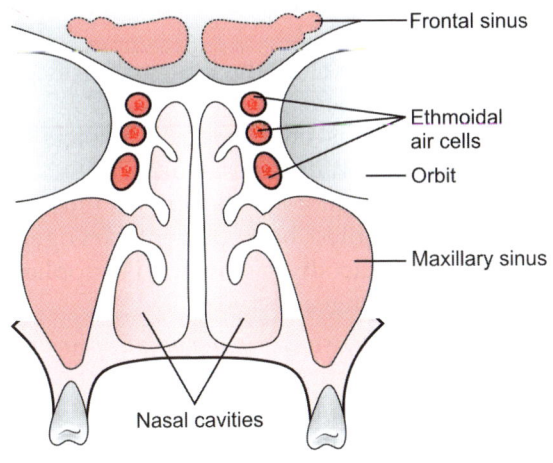

Fig. 6.61: Paranasal air sinuses

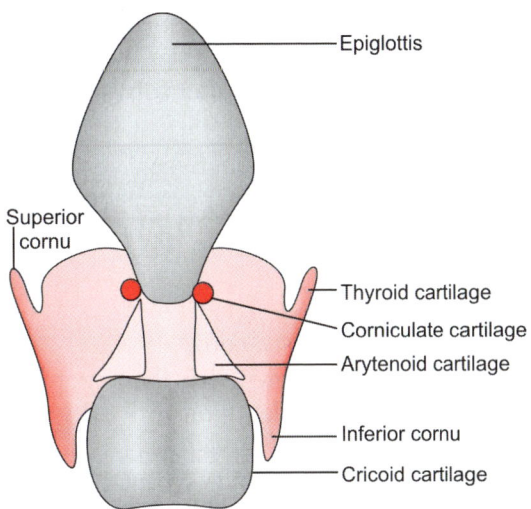

Fig. 6.62: Laryngeal cartilages (seen from behind)

Larynx

- Acts as an air passage.
- Is an organ of phonation (speech).

Laryngeal Skeleton

- Made of cartilages.

Unpaired	*Paired*
Epiglottis	Cuneiform
Thyroid	Corniculate
Cricoid	Arytenoids

Thyroid Cartilage

V- shaped. Anterior prominence of the 2 fused laminae forms Adam's apple or laryngeal prominence. Above this prominence superior thyroid notch is seen. Superior and inferior cornua are other important features (Fig. 6.62).

Cricoid Cartilage

Ring-shaped. Important features are an anterior narrow arch and a broad posterior lamina.

Epiglottis

Leaf-shaped.

Arytenoid

Pyramid-shaped. Its features are an apex, base, muscular and vocal process.

Laryngeal Cavity

It is made of 3 parts: vestibule, ventricle and infraglottic cavity (Fig. 6.63).

Vestibule lies between laryngeal orifice and vestibular folds.

Vestibular Fold

- Also called false vocal cord.

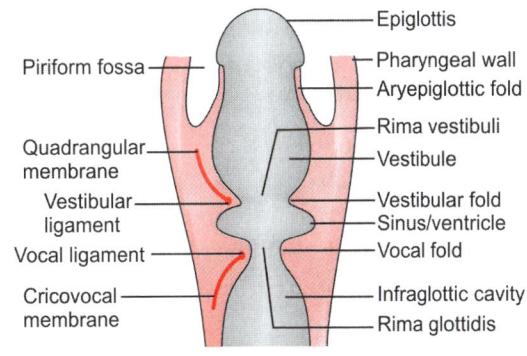

Fig. 6.63: Interior of larynx

- Contains vestibular ligament which is lower margin of quadrangular membrane.
- Space between vestibular folds is rima vestibule.

Ventricle or sinus lies between vestibular and vocal folds. Its upward extension forms saccule of larynx.

Vocal Fold

- Also called true vocal cord.
- Contains vocal ligament. It is the upper free border of conus elasticus (cricothyroid ligament).
- Space between vocal folds is rima glottidis.

Laryngeal Muscles

Extrinsic and intrinsic: Extrinsic move the larynx as a whole and include suprahyoid and infrahyoid muscles which elevate and depress the larynx respectively. Intrinsic move only parts of larynx to alter tension and length of vocal folds and shape and size of rima glottidis.

Intrinsic muscles of larynx include (Fig. 6.64):
- Posterior cricoarytenoid.
- Transverse arytenoids.
- Lateral cricoarytenoid.
- Cricothyroid.
- Thyroarytenoid.
- Aryepiglotticus.
- Oblique arytenoids.
- Vocalis.
- Thyroepiglotticus.

Actions (Fig. 6.65):
1. Muscles which open the glottis: (abductors)
   - Posterior cricoarytenoid.
2. Muscles which close the glottis: (adductors)
   - Transverse arytenoids and lateral cricoarytenoid.
3. Muscles which tense the vocal cords:
   - Cricothyroid

4. Muscles which relax the vocal cords:
   - Thyroarytenoid.
5. Muscles which close the laryngeal orifice:
   - Aryepiglotticus

Cricothyroid is only extrinsic muscle of larynx that lies on its external aspect.

Nerve supply: (motor) All intrinsic muscles of larynx supplied by recurrent laryngeal nerve except cricothyroid which is supplied by external laryngeal nerve.

Blood supply, sensory nerve supply and lymphatic drainage:
- Up to vocal folds—superior laryngeal vessels, internal laryngeal nerve and upper deep cervical lymph nodes.
- Below vocal folds—inferior laryngeal vessels, recurrent laryngeal nerve and lower deep cervical lymph nodes.
  - Superior laryngeal artery is a branch of superior thyroid artery. Superior laryngeal vein drains into superior thyroid vein.
  - Inferior laryngeal artery is a branch of inferior thyroid artery. Inferior laryngeal vein drains into inferior thyroid vein.

APPLIED ANATOMY

- Damage to recurrent laryngeal nerve causes hoarseness of voice.
- Laryngoscopy is a procedure to visualize the interior of the larynx.
- Fractures of laryngeal skeleton may occur as a result of injuries seen in sports, fights or accidents. It is associated with breathing difficulty, problem with speech and hoarseness of voice.
- Laryngeal cancer:
  - Hoarseness of voice is a common symptom.
  - Laryngectomy or removal of larynx may be necessary. In such cases voice rehabilitation is done using esophageal speech or electrolarynx.

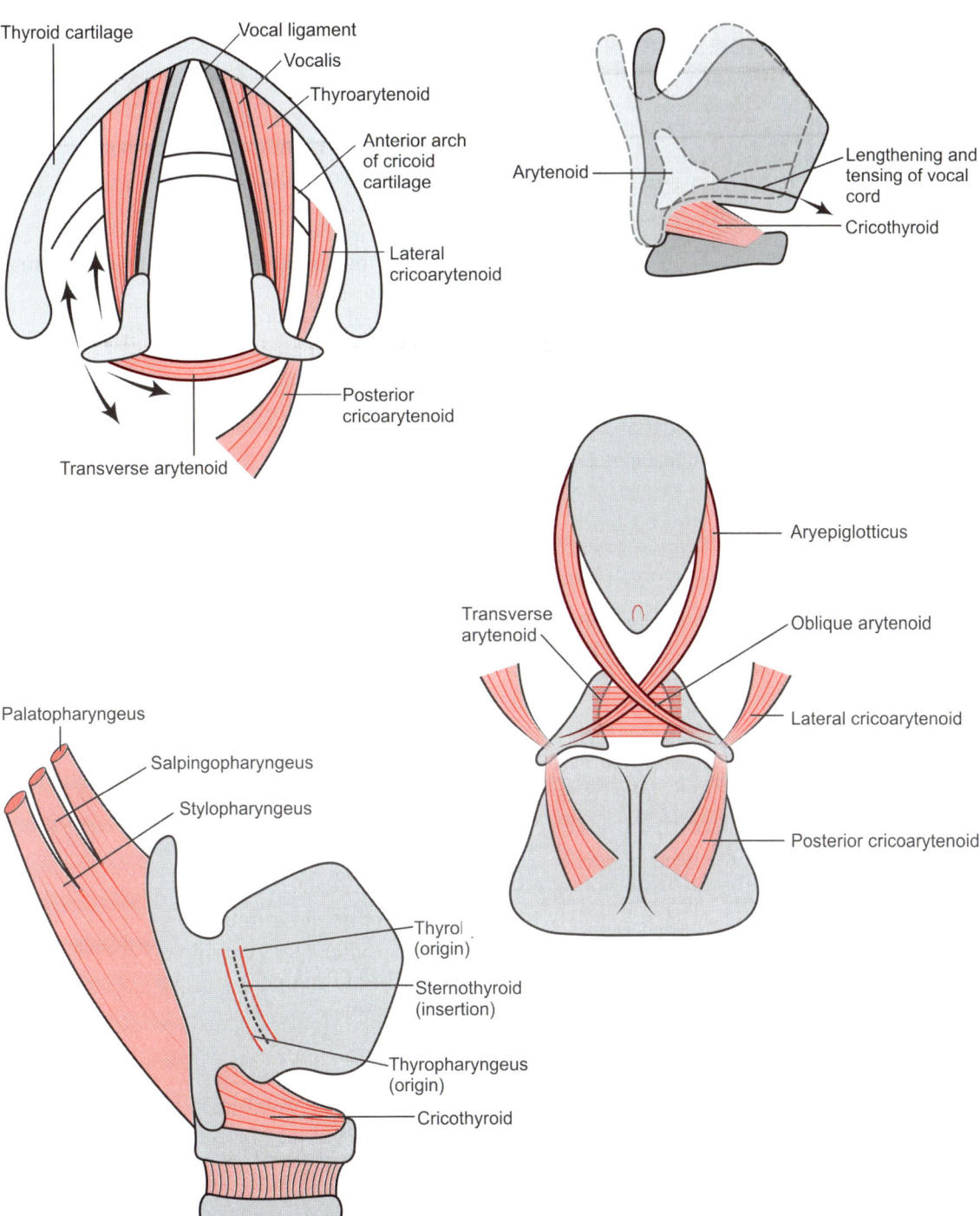

Fig. 6.64: Laryngeal muscles

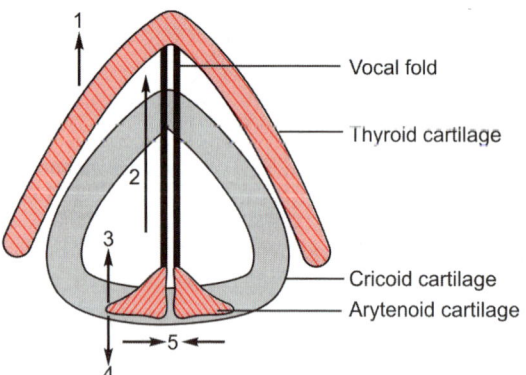

1. Cricothyroid 2. Thyroarytenoid
3. Lateral cricoarytenoid 4. Posterior
cricoarytenoid 5. Oblique and
transverse arytenoids

Fig. 6.65: Actions of laryngeal muscles

CLINICAL ANATOMY

Tracheostomy

- Involves making a surgical incision in the skin of the front of the neck and then making an opening in the front of the trachea.
- This is followed by insertion of a tracheostomy tube to provide an airway, bypassing the upper airway obstruction.
- During this procedure the infrahyoid muscles are retracted laterally and the isthmus of the thyroid is retracted superiorly.
- Care should be taken to avoid injury to the following structures that may be closely related:
  - Inferior thyroid veins
  - Left brachiocephalic vein in children
  - Occasional thyroidea ima artery.

As you journey from the top of the skull to the cerebrum, you come across the following structures:

- Skin
- Connective tissue
- Epicranial aponeurosis
- Loose areolar tissue
- Pericranium
- Outer table of the skull bone
- Diploe containing diploic vessels
- Inner table of the skull bone
- Extradural space (epidural space)
- Endocranium
- Dura mater (at places containing dural venous sinuses)
- Subdural space
- Arachnoid mater
- Subarachnoid space containing the cerebrospinal fluid
- Pia mater
- Cerebrum.

The nervous system is divided into:
1. Central nervous system
2. Peripheral nervous system

Central nervous system is made up of:
1. Brain
2. Spinal cord
   - The brain is safely preserved in the cranial cavity and is surrounded by the meninges of the brain (cranial).
   - The spinal cord is present inside the vertebral canal and is covered by the spinal meninges.

Meninges of the Brain

They are three in number.
1. Dura mater (pachymeninx)—means thick.
2. Arachnoid mater ⎫ Leptomeninges
3. Pia mater   ⎭

Dura Mater

- It is the thick outer layer (Fig. 6.66).
- It is vascular.
- It is made up of two layers, the outer endosteal and inner meningeal.
- These two layers are generally fused together except where they enclose dural venous sinuses.

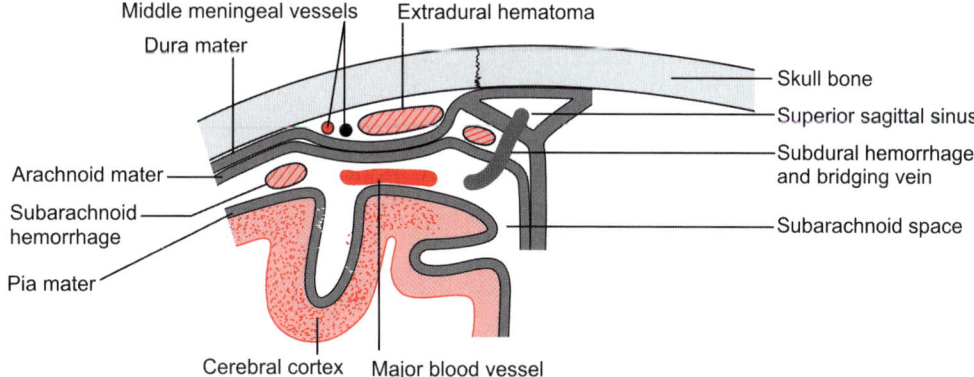

Fig. 6.66: Meninges and meningeal spaces

- Between the inner surface of the bone of the skull and the dura mater, there are meningeal vessels. These vessels supply the diploe of the cranial bone which contains marrow.
- *Dura mater has following important folds:*
  - Falx cerebri
  - Tentorium cerebelli
  - Falx cerebelli
  - Diaphragma sellae

- *Falx cerebri:*
  - It extends from the crista galli anteriorly to the superior surface of the tentorium cerebelli posteriorly (Fig. 6.67).

  - It has an attached border and a free margin.
  - Superior sagittal venous sinus lies along the attached border while the inferior sagittal sinus lies along the free margin.
  - Inferior sagittal sinus joins the great cerebral vein to form the straight sinus which is along the line of attachment of falx cerebri to tentorium cerebelli.

- *Tentorium cerebelli:*
  - It is like a tent above the posterior cranial fossa and forms the roof of the cerebellum (Fig. 6.67).

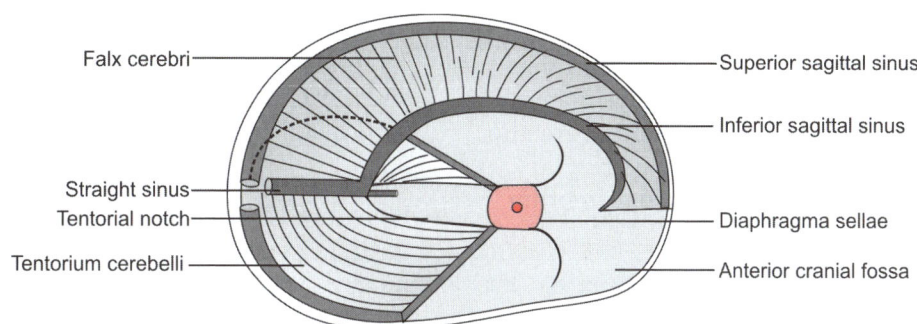

Fig. 6.67: Dural folds and venous sinuses

– It has a free margin and attached margin.
– The free margin is shaped like letter "U". This U-shaped space contains the midbrain.
– The free margin is attached to the anterior clinoid process.
– The attached margin contains two venous sinuses—transverse sinus and superior petrosal sinus.
– The tentorium cerebelli divides the cranial cavity into supratentorial and infratentorial compartments.

- *Nerve supply of dura mater:*
  – Dura mater of the supratentorial compartment is supplied by the branches of trigeminal nerve.

  Therefore, stretching and inflammation of this dura mater results in frontal and parietal headaches.

  – Dura mater of the infratentorial compartment is supplied by the branches of the upper cervical nerves.

  Therefore, involvement of this dura mater results in occipital and posterior neck pains. Acute meningitis of posterior cranial fossa is often associated with neck rigidity. This is brought about by the reflex contraction of the posterior neck muscles.

Arachnoid mater
- It is non-vascular.
- It is a thin fibrous layer which is in direct contact (not fused) with the dura mater.
- Number of trabeculae extend from the arachnoid mater to the pia mater.
- It does not dip into the sulci of cerebrum.

Pia mater
- It is thinner than arachnoid.
- It covers the brain closely.
- It dips into the sulci and lines them.
- It is vascular.

- There is subpial space deep to the pia mater which is continuous with the perivascular space.

Epidural space
- It is a potential space between the periosteum (external periosteal layer of dura) of the skull and the skull bones.
- There are meningeal vessels in this space. Very important meningeal vessels are the middle meningeal artery and middle meningeal vein. Veins are directly applied to the skull. Groove of the meningeal vessels is mainly caused by the veins. These vessels supply the diploe of the cranial bones which contain marrow. They also supply the dura mater.

Epidural hemorrhage (extradural hemorrhage)
- It is caused by the bleeding of middle meningeal vessels commonly. Hematoma is formed in this space.
- Usually, a nuerosurgeon makes a burr hole and removes this hematoma.

Subdural space
- It is a potential space.
- It lies between the dura mater and the arachnoid mater.
- Cerebral veins cross this space on their way to venous sinus. These veins are also called "bridging veins" as they bridge this space between the dura mater and arachnoid mater.
- *Note:* Bridging veins are parts of the cerebral veins lying between the arachnoid and dura (meningeal layer) and connecting cortical surface of brain with a dural sinus.

Subdural hemorrhage
- It is caused by the rupture of cerebral veins (bridging veins).
- In violent jerks as in automobile accidents, due to shearing forces these veins are severed resulting in subdural hemorrhage.

Subarachnoid space

- It is a sponge-like space.
- It lies between the arachnoid mater and pia mater.
- This is traversed by arachnoid trabeculae.
- This contains the cerebrospinal fluid (CSF) and large blood vessels lie in this space. Aneurysm of these vessels may rupture and result in the subarachnoid hemorrhage.

Hydrocephalus

- Increased intracranial pressure due to accumulation of CSF.
- Occurs either due to overproduction or obstruction to drainage of CSF.

Subarachnoid hemorrhage

- Subarachnoid hemorrhage is caused by the rupture of large arteries which results in bloody cerebrospinal fluid.
- *Example:* The berry aneurysm of the anterior communicating artery.
- Following subarachnoid hemorrhage, there is blood mixed cerebrospinal fluid when lumbar puncture is done.

Cerebral hemorrhage (intracerebral hemorrhage)

- Small arteries supplying the brain may rupture resulting in the intracerebral hemorrhage within the brain tissue itself.
- *Example:* Hemiplegia caused by the intracerebral hemorrhage because of involvement of internal capsule.

Spinal Meninges

- It has same three layers as the cranial meninges.
  - Dura mater
  - Arachnoid mater
  - Pia mater

Spinal Dura Mater

- It is shaped like a test tube.

- Its upper margin is attached to the foramen magnum where it is in continuity with the inner layer of the cranial dura mater.
- It terminates at the level of S2 vertebra.
- It is also attached to the posterior longitudinal ligament.
- The outer layer of cranial dura mater is represented by the periosteum of the vertebral canal.
- The space between the periosteum of the vertebral canal and the spinal dura mater is called "spinal epidural space".

Spinal epidural space: It is an actual space. It contains:
1. Internal vertebral venous plexus
2. Loose connective tissue
3. Semiliquid fat
4. Branches of segmental vessels which supply the structures in the vertebral canal.

Internal Vertebral Venous Plexus

- This is a plexus of veins which has no valves (Fig. 6.68).
- It is drained into the segmental veins which are the indirect tributaries of superior vena cava in the upper region and inferior vena cava in the lower region. Therefore, this venous plexus equalizes the pressure between the superior and inferior vena cava.

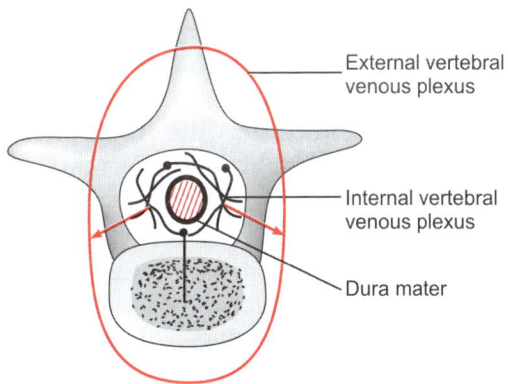

Fig. 6.68: Internal vertebral venous plexus

Should one of the veins be obstructed then the venous blood is shunted to the other vein through the internal vertebral venous plexus.

- This venous plexus also communicates with the intracranial dural venous sinuses.

Cancer cells from pelvis especially from prostate gland are spread to the bodies of the vertebrae through this valveless plexus. Cancer cells are thus spread to these bodies of the vertebrae and even to the skull bones. Hence, patient does not come to the doctor till the advanced stage of disease.

Intervertebral Foramen

- This is bounded by the bodies of the vertebrae and the intervertebral disc anteriorly.
- Superior and inferior vertebral notches of the pedicles form superior and inferior boundaries respectively.
- Articular processes and their associated joints lie posteriorly.
- Structures passing through the intervertebral foramen are:
  1. Corresponding spinal nerve.
  2. Spinal branches of segmental blood vessels.

CLINICAL ANATOMY

- Disc prolapse is the herniation of the nucleus pulposus of the intervertebral disc beyond its confinement. When it occurs posterolaterally into the intervertebral foramen, it commonly compresses the spinal nerve roots, especially common in the lumbar region.
- Even arthritis of joints of vertebral arches and rheumatoid arthritis of the region may result in the involvement of spinal nerve and subsequent referred pain in the area of distribution of the nerve.

Arachnoid Mater

- This is a thin transparent membrane.
- It lines the inner surface of the dura mater throughout.
- It is separated from the dura mater by a potential subdural space.
- Subarachnoid space lies deep to the arachnoid mater. It contains the cerebrospinal fluid (CSF). Arachnoid trabeculae pass from the deep surface of the arachnoid to the pia mater.
- The spinal subarachnoid space is continuous with the cranial subarachnoid space.

Lumbar Cistern

- This is the dilated sac of the subarachnoid space between the L2 and S2 vertebrae.
- This is because the spinal cord terminates at the level of lower border of L1 vertebra but the dura mater and arachnoid extend up to the level of S2 vertebra.
- *It contains:*
  - Cerebrospinal fluid
  - Lower lumbar, sacral and coccygeal nerves
  - Filum terminale (non-nervous filament extending from the lower end of the spinal cord and it is covered by the pia mater).
- Tapping of the cerebrospinal fluid (CSF) from the lumbar cistern is called the lumbar puncture.

Lumbar Puncture

- It is done through a long needle inserted between the spines of L3 and L4 in the adult and through the space between the spines of L4 and L5 in the child (Fig. 6.69).
- This is because the spinal cord terminates at the level of lower border of L1 in the case of the adult and at the level of L3 in the case of newborn.

- A line corresponding to the highest point of iliac crest is marked which corresponds to the spine of L4 vertebra.
- A long needle is inserted just above it (to one side of midline to avoid spinous process) which passes through the following to reach the subarachnoid space:

  Skin → Superficial space → Deep fascia → Erector spinae muscle → Supraspinous ligament → Interspinous ligament → Ligamentum flavum → Epidural space → Dura mater → Subdural space → Arachnoid mater → Subarachnoid space.

Queckenstedt Test

- The spinal and cranial subarachnoid spaces are continuous. Any increase in the volume (pressure) of CSF in cranial subarachnoid space is spread to the spinal subarachnoid space. When internal jugular veins are compressed, it results in increase in pressure in the CSF because of increased pressure in superior sagittal sinus preventing drainage of CSF. This is because IJV is continuous with sigmoid sinus, transverse sinus, and finally superior sagittal sinus.

- If there is any obstruction to the continuity of cranial subarachnoid space with the spinal subarachnoid space, the increase in the pressure of cranial subarachnoid CSF does not raise the CSF pressure in the spinal subarachnoid space. This can be recorded by the manometer attached to the lumbar puncture needle.
- If pressure does not raise in the spinal subarachnoid space following the compression of the internal jugular vein, it is known as "Queckenstedt test positive".
- Lumbar puncture is not done when the Queckenstedt test is positive as it results in the herniation of tonsil of cerebellum into

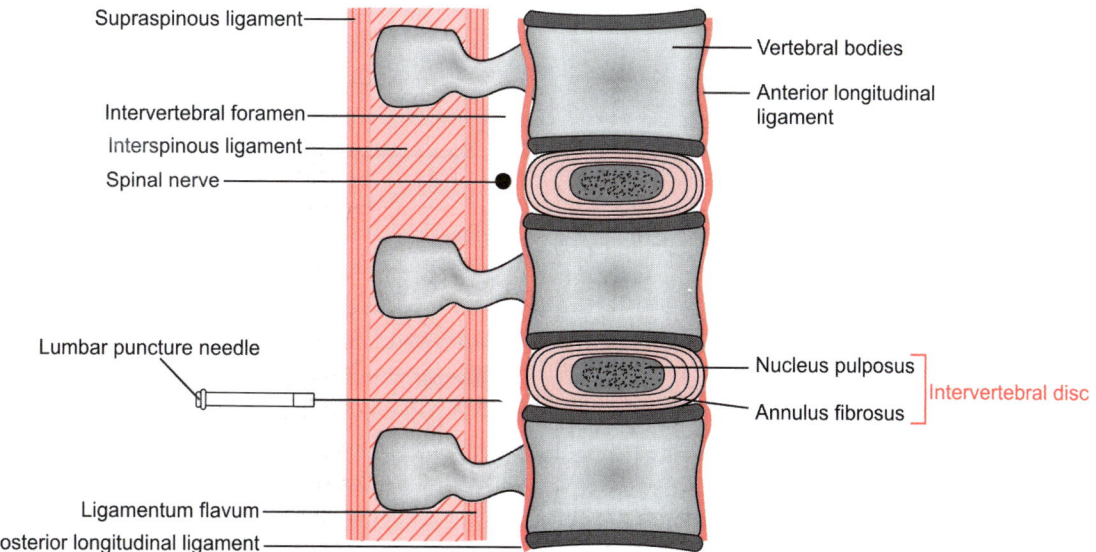

Supraspinous ligament

Intervertebral foramen
Interspinous ligament
Spinal nerve

Lumbar puncture needle

Ligamentum flavum
Posterior longitudinal ligament

Vertebral bodies
Anterior longitudinal ligament

Nucleus pulposus
Annulus fibrosus
Intervertebral disc

Fig. 6.69: Lumbar spine

the foramen magnum and subsequent compression of the medulla oblongata. Since medulla oblongata consists of vital respiratory and cardiac centres, it may result in death.

- When the Queckenstedt test is positive, cisternal puncture is done through the foramen magnum.

Pia mater

- This is the vascular inner layer of spinal meninges.
- It covers the spinal cord closely.
- It covers the filum terminale.
- On either side of the pia mater, there is a longitudinal thickening which has teeth-like 21 pairs of processes. This is called ligamenta denticulata.

Importance of ligamenta denticulata:

- The teeth-like processes of this ligament connect the pia mater with the dura mater (Fig. 6.70).

- These processes lie between the ventral and dorsal roots.
- They help to hold the spinal cord in its position.
- They serve as a guide to the surgeon to identify the dorsal and ventral roots.

Dural Venous Sinuses

- The dura mater is made up of two layers but two layers are fused together except at the places where they are split to enclose the dural venous sinuses. Dural venous sinuses are the venous spaces between the two layers of dura mater (Fig. 6.71).
- They are called the intracranial dural venous sinuses.

Characteristics of these sinuses:

- They are the spaces between the two layers of dura mater.
- They have no muscular wall.
- They have no valves.
- They are lined by endothelium.

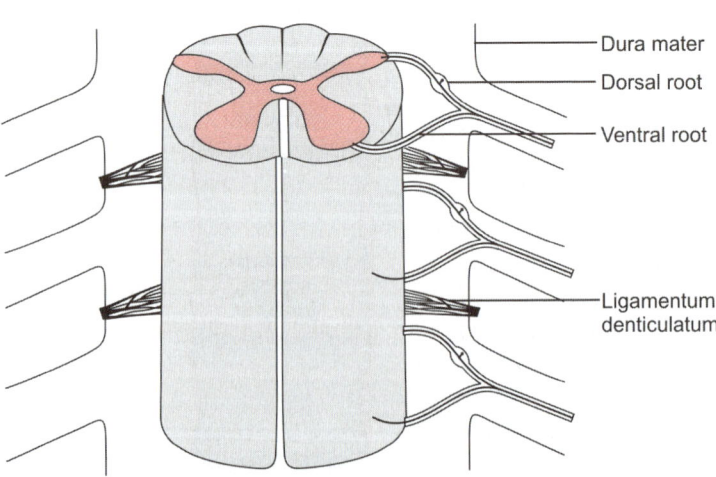

Fig. 6.70: Ligamentum denticulatum

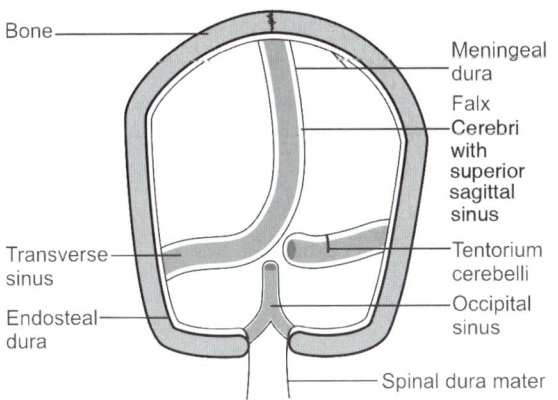

Bone — Meningeal dura — Falx Cerebri with superior sagittal sinus — Transverse sinus — Endosteal dura — Tentorium cerebelli — Occipital sinus — Spinal dura mater

Fig. 6.71: Dural folds and sinuses

- These sinuses are divided into paired and unpaired sinuses:

Paired	Unpaired
Sphenoparietal	Anterior intercavernous
Cavernous	Posterior intercavernous
Superior petrosal	Superior sagittal
Inferior petrosal	Inferior sagittal
Transverse	Straight
Sigmoid	Occipital

- Venous sinuses present along the attachment of the tentorium cerebelli
  - Superior petrosal sinus
  - Transverse sinus
- Venous sinus at the junction of tentorium cerebelli with the falx cerebri—straight sinus.
- Venous sinus along the superior attachment of the falx cerebri—superior sagittal sinus.
- Venous sinus along the lower free margin of the falx cerebri—inferior sagittal sinus.
  - *Note:* The superior sagittal sinus lies between the two layers of the dura mater (meningeal and endosteal) while the inferior sagittal sinus lies within the inner (meningeal) layer of the dura mater.

- Venous sinus along the falx cerebelli attachment to internal occipital crest in midline of the posterior cranial fossa— occipital sinus.
- Cavernous sinus lies on either side of the body of the sphenoid bone.
- Sphenoparietal sinus lies along the lesser wing of the sphenoid.
- Superior petrosal sinus lies along the upper border of the petrous temporal bone.
- Inferior petrosal sinus lies along the lower border of the petrous part of the temporal bone.

- Sigmoid sinus is S-shaped sinus which continues as the internal jugular vein in the jugular foramen. It is closely related to the mastoid antrum. Therefore, infection from this area may spread to sigmoid sinus.

Cavernous Sinus

- This is a paired sinus in the middle cranial fossa.
- It lies on either side of the body of the sphenoid bone (Fig. 6.72).
- It extends from the apex of the petrous part of the temporal bone to the medial end of the superior orbital fissure.

Relations

- *Lateral:* Temporal lobe of the cerebrum.
- *Medial:* Hypophysis and sphenoidal air sinus.
  In the thickness of the lateral wall the following structures are present:
1. Oculomotor nerve
2. Trochlear nerve
3. Ophthalmic division of trigeminal nerve
4. Maxillary division of trigeminal nerve
  (These structures lie between the dura mater and the endothelium of the sinus).
Two structures lie inside the cavernous sinus:
- The internal carotid artery.
- Abducent nerve.
  (These two structures are also separated from the blood in the cavernous sinus by the

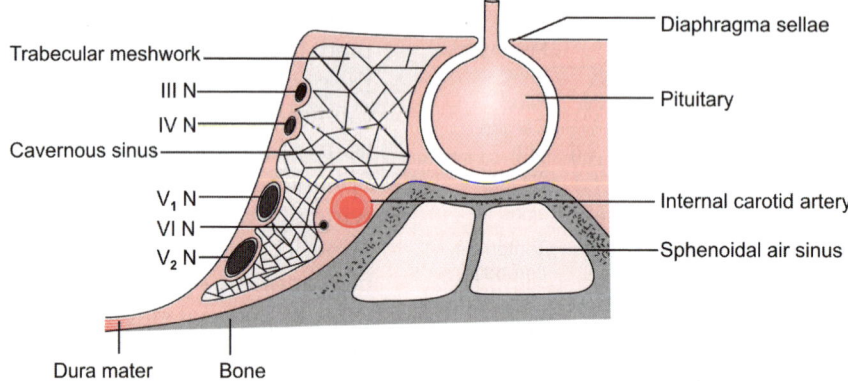

Fig. 6.72: Cavernous sinus

endothelium. Abducent nerve lies inferolateral to the internal carotid artery).

Following veins drain into the cavernous sinus:
- Superior ophthalmic vein.
- Inferior ophthalmic vein.
- Sphenoparietal sinus.
- Superficial middle cerebral vein.

Following sinuses drain blood away from the cavernous sinus:
- Superior petrosal sinus.
- Inferior petrosal sinus.
- Emissary veins.

Emissary veins pass through the foramen ovale and foramen lacerum and connect the cavernous sinus with the veins outside the cranium (pterygoid venous plexus). These veins serve to equalize the pressure. They may also carry infection from extracranial source to cavernous sinus resulting in the cavernous sinus thrombosis.

Pulsating tumor of the eyeball: When the internal carotid artery is injured, the arterial blood gets mixed with the venous blood of the cavernous sinus; a communication is established between cavernous sinus and internal carotid artery and with each heart beat, the eyeball pulsates.

PITUITARY GLAND

- Also called epiphysis cerebri.
- 12 mm transversely and 8 mm antero-posteriorly.
- 500 mg weight.
- 2 parts differing in origins:
  - Anterior lobe or adenohypophysis made of pars anterior, pars intermedia and pars tuberalis.
  - Posterior lobe or neurohypophysis made of pars nervosa, infundibulum and median eminence.
- *Important relations:*
  - Lies in hypophyseal fossa of sphenoid.
  - Superiorly, diaphragma sella and optic chiasma.
  - Inferiorly, sphenoid air sinus.
  - Laterally, cavernous sinus.
- *Blood supply:*
  - Arteries—superior and inferior hypophyseal arteries; branches of internal carotid artery.
  - Hypophyseal veins drain into cavernous sinus.
- *Important features:*
  - Hypophyseal portal vessels (Fig. 6.74).
  - Hypothalamohypophyseal tract carrying hormones from supraoptic and para-ventricular nuclei of hypothalamus to posterior pituitary.

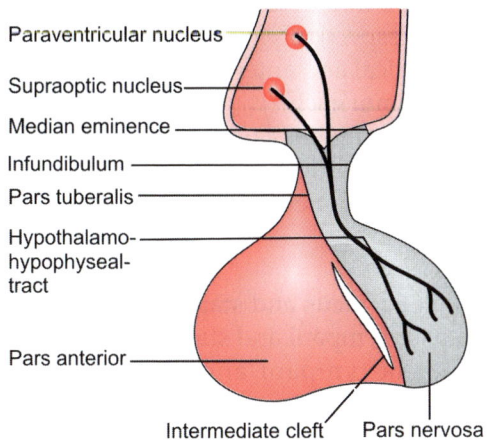

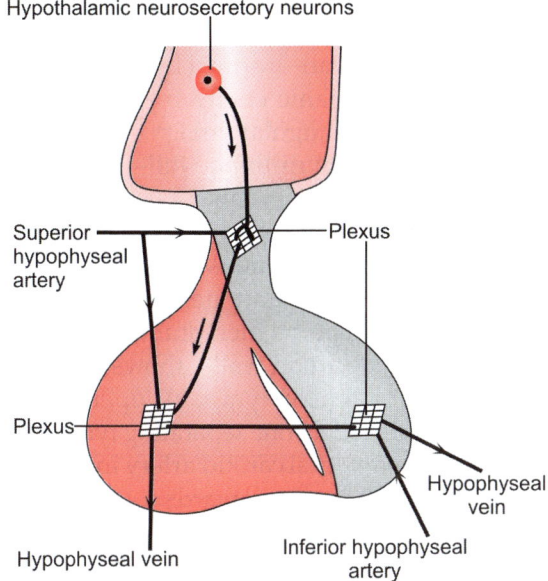

Fig. 6.73: Hypothalamohypophyseal tract

Fig. 6.74: Hypophyseal portal system

1. Pituitary tumors can cause pressure effects on optic chiasma owing to close relation and cause visual field defects.
2. Common approach to pituitary for surgery is trans-sphenoidal approach by nasal route.

EAR

Divided into:
1. External
2. Middle and
3. Internal ear.

External Ear

- External ear is separated from middle ear by tympanic membrane.
- It is made of auricle and external acoustic meatus (Fig. 6.75A).

External acoustic meatus:
- It is S-shaped.
- Lateral 1/3rd is cartilaginous and medial 2/3rd is bony.

- Otoscope is a device used to visualize the external acoustic meatus and tympanic membrane.
- Impacted ear wax may cause pain and conduction deafness.

Tympanic Membrane

- Oval membrane.
- ~1 cm in diameter.
- Covered externally by skin and on inner aspect by mucous lining.
- Has a concave lateral surface directed downwards and forwards.
- Its anterosuperior part between anterior and posterior malleolar folds is flaccid called pars flaccida and rest is tense called pars tensa (Fig. 6.75B).
- The point at tip of handle of malleus is called umbo.
- When illuminated by light a cone of light is seen in the anteroinferior quadrant with the apex of cone at the umbo.

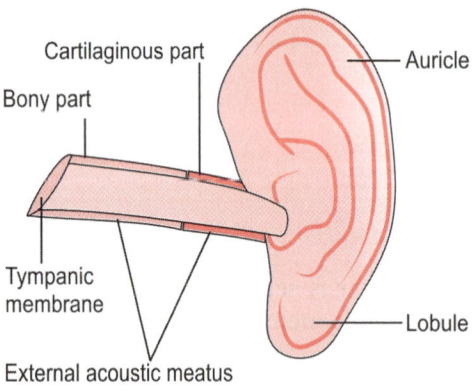

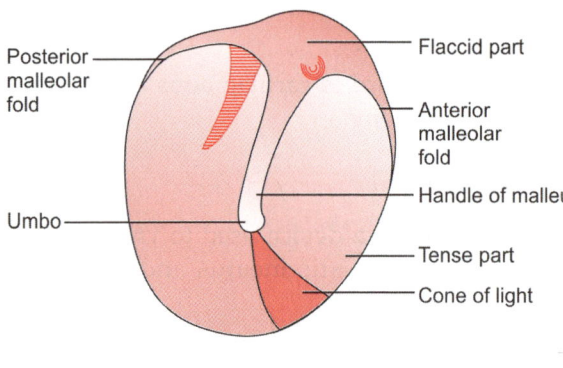

B

Fig. 6.75: A. External ear, B. Tympanic membrane (lateral aspect)

• Perforation of tympanic membrane occurs with infections of middle ear. Small perforations heal spontaneously but large ones need surgical repair.

Middle Ear

• Cavity filled with air.
• Located in petrous temporal bone.
• Contains ear ossicles.
• Communicates with nasopharynx through auditory tube.
• Communicates with mastoid air cells through aditus of antrum.
• Shaped like dumbbell; because medial and lateral walls are separated by a distance of

6 mm, 2 mm and 4 mm at roof, centre and floor respectively.
• Its vertical and anteroposterior dimensions are 15 mm each.
• Part of tympanic cavity situated above level of tympanic membrane is called epitympanic recess.

Contents

1. Malleus, incus and stapes (3 ossicles).
2. Tensor tympani and stapedius (2 muscles).
3. Chorda tympani and tympanic plexus (3 nerves).

Boundaries (Fig. 6.76B)

• *Roof:* Tegmental wall—formed by tegmen tympani separating tympanic cavity from middle cranial fossa.
• *Floor:* Jugular wall—formed by bone which separates tympanic cavity from superior bulb of internal jugular vein.
• *Medial wall:* Labyrinthine wall—separates tympanic cavity from inner ear and shows promontory.
• *Lateral wall:* Membranous wall—separates tympanic cavity from external ear and is formed by tympanic membrane.
• *Anterior wall:* Carotid wall—shows opening of canal for tensor tympani, opening of auditory tube and bone separating tympanic cavity from internal carotid artery in carotid canal from above downwards.
• *Posterior wall:* Mastoid wall—shows aditus to mastoid antrum through which epitympanic recess communicates with mastoid antrum. Pyramid is a cone-shaped projection through the mouth of which the stapedius muscle emerges and inserts into neck of stapes.
  – *Other important features on medial wall:*
    ♦ Promontory
    ♦ Round window (fenestra cochlea) closed by secondary tympanic membrane

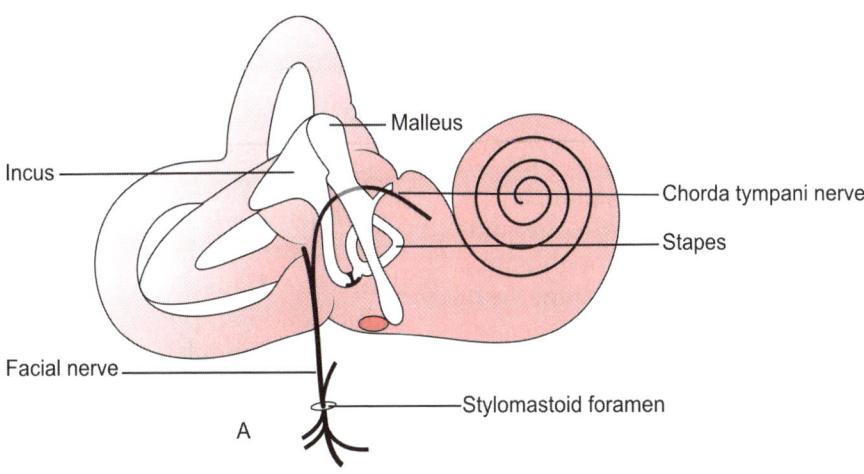

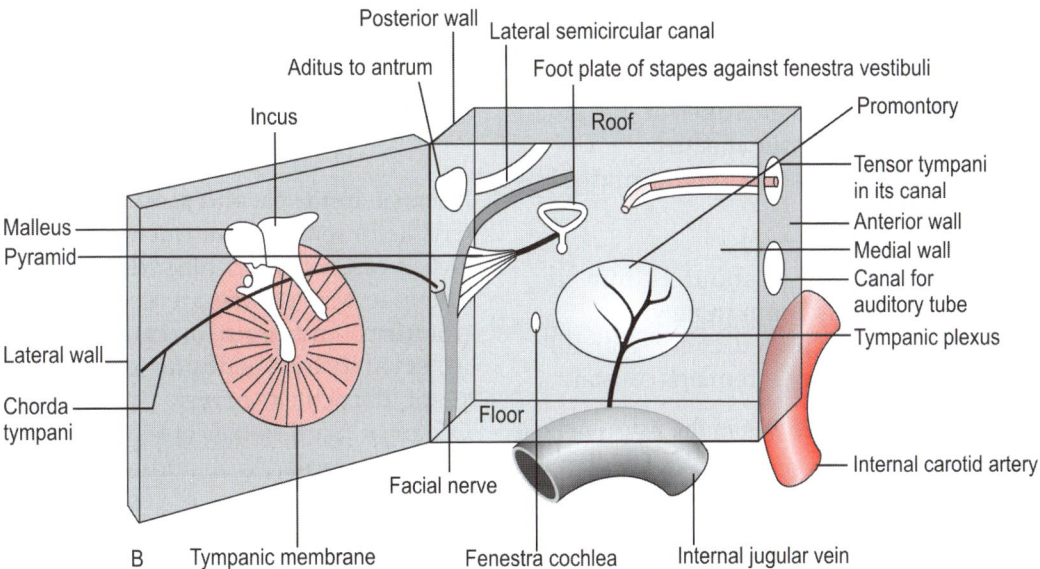

Fig. 6.76: A. Ear ossicles and chorda tympani, B. Walls of tympanic cavity (lateral wall has been opened like the lid of a box)

♦ Oval window (fenestra vestibule) closed by footplate of stapes.

Arterial supply: Branches of maxillary, posterior auricular, middle meningeal and internal carotid artery.

Mastoid Antrum

- Air-filled space in mastoid process of temporal bone.
- 1 cm in diameter with capacity of 1 ml.
- Bounded above by tegmen tympani, below by mastoid air cells, anteriorly communicates with tympanic recess through aditus and behind it is separated by bone from sigmoid sinus.

- Infection from it (mastoiditis) can spread above to brain and posteriorly to sigmoid sinus causing sigmoid sinus thrombosis due to its close relationship.

Suprameatal Triangle

- Boundaries:
  - *Superior:* Supramastoid crest.
  - *Anteroinferiorly:* Posterosuperior margin of the external acoustic meatus.
- It forms the lateral wall of the matoid antrum.
- It lies deep to cymba concha.
- In adults; bone here is about 12 mm in thickness; while it is 2 mm in newborn.
- One mm of bone is added every year till about 12 years and then it remains constant.

- In mastoid operations this is the approach area.

Auditory Tube

- Also called eustachian tube.
- Posterolateral 1/3rd is bony; rest is cartilaginous.
- Equalizes pressure in tympanic cavity with atmospheric pressure.

- The tube acts as a pathway for spreading of infections from nasopharynx to the middle ear.
- It gets blocked with infections.

Internal Ear

- 2 components—bony and membranous labyrinth (Fig. 6.77A).
- Bony or osseous labyrinth includes semicircular canals, vestibule and cochlea. Filled with perilymph.
- Membranous labyrinth includes semicircular ducts, utricle, saccule, cochlear duct, endolymphatic duct and sac. Filled with endolymph.

The parts of membranous labyrinth contained in bony labyrinth are as follows:

Semicircular canals (semicircular ducts), vestibule (utricle, saccule) and cochlea (cochlear duct).

Ampullae are dilated regions of semicircular ducts located near their junction with utricle.

Epithelial lining of membranous labyrinth is specialized to form sensory structures called:

1. Maculae in utricle and saccule.
2. Cristae in semicircular ducts.
3. Organ of Corti in cochlear duct.
- Maculae and cristae are concerned with position and equilibrium sense and innervated by vestibular component of vestibulocochlear nerve.
- Organ of Corti is concerned with hearing and is concerned with auditory or hearing or cochlear component of vestibulocochlear nerve (Fig. 6.77B).

CLINICAL ANATOMY

- Any pathology of internal ear results in tinnitus (ringing), vertigo (dizziness) or sensorineural hearing loss depending on the site of involvement.

ORBIT

- Is a pyramidal cavity located on either side of the root of the nose.

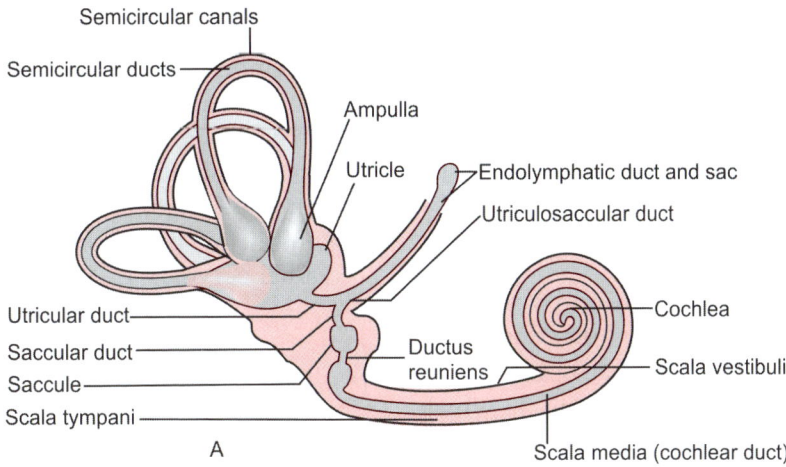

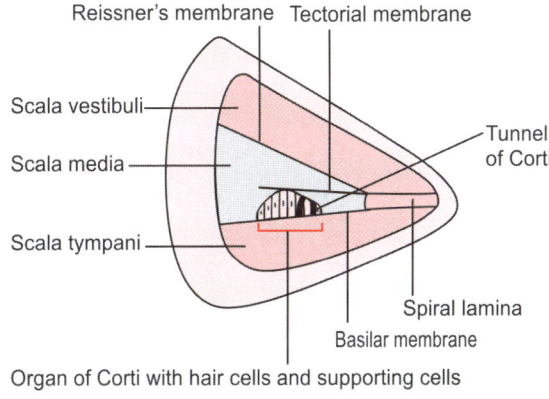

Fig. 6.77: A. Bony and membranous labyrinth, B. Organ of Corti

- It contains the eyeball.
- The eyeball is surrounded by a fascial sheath known as Tenon's capsule. The thickened lower part of the fascial sheath forms the suspensory ligament of the eyeball.
- Orbital fascia on the other hand lines the bony orbit forming its periosteum.
- Orbital septum is a weak membrane that

runs from the margins of the orbit to the tarsal plates.
- Medial and lateral palpebral raphae connect the tarsal plates to the medial and lateral margins of the orbit respectively.

EYE

- Consists of 3 coats: fibrous coat, vascular coat and nervous coat (Fig. 6.78B).

- Fibrous coat
  - Anterior 1/6th is cornea.
  - Posterior 5/6th is sclera.
  - Both meet at sclerocorneal junction or limbus where aqueous humor drains by way of canal of Schlemm and sinus venosus sclerae.
- Vascular coat
  - Has 3 parts from behind forwards namely choroid, ciliary body and iris.
  - Choroid has rich blood vessels.
  - Ciliary body has ciliary muscle which helps in accommodation.
  - Iris has 2 muscles namely sphincter pupillae supplied by parasympathetic and dilator pupillae supplied by sympathetic which bring about constriction and dilation of pupil respectively.
- Nervous coat
  - Or retina is made of 10 layers and is responsible for photoreception and visual impulse generation.

EXTRAOCULAR MUSCLES

- Lie outside eyeball; within orbits.
- They include: 4 recti (superior, inferior, medial and lateral); 2 obliques (superior and inferior) and levator palpebrae superioris which elevates the upper lid (Figs 6.79, 6.80 and 6.81A).
- The 4 recti arise from the common tendinous annular ring (Fig. 6.78A).
- The 4 recti are inserted into the sclera a little behind the sclerocorneal junction.
- The superior oblique after passing through trochlea runs posterolaterally to be inserted into posterosuperior lateral quadrant of sclera behind coronal equator of the eye.
- The inferior oblique runs posterolaterally from its origin to be inserted into posteroinferior lateral quadrant of sclera behind coronal equator of the eye.

Nerve Supply

- Remember mnemonic $LR_6(SO_4)_3$.
- Lateral rectus is supplied by abducent nerve (6th cranial nerve).
- Superior oblique is supplied by trochlear nerve (4th cranial nerve).
- Remaining by oculomotor nerve (3rd cranial nerve) (Fig. 6.85).

Actions (Figs 6.81B and 6.82)

1. *Superior oblique:* Depression, abduction and intorsion.
2. *Inferior oblique:* Elevation, abduction and extorsion.
3. *Superior rectus:* Elevation, adduction and intorsion.
4. *Inferior rectus:* Depression, adduction and extorsion.
5. *Medial rectus:* Adduction.
6. *Lateral rectus:* Abduction.

APPLIED ANATOMY

1. When VI nerve is injured, due to lateral rectus palsy, the eye cannot be abducted.
2. When IV nerve is injured, there is inability to depress the adducted eye. Patient cannot see the tip of the nose. Difficulty in walking downstairs because of diplopia (double vision) on looking downwards.
3. When III nerve is injured, drooping of upper lid due to paralysis of levator palpebrae superioris and eye is down and out because of unopposed lateral rectus and superior oblique.

Veins of orbit: Superior and inferior ophthalmic veins drain into the cavernous sinus.

Arteries of orbit: Ophthalmic artery is the main artery.

Branches of ophthalmic artery (Fig. 6.83):
- Central artery of retina

1. Lacrimal nerve, 2. Frontal nerve, 3. Trochlear nerve
4. Superior and inferior divisions of oculomotor nerve
5. Nasociliary nerve, 6. Abducent nerve

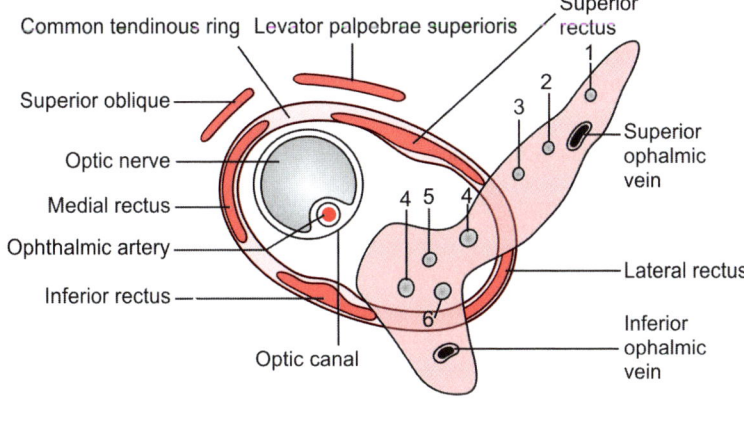

A

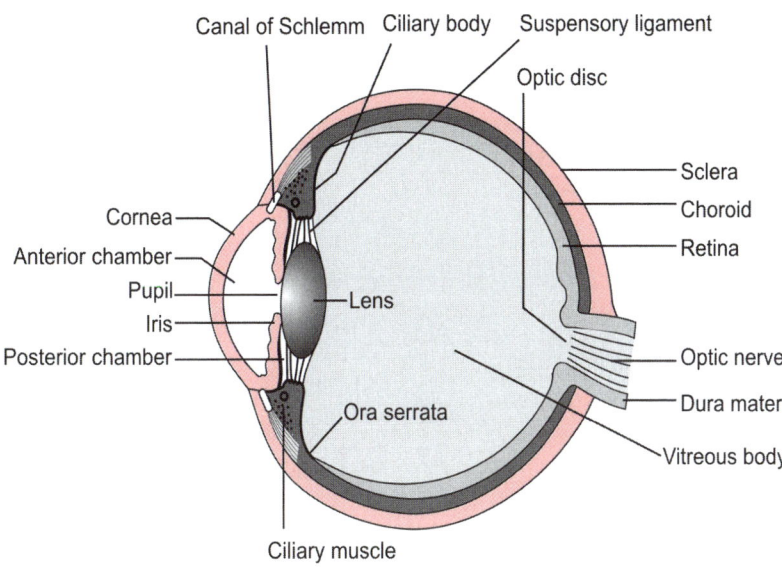

B

Fig. 6.78: A. Superior orbital fissure, B. Structure of eye

- Supraorbital
- Supratrochlear
- Lacrimal
- Dorsal nasal
- Short and long ciliary

- Anterior and posterior ethmoidal
- Muscular

Nerves of orbit:
- Optic
- Oculomotor

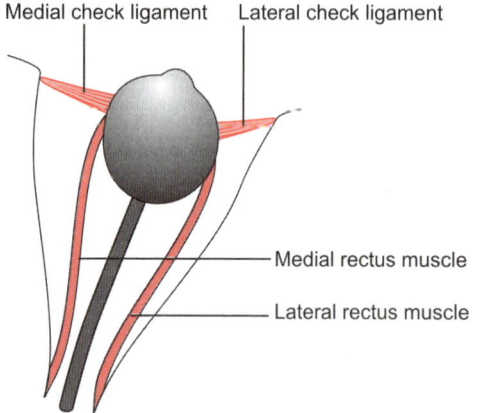

Fig. 6.79: Medial and lateral recti

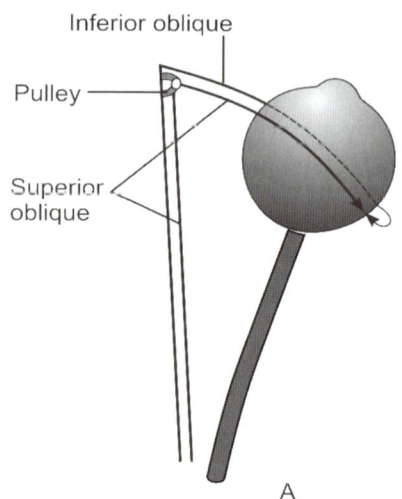

A

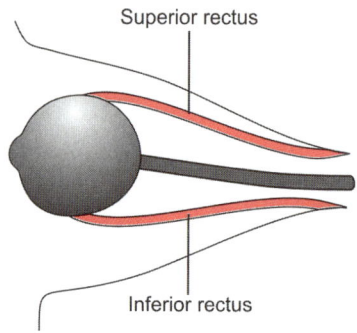

Fig. 6.80: Superior and inferior recti

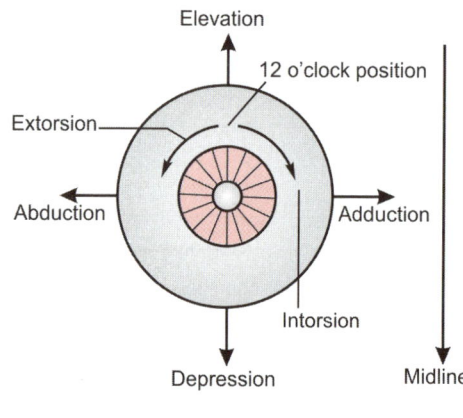

B

Fig. 6.81: A. Superior and inferior oblique, B. Movements of eyeball

- Trochlear
- Abducent
- Ophthalmic branch of V nerve
- Sympathetic
- Ophthalmic nerve divides anterior part of cavernous sinus into frontal, lacrimal and nasociliary nerves (Fig. 6.84).
- Frontal nerve divides into supratrochlear and supraorbital.
- Nasociliary nerve gives long ciliary, infratrochlear, anterior and posterior ethmoidal branches.

- Anterior ethmoidal gives 2 internal nasal and 1 external nasal branch.

Ciliary Ganglion

- Situated between optic nerve and lateral rectus muscle.
- Short ciliary nerves arise from it.
- Sympathetic fibers pass through it without relay (Fig. 6.86).

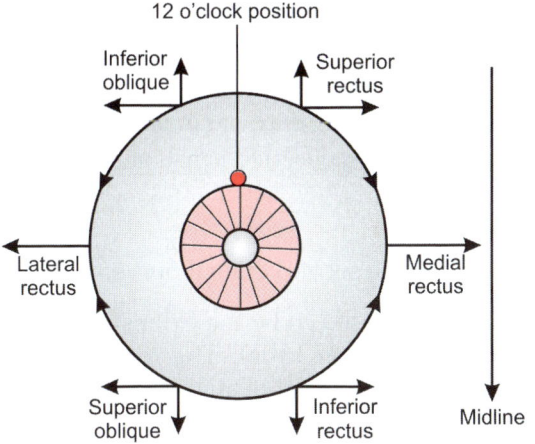

Fig. 6.82: Actions of extraocular muscles

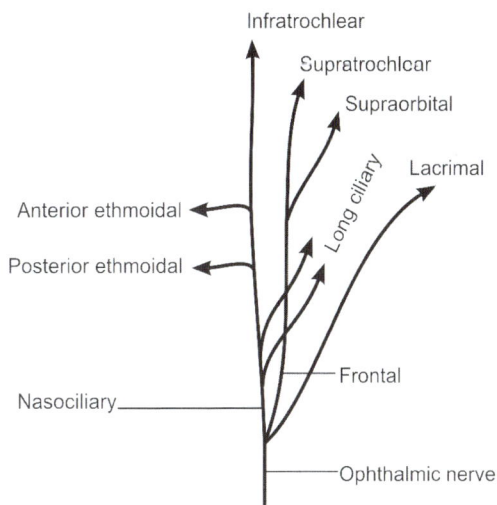

Fig. 6.84: Branches of ophthalmic nerve

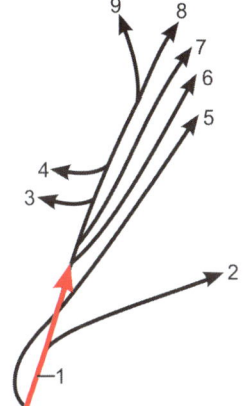

1. Main trunk
2. Lacrimal
3. Posterior ethmoidal
4. Anterior ethmoidal
5. Central artery of retina
6. Posterior ciliary
7. Supraorbital
8. Supratrochlear
9. Dorsal nasal

Fig. 6.83: Branches of ophthalmic artery

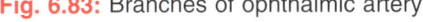

Fig. 6.85: Branches of oculomotor nerve

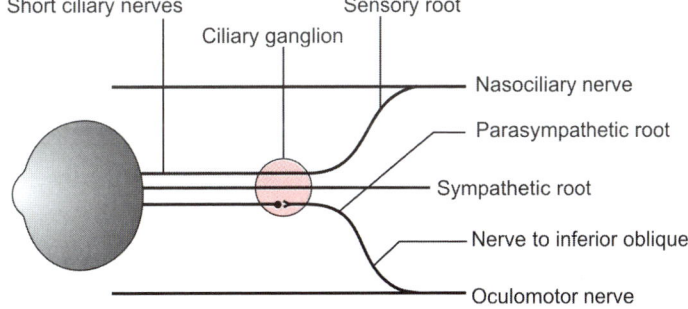

Fig. 6.86: Ciliary ganglion

- Preganglionic parasympathetic fibers originating in Edinger Westphal nucleus relay in it and reach it via the nerve to inferior oblique branch of inferior division of oculomotor nerve.
- Sensory root comes from nasociliary nerve.

Cranial Nerves

Brainstem includes three parts:
a. Midbrain.
b. Pons.
c. Medulla oblongata.

  Third and fourth cranial nerves are attached to the midbrain.

  Fifth to eighth cranial nerves are attached to the pons.

  Ninth to twelfth cranial nerves are attached to the medulla oblongata.

Remember:

2 Cranial nerves—to the forebrain
2 Cranial nerves—to the midbrain
4 Cranial nerves—to the pons
4 Cranial nerves—to the medulla oblongata.

Olfactory Nerve

- This is the first cranial nerve.
- It passes through the cribriform plate of ethmoid bone on either side of the crista galli.
- Olfactory bulb carries the cell body of the second order neurons and this nerve is a direct continuation of the brain. It is directly connected with the cerebrum. It is surrounded by the meninges. Therefore, CSF in the subarachnoid space accompanies the nerve up to the cribriform plate.

  That is the reason why CSF leaks through the nose in the fractures of the ethmoid bone. This is called CSF rhinorrhea.
- It carries special sense of smell.

- As age advances the acuity of sense of smell decreases because the number of olfactory neurons decreases.
- Anosmia—no sense of smell.
- Parosmia—perverted sense of smell.

Optic Nerve

- This is the second cranial nerve.

- It is supposed to be the extension of brain tissue (neural tube). The myelin of this nerve is given by the oligodendrocytes and this is the important nerve involved in multiple sclerosis.
- It is surrounded by the meninges and the subarachnoid space. Therefore, any increase in the CSF pressure results in papilledema, the bulging of the optic disc.
- Injury to the optic nerve results in visual field defects.

Oculomotor Nerve

- It is the third cranial nerve.
- Its nuclei lie in the floor of the cerebral aqueduct at the level of superior colliculus of midbrain (Fig. 6.87).
- Its parasympathetic nucleus is called the Edinger-Westphal nucleus.
- It emerges from midbrain to pass between posterior cerebral and superior cerebellar arteries to enter interpeduncular fossa.
- It pierces the dura mater in front of the decussation of free and attached borders of tentorium cerebelli.
- It lies in the lateral wall of the cavernous sinus.
- It passes through the superior orbital fissure and it supplies the following muscles:
  1. Superior rectus
  2. Inferior rectus
  3. Medial rectus
  4. Inferior oblique
  5. Levator palpabrae superioris

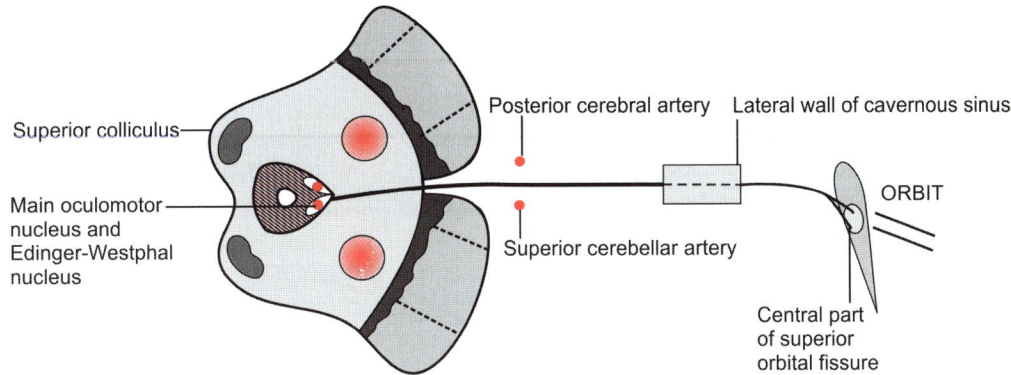

Fig. 6.87: Oculomotor nerve

CLINICAL ANATOMY

In oculomotor paralysis, the only two muscles of the eyeball which are not paralyzed are the lateral rectus muscle (supplied by the abducent nerve) and the superior oblique muscle (supplied by the trochlear nerve). Lateral rectus abducts the eyeball and superior oblique bends the front of the eyeball downwards and rotates it medially. The symptoms in the oculomotor palsy are:

1. Down and out position of the eyeball.
2. Ptosis (paralysis of levator palpebrae superioris).
3. Dilatation of pupil (oculomotor carries parasympathetic constrictor fibers to sphincter pupilla).
4. Diplopia (because the axes of the two eyeballs do not agree with each other).

• What are the afferent and efferent limbs of pupillary light reflex?
  – *Afferent:* Optic nerve.
  – *Efferent:* Oculomotor nerve.

Trochlear Nerve

• It is the fourth cranial nerve.
• Its nucleus is placed in floor of the cerebral aqueduct of the midbrain at the level of inferior colliculus (Fig. 6.88).

• It is the only cranial nerve which emerges on the dorsal aspect of brainstem and the nerves of the 2 sides decussate in the tectum.
• Winds around cerebral peduncles and passes between posterior cerebral and superior cerebellar arteries.
• It lies in the lateral wall of the cavernous sinus.
• It enters the orbit through the superior orbital fissure.
• It supplies only one muscle—superior oblique.

CLINICAL ANATOMY

When the superior oblique of one side is paralyzed, it results in misalignment of the eye called hypertropia. This results in diplopia. In order to avoid diplopia, the patient turns the head away from the affected eye side. For example, when the right trochlear has palsy, the head is held down and tilted to the left. (Remember the head always moves in the direction of action normally served by the affected muscle). In the clinical scenarios given for the involvement of trochlear nerve, remember the patient complains diplopia when he reads a book or looks down while climbing stairs.

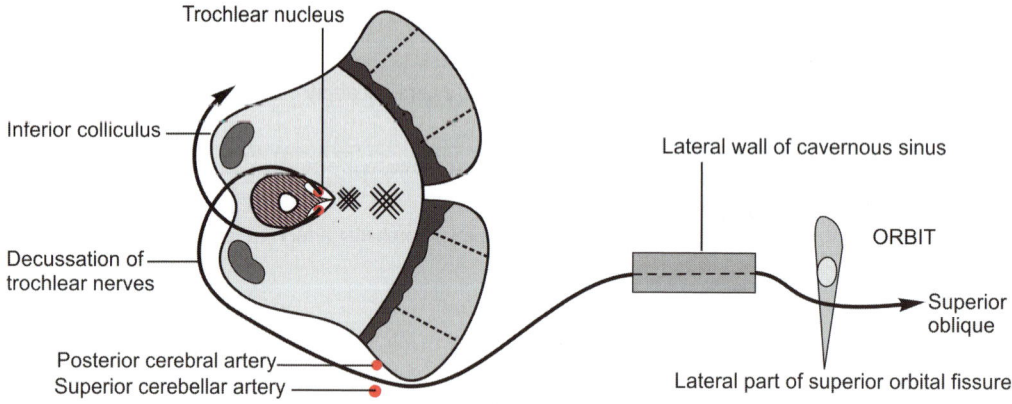

Fig. 6.88: Trochlear nerve

Trigeminal Nerve

- It is the fifth cranial nerve.
- Trigeminal ganglion is a sensory ganglion in the course of trigeminal nerve (Figs 6.89 and 6.90).
- It is divided into three parts:
  1. Ophthalmic
  2. Maxillary
  3. Mandibular

- Ophthalmic nerve divides into three branches and these branches pass through the superior orbital fissure.
  - Maxillary nerve passes through the foramen rotundum.
  - Mandibular nerve passes through the foramen ovale.
  - Mandibular nerve supplies the muscles of mastication. When there is a tumour

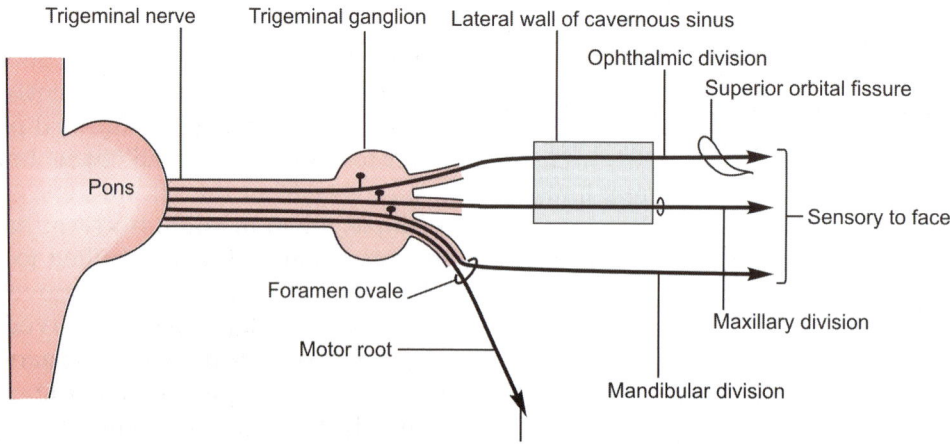

Fig. 6.89: Trigeminal nerve

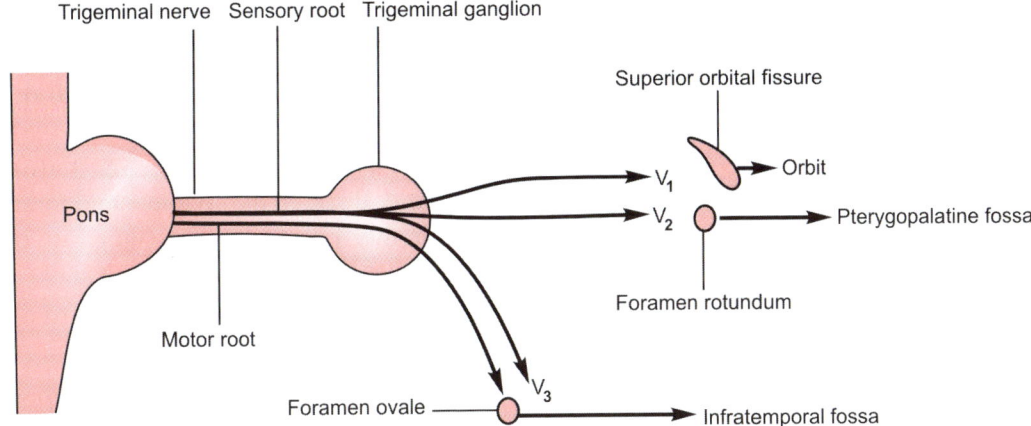

Fig. 6.90: Trigeminal nerve

close to the foramen ovale, the muscles of mastication of that side are paralyzed.

- Motor nucleus and principle sensory nucleus lie in the upper part of pons.
- What are the afferent and efferent limbs of corneal reflex?
  – *Afferent:* Ophthalmic nerve.
  – *Efferent:* Facial nerve.

- Infraorbital nerve block:
  – Infraorbital foramen is site of injection.
  – Used in dentistry for repairing maxillary incisor teeth.
  – Accidental injection of anesthetic into orbit, which is in close relation to the injection site results in transient paralysis of extraocular muscles.
- Inferior alveolar nerve block:
  – Mandibular foramen is site of injection.
  – Used in dentistry for repairing mandibular teeth.
  – Accidental injection of anesthetic (into parotid gland) further posterior to the actual injection site results in transient paralysis of facial muscles due to involvement of facial nerve branches.

- Similarly, mental nerve block is given into the mental foramen (to anesthetize ipsilateral lower lip and chin) and buccal nerve block is given into the mucosa behind the lower 3rd molar tooth (to anesthetize ipsilateral cheek).
- What is tic douloureaux (trigeminal neuralgia)?
  – It is a severe stabbing pain to one side of the face. It may be triggered by any point over the distribution of the branches of the trigeminal nerve.
  – Compression of trigeminal nerve by a tumor or an arteriovenous anastomosis may be responsible to produce this. It is more common in patients of multiple sclerosis.

Abducent Nerve

- It is the sixth cranial nerve.
- It is the longest cranial nerve within the cranial cavity.
- It is often involved in the central herniation of the brain.
- It makes a steep ascent on clivus of skull and crosses the apex of petrous temporal

bone where it can be subjected to pressure of raised intracranial tension (Fig. 6.91).
- It lies in the lateral wall of the cavernous sinus.
- It passes through the superior orbital fissure and it supplies the lateral rectus muscle.

Facial Nerve

- It is the seventh cranial nerve (Fig. 6.92).
- Its nucleus lies in the lower part of the pons.
- It exits the interior of the skull by passing through the internal acoustic meatus.

- It runs within the petrous part of the temporal bone.
- It is closely related to the medial and posterior walls of the middle ear.
- It gives following branches before it emerges through the stylomastoid foramen:
  - Greater petrosal nerve (when involved loss of lacrimal secretion).
  - Nerve to stapedius (when involved hyperacusis).
  - Chorda tympani nerve (loss of sensation of taste from the anterior two-thirds; but taste sensation is not completely lost because taste is perceived from the posterior 1/3rd).
- After emerging through the stylomastoid foramen, it supplies all the following muscles:
  - Posterior belly of digastric
  - Stylohyoid

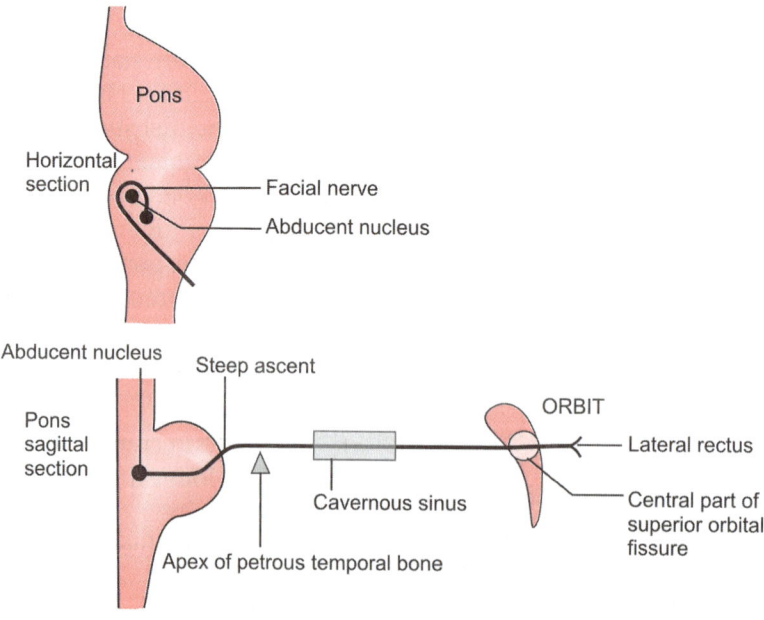

Fig. 6.91: Abducent nerve

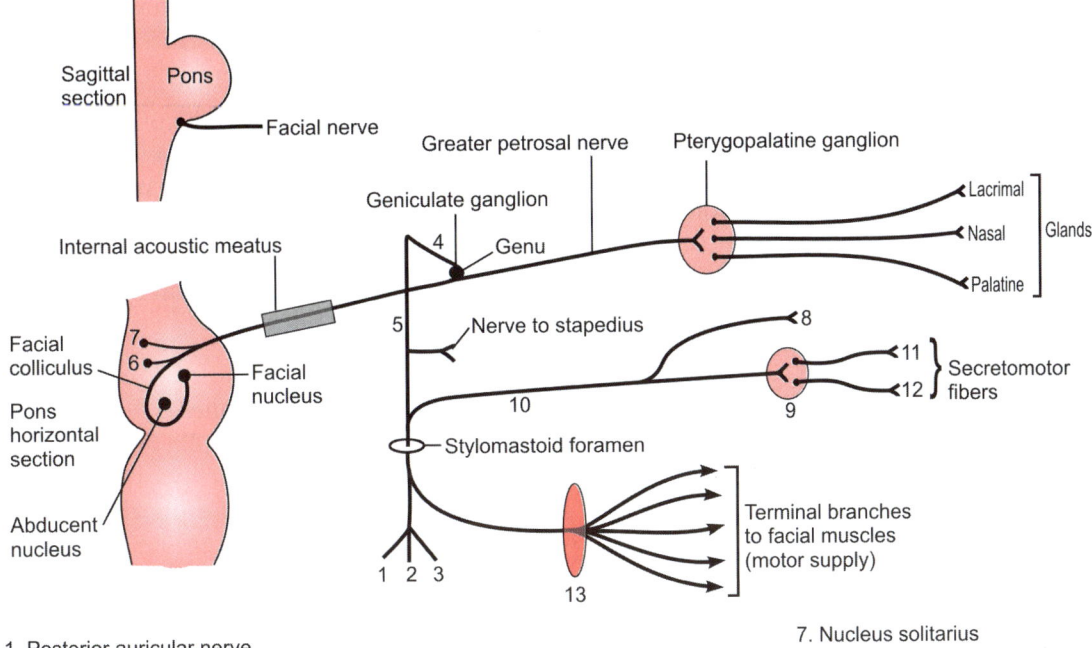

1. Posterior auricular nerve
2. Nerve to posterior belly of digastric
3. Nerve to stylohyoid
4. Horizontal part of facial nerve
5. Vertical part of facial nerve
6. Superior salivatory nucleus

7. Nucleus solitarius
8. Tongue (taste) anterior 2/3rd
9. Submandibular ganglion
10. Chorda tympani nerve
11. Submandibular gland
12. Sublingual gland
13. Parotid gland

Fig. 6.92: Facial nerve

– Posterior auricular muscles and occipital belly of occipitofrontalis.

• It enters the parotid gland and divides into its 5 terminal branches (temporal, zygomatic, buccal, mandibular, cervical) within the substance of the parotid.

• All the muscles of facial expression including buccinator are supplied by it (when buccinator is paralyzed, food is collected in the vestibule of the mouth between teeth and cheek).

• If the facial nerve is cut anywhere along its course, it is known as lower motor neuron palsy of facial nerve or Bell's palsy.

• Depending on the site of lesion in the course of facial nerve the symptoms may be one or more of the following (the more proximal/higher the lesion, the more will be the symptoms; the more distal/lower the lesion, the fewer will be the symptoms):
  – Altered lacrimal secretion (greater petrosal nerve involved).
  – Hyperacusis (impaired hearing due to excessive acuteness) (nerve to stapedius involved).
  – Loss of taste from anterior 2/3rd of tongue (chorda tympani nerve involved).
  – Altered salivary secretion (chorda tympani nerve involved).
  – Paralysis of facial muscles.

Note: Geniculate ganglion contains pseudounipolar cells. Their processes form taste fibers.

Vestibulocochlear Nerve

- It is the eighth cranial nerve.
- It is attached to the cerebellopontine angle along with the facial nerve.
- It enters the internal acoustic meatus along with the facial nerve (Fig. 6.93).
- Vestibular component is linked to equilibrium and cochlear component to hearing. The fibers of vestibular and cochlear nerve are axons of vestibular and cochlear ganglia respectively.
- Remember the mnemonic "seven up". (Seventh cranial nerve is superior and vestibulocochlear nerve is inferior in the internal acoustic meatus).

- Involvement of the nerve results in sensorineural hearing loss.

- Vestibular schwannoma is a very common condition which involves this nerve and the symptoms are:

  - Vertigo, nausea, tinnitus and loss of unilateral hearing. As the schwannoma expands it involves facial nerve first and later trigeminal nerve.
  - It is the tumor of the Schwann cells which give myelin to the cranial nerve.

Glossopharyngeal Nerve

- It is the ninth cranial nerve.
- It is attached to the medulla posterior to the olive.
- It emerges through the jugular foramen (Fig. 6.94).
- In the neck it passes deep to styloid process between the internal jugular vein and internal carotid artery.
- It passes between the internal and external carotid arteries.

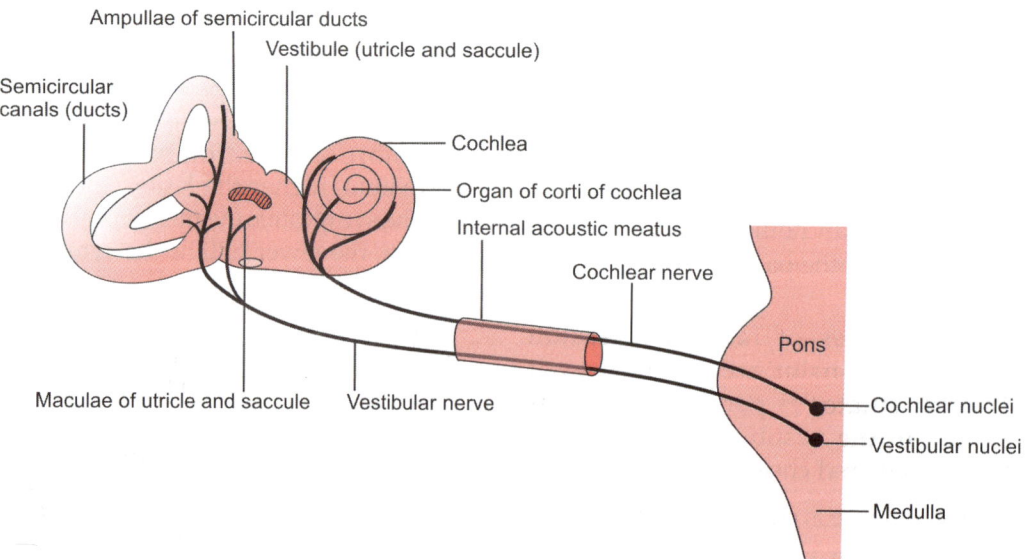

Fig. 6.93: Vestibulocochlear nerve

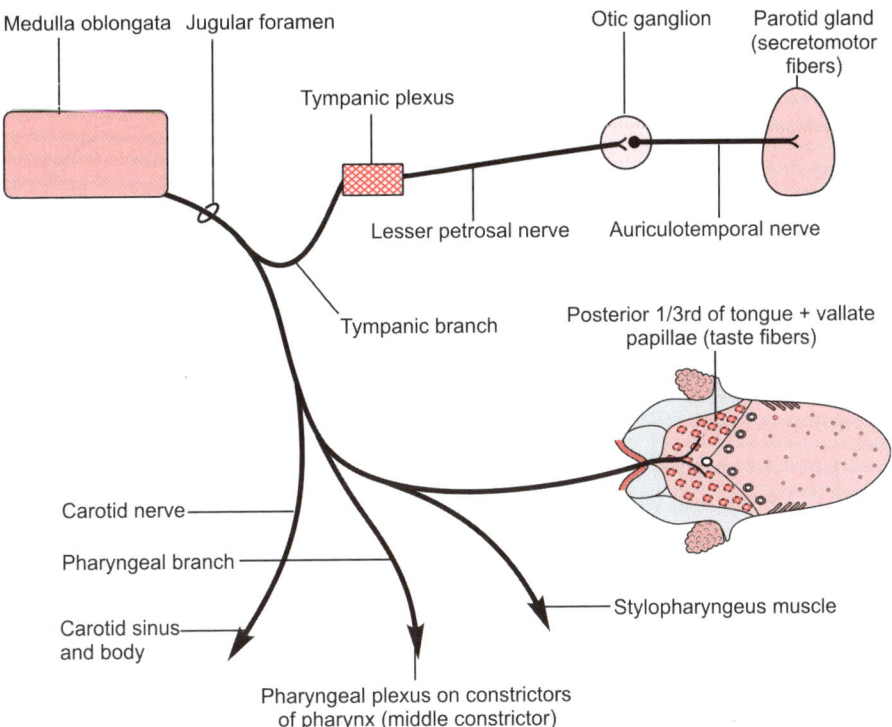

Fig. 6.94: Glossopharyngeal nerve

- It supplies only one muscle: stylopharyngeus.
- It gives branches to the carotid sinus and carotid body.
- It supplies sensory fibers to the posterior one-third of the tongue and pharynx.

- *Gag reflex:*
  - When something touches the back of the throat, there is contraction of throat. This is called gag reflex.
  - The afferent limb of the gag reflex is glossopharyngeal nerve ending in nucleus solitarius.
  - The efferent limb of gag reflex is vagus nerve from the nucleus ambiguous.
  - Absence of gag reflex indicates damage to the glossopharyngeal nerve or vagus nerve.

  - The reflex is elicited by stroking of the posterior pharynx with a cotton-tipped swab.
- Superior ganglion has no branches.
- Inferior ganglion (petrosal ganglion) carries taste sensation to nucleus solitarius.

- *Lesion of the nerve results in:*
  - Loss of taste from posterior 1/3rd of the tongue.
  - Ipsilateral loss of gag reflex.
- *Glossopharyngeal neuralgia:*
  - It is unilateral. It is rarer than the trigeminal neuralgia.
  - It is characterized by severe pain in throat, tongue and ear.

– Likely to be due to irritation of 9th nerve by tumors, infection of throat and blood vessels pressing on 9th nerve.
– Triggering factors include coughing, laughing, chewing, speaking and swallowing.

Vagus Nerve

- It is tenth cranial nerve.
- It is important for speech and swallowing and also for the visceral control of organs in thorax and abdomen.
- Superior (jugular) vagal ganglia carry general somatic sensation to the nucleus of spinal tract of the trigeminal nerve from the external acoustic meatus and tympanic membrane of the ear.
- Inferior (nodose) vagal ganglia carry special visceral sensation to nucleus solitarius and general visceral sensation to nucleus solitarius and dorsal nucleus of vagus (mainly).
- It emerges through jugular foramen (Fig. 6.95).
- It lies in the carotid sheath posterior to and between internal jugular vein and internal carotid artery initially and then between internal jugular vein and common carotid artery.
- Apart from various visceral branches it gives pharyngeal branch to pharyngeal plexus, superior laryngeal nerve, recurrent laryngeal nerve, cardiac branches to cardiac plexus.
- Superior laryngeal nerve divides into external (to cricothyroid) and internal (mucus membrane of larynx upto the level of vocal cords).
- Recurrent laryngeal nerve supplies all intrinsic muscles of larynx except crico-thyroid and mucus membrane below level of vocal cords.

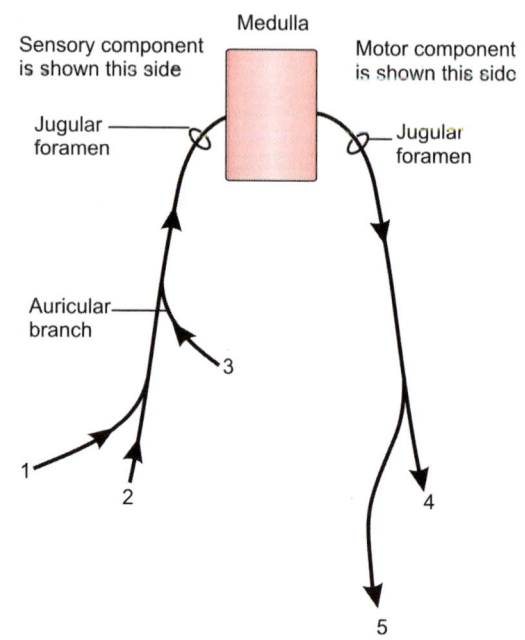

1. General sensations from thoracic and abdominal viscera
2. Taste fibers from posteriormost part of tongue and epiglottis
3. External ear
4. Thoracic and abdominal viscera except terminal part of GIT supplied by sacral segments of spinal cord
5. All muscles of pharynx except stylopharyngeus. All muscles of palate except tensor palati. Laryngeal muscles (by fibers from cranial root of accessory nerve joining vagus)

Fig. 6.95: Vagus nerve

CLINICAL ANATOMY

- Damage to vagus results in:
  - Dysphagia.
  - Hoarseness of voice and cadeveric (between abducted and adducted) position of the vocal cord on the affected side.
- When vagus is involved along with the glossopharyngeal nerve there is loss of gag reflex and the uvula is deviated to the normal side.

Accessory Nerve

- It is the eleventh cranial nerve.
- There are two components of this nerve:
  1. Spinal part
  2. Cranial part
- Spinal part enters the cranial cavity through the foramen magnum and joins the cranial part as it exits the skull through the jugular foramen (Fig. 6.96).
- The cranial part then joins the vagus.
- The spinal part passes backwards between internal jugular vein and internal carotid artery crossing deep to the posterior belly of digastric.
- It pierces sternomastoid and emerges from its posterior border (above its middle).
- It crosses posterior triangle roof and ends in trapezius 5 cm above clavicle.
- It supplies two muscles:
  i. Sternomastoid
  ii. Trapezius

- When sternomastoid is paralyzed, there is weakness in turning the head to the opposite side. When trapezius is paralyzed there is drooping of the shoulder.
- The spinal part of the nerve is prone to injury in cervical lymph node biopsy, internal jugular vein puncture and other such procedures.

Vernet's Syndrome

- Is paralysis of motor components of IX, X and XI cranial nerves in posterior fossa.
- Loss of gag reflex.
- Deviaton of uvula to the normal side.
- Ipsilateral paralysis of sternomastoid and trapezius.
- Dysphagia and hoarseness of the voice.
- Ipsilateral vocal cord palsy.

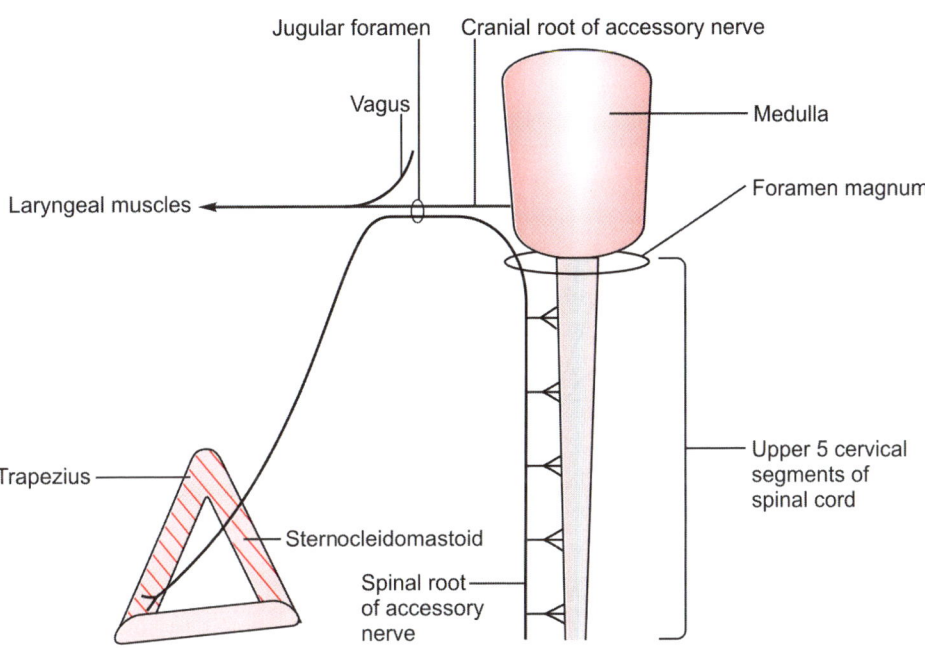

Fig. 6.96: Accessory nerve

Hypoglossal Nerve

- It is the twelfth cranial nerve.
- It exits through the anterior condylar canal (hypoglossal canal) (Fig. 6.97).
- It descends deep to stylohyoid and posterior belly of digastric.
- In carotid triangle it curves across the internal and external carotid artery and loop of lingual artery origin.
- It then runs superficial to hyoglossus and deep to mylohyoid muscles.
- It supplies all the muscles of the tongue except palatoglossus.
- Fibers of C1 are distributed to thyrohyoid and geniohyoid through hypoglossal nerve.

CLINICAL ANATOMY

When the nerve is injured the tongue deviates to the paralyzed side. This is because when you ask to protrude the tongue the genioglossus acts and the normal side protrudes and the side of lesion cannot keep pace with it so the tongue moves towards the paralyzed side. It is like cart loosing one of its wheels, the cart is turned to the side of the fallen wheel.

Constriction of the Pupil

- It is a parasympathetic activity.
- The nucleus is the Edinger-Westphal nuleus of the oculomotor nuclei.
- The preganglionic parasympathetic fibers terminate in the ciliary ganglion.
- The postganglionic neurons from the ciliary ganglion end in sphincter pupillae which constricts the pupil.

Cervical Sympathetic Chain

- Lies in neck embedded in posterior wall of carotid sheath.
- Has 3 ganglia: superior, middle, inferior (Table 6.1, Fig. 6.98).

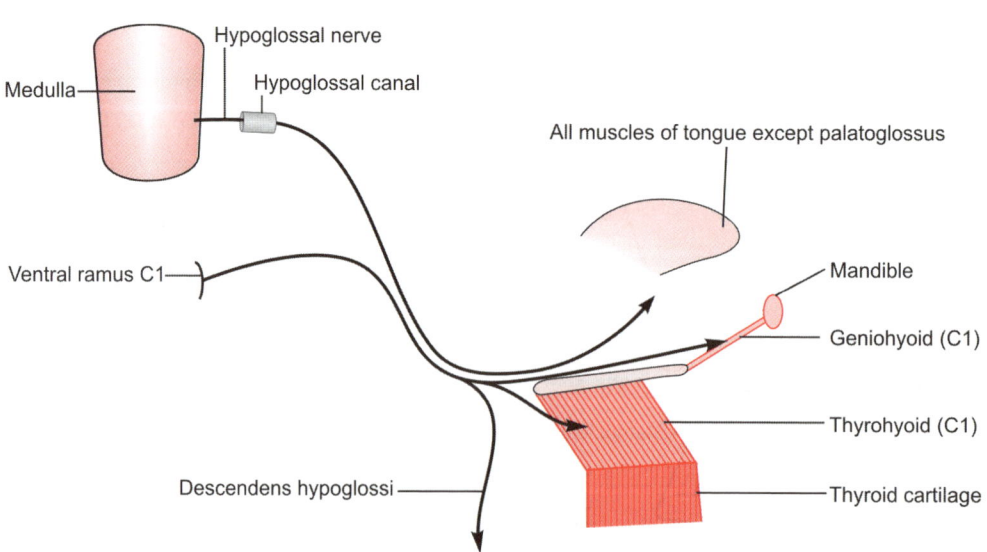

Fig. 6.97: Hypoglossal nerve

	Ganglion Superior	Middle	Inferior
	Table 6.1: Cervical sympathetic chain ganglia		
Position	Lies opposite C2, 3 vertebra.	Lies opposite C6 vertebra.	Lies opposite neck of I rib
Branches	Gray rami communicans to C1–4	Gray rami communicans to C5, 6	Gray rami communicans to C7, 8
	Cardiac branch to cardiac plexus	Cardiac branch to cardiac plexus	Cardiac branch to cardiac plexus
	Internal carotid nerve to internal carotid artery	To inferior thyroid artery	To subclavian artery
	To external carotid artery and its branches	Ansa subclavia	To vertebral artery
	Communicating to 9th, 10th and 12th cranial nerves		
	Pharyngeal branch to pharyngeal plexus		

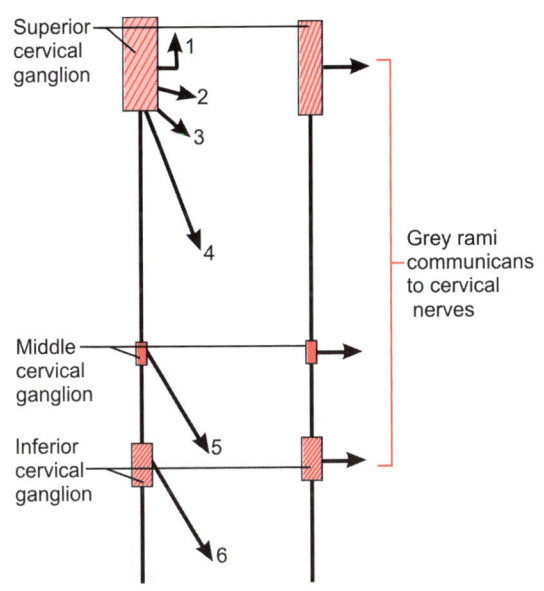

1. To internal carotid plexus, 2. To carotid sinus and carotid body, 3. To external carotid plexus, 4. Superior cardiac nerve, 5. Middle cardiac nerve, 6. Inferior cardiac nerve

Fig. 6.98: Cervical sympathetic chain

Craniovertebral Joints

- Include atlanto-axial and atlanto-occipital joints (Fig. 6.99A).
- *Atlanto-axial joints:*
  - It includes 3 joints namely: 1 median atlanto-axial joint and 2 lateral atlanto-axial joints between atlas and axis.
  - Side to side rotation (as in saying 'no') of head movement occurs here.
  - Lateral atlanto-axial joints are plane type occurring between inferior articular facet of atlas and superior articular facet of axis.
  - Median atlanto-axial joint is pivot type occurring between dens of axis and anterior arch of atlas.
- Transverse ligament of atlas keeps dens in place.
- *Atlanto-occipital joints:*
  - Occur between kidney-shaped articular facets of occipital condyles and superior articular facets of atlas.

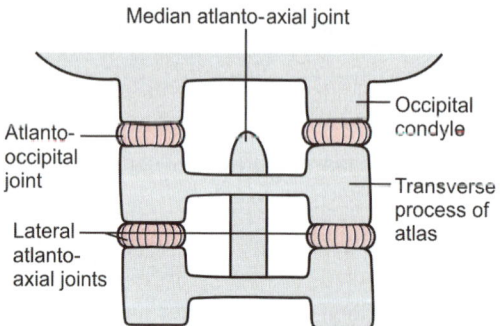

Fig. 6.99A: Atlanto-occipital and atlantoaxial joints

- 2 in number.
- Ellipsoid type.
- Nodding ('yes') movement occurs at this joint involving flexion and extension.

Note:

1. Anterior atlanto-occipital membrane connects upper border of anterior arch of atlas with anterior margin of foramen magnum of occipital bone.

2. Posterior atlanto-occipital membrane connects upper border of posterior arch of atlas with posterior margin of foramen magnum of occipital bone.

3. Ligaments connecting axis with occipital bone include (Fig. 6.99B):

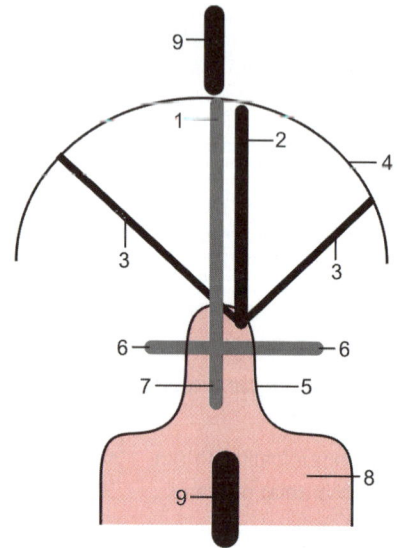

1. Upper band of cruciate ligament (posterior to apical ligament), 2. Apical ligament, 3. Alar ligament, 4. Inner aspect of basilar part of occipital bone, 5. Dens, 6. Transverse ligament, 7. Lower band of cruciate ligament, 8. Body of axis, 9. Membrana tectoria (cut)

Fig. 6.99B: Ligaments of craniovertebral joints

- Apical ligament
- Alar ligaments
- Cruciate ligament and
- Membrana tectoria.

Index